COVID-19 Unmasked

The News, the Science, and Common Sense

Other Related Titles from World Scientific

Computational Modeling of the COVID-19 Disease: Numerical ODE Analysis with R Programming
by William E Schiesser
ISBN: 978-981-122-287-0

The COVID-19 Epidemic in China
by Lawrence J Lau and Yanyan Xiong
ISBN: 978-981-122-250-4
ISBN: 978-981-122-419-5 (pbk)

Impact of COVID-19 on Asian Economies and Policy Responses
edited by Sumit Agarwal, Zhiguo He and Bernard Yeung
ISBN: 978-981-122-937-4

COVID-19 Unmasked

The News, the Science, and Common Sense

Winfried Just

Ohio University, USA

World Scientific

NEW JERSEY · LONDON · SINGAPORE · BEIJING · SHANGHAI · HONG KONG · TAIPEI · CHENNAI · TOKYO

Published by

World Scientific Publishing Co. Pte. Ltd.

5 Toh Tuck Link, Singapore 596224

USA office: 27 Warren Street, Suite 401-402, Hackensack, NJ 07601

UK office: 57 Shelton Street, Covent Garden, London WC2H 9HE

Library of Congress Cataloging-in-Publication Data
Names: Just, W. (Winfried) author.
Title: COVID-19 unmasked : the news, the science, and common sense /
    Winfried Just, Ohio University, USA.
Description: New Jersey : World Scientific, [2021] | Includes bibliographical references.
Identifiers: LCCN 2021001165 | ISBN 9789811233593 (hardcover) |
    ISBN 9789811235610 (paperback) | ISBN 9789811233609 (ebook) |
    ISBN 9789811233616 (ebook other)
Subjects: LCSH: COVID-19 (Disease) | COVID-19 (Disease)--Forcasting. | COVID-19 (Disease)--
    Social aspects. | COVID-19 (Disease)--Economic aspects. | COVID-19 (Disease)--Epidemiology.
Classification: LCC RA644.C67 J87 2021 | DDC 362.1962/414--dc23
LC record available at https://lccn.loc.gov/2021001165

British Library Cataloguing-in-Publication Data
A catalogue record for this book is available from the British Library.

DISCLAIMER: The contents of this book reflect the scientific views of the author on the effects of preventive measures against the spread of COVID-19 from a mathematical modeling perspective. This perspective is supported by, but not necessarily shared in all details, by the publisher. While the text contains a number of practical recommendations for protecting oneself against contracting the disease, no combination of such steps can ensure 100% protection against infection. Moreover, readers will still need to meticulously follow all rules and guidelines of health authorities in their jurisdictions.

Design of figures: Winfried Just
Color illustrations: Kevin Justus
Histograms: Daniel Ntiamoah

For any available supplementary material, please visit
https://www.worldscientific.com/worldscibooks/10.1142/12191#t=suppl

Contents

Dedication

I dedicate this book to the loving memory of my maternal grand-mother, a courageous woman with a big heart and an abundance of practical wisdom.

And I dedicate it to all nurses who daily risk their own health and lives caring for patients with infectious diseases.

In her days, grandma Trudel was one of them.

Acknowledgments

This book owes its existence to countless wonderful people who helped me become its author. My teachers, my students, my colleagues, my friends, my family. My deepest gratitude is to my wife Ewelina for bringing so much joy to my life. Without her support and understanding, I would not have been able to find the time and energy that it took to complete this project.

A number of people directly contributed to this book. Most notably Ohio University students Daniel Ntiamoah and Kevin Justus, who made most of the figures. I received important critical feedback on earlier versions from anonymous reviewers and from my former student Mason Korb. The anonymous technical editor and Ohio University students Dylan Denner and Daniel Ntiamoah provided enormous help with meticulously proofreading earlier versions and making numerous constructive suggestions for improvements. I am greatly indebted to all these contributors.

Last but not least, my heartfelt thanks go to Rochelle Kronzek, Yolande Koh, and Joy Quek of World Scientific. Without Rochelle's strong support and encouragement of this project, writing this text would not have been possible. And her many specific suggestions greatly helped me improve the selection of examples as well as the writing of many passages. Yolande and Joy lent their superb technical expertise and great dedication to turning the manuscript into a book.

With all the help and support I got, I think this book really has many authors. The responsibility for its shortcomings is still exclusively my own.

Who may want to read this book?

The COVID-19 pandemic is in the news every day. We read stories of people getting sick and dying, of people losing their jobs, of people refusing to wear masks. We are bombarded with facts and numbers that change daily. How can we keep up with this deluge of information and data? How can we tell which snippets of information are most important and trustworthy?

We read: "Scientists recommend", "Experts warn", "A new model predicts". New scientific findings are reported every week, sometimes in barely comprehensible jargon. Different models give different projections. How do scientific experts come up with their recommendations?

We worry about getting infected, losing our income, and about the future of society. If we want to protect ourselves and others from the disease and its economic repercussions, we need to make sense of the scientific information. What do the predictions of scientists really mean for us, for our friends, and our families? And how to make rational decisions? How to have sensible conversations about the pandemic, both with those who broadly share our own views and those with whom we disagree?

If such questions are on your mind, this book may be for you.

Alice, a student of epidemiology, will explain the science to her fellow students Bob, Cindy, and Frank. They have a lot of questions for Alice, some perhaps similar to the ones you are struggling with. And they have the same concerns that we all share to varying degrees: What the pandemic is doing to our health, our economy, and our cherished freedoms. In their conversations, the students will discover how the science relates to these questions.

In the particular story that ties these dialogues together, the students talk about the planned re-opening of their university for the upcoming fall semester. It could have been a story about sending kids back to school, about whether it is safe to go on a vacation, or countless other difficult decisions we need to make. If we want to decide wisely, we need to understand how COVID-19 infections spread among people.

This book focuses on epidemiology, the science of how infections spread and how the spread can be mitigated. The science of how many infections can be prevented by certain kinds of actions. This is what we need to understand if we want to act wisely, as individuals and as a society. Every such action relates to medical, economic, and political aspects of the COVID-19 pandemic. The conversations between Alice and her fellow students refer to this broader context, but this is not a book about medicine, economics, or political science. These aspects of the COVID-19 pandemic are left to different books by other authors.

The aim of this book is to empower you to think about the COVID-19 pandemic like an epidemiologist. About the various preventive measures, what they are trying to accomplish, what the obstacles are. About what is likely to be most effective in the long run at moderate economic and personal cost. About the likely consequences of your personal decisions. About how to best protect yourself and others while allowing all of us to lead lives that are as close as possible to normal.

Thinking like an epidemiologist is not as difficult as it may sound. It only requires three things:

The first is focusing on the big picture. Epidemiology studies how diseases spread among large groups of people, such as the populations of entire countries. By now you have probably read and heard countless stories about how patients suffer from COVID-19 infections. You may even have experienced the suffering yourself or seen it up close in a family member or a friend. Every single case of severe infection or death is a personal tragedy. But we cannot understand how the infection spreads through a population by keeping our focus on individual cases. With such a narrow focus, we would lose sight of the forest for the trees. In this book we will take a bird's-eye view and try to understand the forest.

The second key to thinking like an epidemiologist is becoming familiar with a few basic concepts like contacts, reproduction numbers, and models. We all know about contacts, and you have probably already read somewhere about reproduction numbers and models. Alice will explain in detail what these concepts mean in epidemiology.

The third key is using these concepts to make connections between the various preventive measures like social distancing, wearing masks, or contact tracing on the one hand, and the future spread of the infection on the other. We all have been reading about these a lot, perhaps an article about social distancing here, another article about contact tracing there. When we look at these preventive measures through the lens of epidemiology, we can understand how they all work together. How they can make sure that this pandemic will not spiral out of control and will be over in the not-so-distant future. And how they may fail to achieve this goal.

This book is about making sense of the deluge of COVID-19 data and facts, about connecting the dots. Perhaps you will find in these pages the particular fact or story that most intrigues you. But there are just too many stories happening all over the world. And perhaps you will find a direct answer the particular question that is bothering you most. But there are just too many questions. You definitely will learn how to make sense of various tidbits of information, how to put the numbers in various charts and data sets into their proper context, how to spot fallacious arguments and misinterpretations of data. Chances are that, equipped with this knowledge, you will be able to figure out yourself the answers to your most pressing questions. If this book will help you in making rational decisions and informed choices based on your own common sense, it will have achieved its goal.

The book is organized into 29 short chapters. Alice answers specific questions from her fellow students in her online chatroom and shows how the science relates to our everyday concerns. Most of these conversations happen over the summer of 2020 and are based on data and contemporary events for this time period. For greater transparency, each chapter covers a separate topic, but occasionally one meeting of the students has been split up into separate chapters.

While some chapters present slightly more advanced material than others, you will not need a scientific background to follow Alice's explanations. The technical concepts are explained at a slow pace in small steps, and the occasional calculations presented here require only high-school mathematics. If you prefer, you can simply skip the calculations.

Many conversations do not need to be read in a specific order, and you can often jump ahead to the topics that interest you most. But there are some dependencies. You probably want to read Chapters 2 and 3 to find out who the characters are and what they are most concerned about. Chapter 4 introduces key concepts that will be used throughout the remainder of the book. The end of Chapter 3, as well as Chapters 6, 7, 8, and 25 cover some basics on interpreting charts and graphs. Chapters 9, 10, 11, and 13 form a sequence. They cover in detail reproduction numbers and give us a way of thinking about the overall strategy for mitigating the spread of COVID-19. After reading these chapters, you will be able to think about the spread of COVID-19 like an epidemiologist. Many of the subsequent chapters reference reproduction numbers, but the dependence is not as strong as the dependence on Chapter 4. If you really want to, you could skip Chapters 11 and 13 and still follow most of the later discussions. For easier reference, the crucial material of Chapters 4, 9, and 10 is summarized at their ends in the form of bullet points. Chapters 15, 16, and 19 form a natural sequence. Chapters 17 and 18 both depend on Chapter 16. Chapters 20, 21, Chapters 23, 24, and Chapters 26, 27 also form sequences.

The endnotes for the chapters give some additional scientific information and pointers to sources where you can read more about the chapter's topic. COVID-19 is a very recent and rapidly evolving threat. Scientific research on the pandemic progresses at a frantic pace. New findings are published daily. As we learn more, some of the earlier findings and predictions become outdated. The chapter endnotes can give only a snapshot in time of the literature on the subject. And certainly not of the entire literature; only of selected items that connect directly to the dialogues. As this book is aimed at a general audience, our selection gives higher preference to easily accessible web-based sources and newspaper articles than to technical research papers.

You will find a lot of data in this book. Please keep in mind that these are historical data for the times when the conversations took place or when the chapter endnotes were written. The COVID-19 pandemic is still ongoing, and the situation changes daily. If you see a reference to a publicly available source in the book, by the time you click on the URL, the numbers will have changed from the ones quoted here. Numbers of infections, mortality estimates, hospitalization rates are all likely to change as the pandemic—together with our knowledge of it and our control over it—evolves. The same applies to policies on testing and quarantining, which will differ by country and region. The book only gives some information based on a particular time and for particular locations. For practical day-to-day decisions, you will need to rely on the latest updates for your region and follow the particular recommendations of your local health authorities.

The historical information about facts and numbers given in this book is often fairly sketchy. You may want to know more about the details, and the chapter endnotes give you pointers to easily accessible sources where you can find them. The data quoted here mainly serve as a necessary backdrop for the primary goal of this book: To show you how to make sense of the information. The facts on the ground, the numbers, and the policies all keep changing. But the methods for drawing conclusions from the information remain the same; anytime, everywhere in the world. It is the fervent hope of the author that this book will help you in drawing your own conclusions, for your benefit, the benefit of your loved ones, and your community.

List of Endnotes

Chapter 1

The COVID-19 epidemic and our response to it

For decades, there had been warnings of imminent pandemics.[1]
Pathogens constantly mutate. New species of viruses appear all the time. In our interconnected world, millions of people travel to different countries each day. Therefore, scientists had predicted that one day a new deadly virus would emerge, would spread from continent to continent, infect hundreds of millions of people, kill millions, and fundamentally change how we could go about our daily lives.

Many people understood the danger; all of us hoped that this would not happen any time soon.

Mother Nature fired a few warning shots. The SARS outbreak in 2002–2004 infected 8,422 people from 29 different countries and claimed at least 916 lives before it was contained [1]. The 2009 H1N1 pandemic, commonly known as the swine flu, may have caused on the order of half a million deaths worldwide [2]. The Ebola outbreak in 2013–2016 originated in West Africa, but reached countries as far away as Europe and the United States. During this outbreak, 28,652 people were infected and 11,325 lost their lives. But thanks to vigorous interventions and strong international cooperation, it was relatively quickly brought under control [3]. The tolls of SARS, the swine flu, Ebola, and a number of other disease outbreaks over the last couple of decades were large, but not nearly as huge as they might have been without swift, decisive, and competent action. We had been lucky.

Then our luck run out. In December 2019, cases of "pneumonia of an unknown cause" were being reported in the city of Wuhan, in the Chinese province of Hubei. It took several weeks, until January 20 of 2020, before the Chinese National Health Commission confirmed human-to-human transmission of the virus that caused these infections. On January 23, a lockdown was imposed on Wuhan and other cities in Hubei province. It drastically restricted people's freedom of movement and ultimately succeeded in stopping the spread of the disease in Wuhan.

But by January 23, the virus had already spread to other provinces of China and abroad. In February, South Korea already had a large outbreak of COVID-19, the disease caused by this virus.[2]

By late February, Italy had exploding numbers of new COVID-19 cases that quickly overwhelmed the health care system in some regions of the country. At the time of this writing, December 23, 2020, over 78 million COVID-19 infections have been reported in 220 countries and territories, and over 1.7 million people have died from the infection worldwide [4].

The pandemic has caused severe disruptions to the world economy and has drastically altered social life almost everywhere.

Most countries decided to impose severe and lengthy lockdowns at great economic cost. Many of them had succeeded in bringing down new infections to very low levels by early summer so that people could again lead reasonably normal lives. Notable examples are China, South Korea, and Italy, all of whom had experienced large outbreaks early in the course of the infection. Other countries took less decisive action and continued to see high numbers after the lockdowns were lifted. But even some of the countries who most successfully dealt with their early outbreaks experienced second peaks of new infections at some later time. As the year 2020 draws to a close, millions of people in several countries are again living under lockdown.

The infections are caused by a new species of coronavirus that is quite similar to the one that caused the SARS outbreak in 2002–2004. For this reason, the virus was named SARS-CoV-2, which stands for Severe Acute Respiratory Syndrome-CoronaVirus-2. The virus is mainly transmitted directly from person to person through tiny droplets in a person's breath that travel through the air. Indirect transmission through touching contaminated surfaces may also occur.

Infection manifests itself first through flu-like symptoms that are usually mild. A large proportion of carriers of COVID-19 remain entirely asymptomatic, but can still infect others. But in many cases, the initially mild symptoms progress to severe respiratory illness that requires hospitalization and ICU treatment with the use of a ventilator. COVID-19 is much more contagious and appears to be between 5 to 10 times deadlier than the seasonal flu. Mortality is highest among older people and those with pre-existing conditions such as hypertension, diabetes, or cardiovascular disease. Even people who survive and recover from a COVID-19 infection may suffer long-term effects, including neurological diseases.

There is currently no cure for COVID-19, although some drugs are known to increase chances of survival to some limited extent. Vaccines have recently been approved in a number of countries. Studies have shown them to be highly effective, but it may take at least until mid-2021 before sufficiently many people can be vaccinated so that the populations of entire countries will be protected.

As we go into 2021, there is great hope that vaccinations will curb the spread of COVID-19, mixed with fear of new mutant strains of the coronavirus. Nobody knows for how much longer we will need to wear masks and continue social distancing. Our lives may never be quite the same again.

Endnotes

[1] The book [5] by Pulitzer-winning journalist Laurie Garrett is an example of the extensive literature on the topic. It appeared a quarter of a century ago.

[2] COVID-19 is an acronym that stands for COronanaVirus Disease 2019 and is usually rendered in capital letters. But as it occurs so frequently in this text, for the dialogues the author adopted the spelling Covid-19 of some media outlets that is easier on the eyes.

References

[1] Chan-Yeung M, Xu RH. SARS: epidemiology. Respirology 2003 Nov 14 [cited 2020 Dec 23]; 8(1):S9–S14.
https://onlinelibrary.wiley.com/doi/full/10.1046/j.
1440-1843.2003.00518.x
DOI: 10.1046/j.1440-1843.2003.00518.x

[2] Centers for Disease Control and Prevention; Influenza (Flu). 2009 H1N1 Pandemic (H1N1pdm09 virus). [cited 2020 Dec 23]. https://www.cdc.gov/flu/pandemic-resources/2009-h1n1-pandemic.html

[3] Centers for Disease Control and Prevention; Ebola (Ebola Virus Disease). 2014-2016 Ebola Outbreak in West Africa. [cited 2020 Dec 23]. https://www.cdc.gov/vhf/ebola/history/2014-2016-outbreak/index.html

[4] Worldometers.info. Dover, Delaware, U.S.A. COVID-19 coronavirus pandemic. [cited 2020 Dec 23].
https://www.worldometers.info/coronavirus/

[5] Garrett, L. The Coming Plague: Newly Emerging Diseases in a World Out of Balance. New York: Farrar, Straus and Giroux; 1994. 750p.

Chapter 2

What are scientists up to?

In March 2020, when the Covid-19 pandemic struck, universities around the world had sent students home and offered instruction only online. By early summer 2020, many were considering plans to re-open in the Fall Semester for face-to-face instruction. Ohio University announced such plans in June 2020, and the following ad appeared on social media:[3]

Hi all Bobcats[4] out there!

We will be back on campus in the fall. I'm so excited about this! But how can we make sure we will stay healthy? Why are we being asked to take all these precautions? Are they really necessary? How can we socialize, meet people, and still be safe? Is that even possible?

I'm Alice, a graduate student of epidemiology here at OU and can perhaps answer some of your questions about the science behind the recommended preventive measures. Please join me via zoom in my chatroom if you'd like to talk about this.

Alice's chatroom came online on June 28, 2020, and three of her fellow students showed up. The students started their first meeting with a discussion of the role of science and scientists[5] and then kept meeting via zoom over the summer.

Bob: Hi! I'm Bob, from Cincinnati, Ohio and a business major.

Alice: Nice to meet you, Bob! I'm Alice. What brings you here?

Bob: There's a lot of info about Covid-19 in the press and in social media. Too much to keep up with. And one article often contradicts the next. Your invite says that you study epidemiology, I thought that you could perhaps clear up a few things for me.

Cindy: Hi, Alice and Bob! So glad to meet you. I'm Cindy from Circleville, Ohio. Bob, you're right, the info on social media is so confusing. Alice, please help us to make sense of it all!

Bob: Nice to meet you, Cindy.

Alice: Welcome to my chatroom, Cindy.

Cindy: I study healthcare administration and have an internship lined up for September. That's in patient records at our student health center. Not sure whether they'll still let me do this. But perhaps I should cancel it myself. I'm so scared of getting infected with Covid-19! And then I may perhaps infect others.

Bob: Sounds like this internship will be very important for your degree. Don't miss out on the opportunity; just be extra careful while you work in that building.

I'm most worried that this corona thing will totally wreck the economy. I'll graduate next spring. But with so many companies laying people off and not hiring anyone, how am I going to find a decent job?

Alice: Let's hope things will get better by then. Perhaps you can teach us some things about the economic impact of the pandemic, Bob.

Frank: Yeah, this lockdown has already done way too much damage. As you wrote in your ad: Are all these precautions really necessary? Glad somebody wants to seriously talk about this.

I'm Frank, by the way, mechanical engineering major, from Vinton county, Ohio. Hi all!

Cindy: Hi Frank!

Bob: Nice to meet you, Frank!

Alice: Welcome to my chat room, Frank. I'm a graduate student in epidemiology, the science of how infectious diseases spread. I'll try to explain what scientists know about Covid-19 and how it relates to the preventive measures that we all should take.

Frank: I don't trust those scientists.

Alice: Why don't you trust scientists, Frank?

Frank: Well, as an engineering student, I trust physicists. But not epidemiologists. How can they know what's going to happen if every single new infection depends on who accidentally got too close to whom? I think they just make things up. And then try to boss us around and tell everybody what to do and what not to do. That's not how it's supposed to be in a free country.

Alice: What if I told you that biologists know that deer tend to come out around dusk? And then recommended that you drive extra carefully at that time of the day, slow down a bit, and watch out for them. Would that be unreasonable advice?

Frank: No, not that one. My grandpa told me the same thing many times, and he would have known. I don't need no biologists or other scientists for that.

Alice: How did your grandpa know?

Frank: He was a great hunter and outdoorsman who observed the deer and other animals all his life. And he learned a lot from his fellow hunters by listening to their stories.

Alice: Seems your grandpa had a lot of wisdom.

Frank: You can say that.

Alice: Now suppose there suddenly appeared a new species of large mammals in Ohio, called ... ummm ... cornuses. What would you do to avoid hitting them on the road?

Frank: Come on, Alice! There are no cornuses!

Cindy: Hold on, Frank. Maybe Alice has a good story to tell?

Bob: I thought Alice wanted to talk with us about science. About facts, not stories.

Alice: Yes, Bob, scientists study facts. But sometimes we have to ask ourselves What-If questions and think through a hypothetical scenario. Then we can understand the consequences if something similar were to happen in real life.

Cindy: So, about these cornuses, we would need to know whether they also come out at dusk or instead prefer sunbathing at noon in the middle of the road, right?

Bob: OK, I get it. We would need to ask somebody about cornuses. What would your grandpa tell us about them, Frank?

Frank: There are no cornuses!

Cindy: Come on, Frank, just play along!

Frank: Alright, if you absolutely want me to play this game: There were no cornuses in grandpa's days, so he would not have known.

Cindy: So who would you ask then?

Frank: Somebody who spends time outdoors observing wildlife, including your cornuses.

Alice: And that is exactly what scientists do. They and their students like me observe how the real world works by collecting data. Then they share and discuss the data with their colleagues.

If there were cornuses, scientists would learn about the dangers they pose. Pretty much in the same way your grandpa learned about the dangers posed by deer, Frank.

Frank: I see your point. But there are no cornuses.

Alice: Not cornuses, but a new species of coronavirus that causes Covid-19. It was unknown until late 2019, and it poses a major threat to humans. Scientists are collecting data on it so that we can better understand what, exactly, it does to people and how it spreads among us.

Unlike deer, we cannot observe viruses directly with our senses; we need sophisticated equipment like powerful microscopes and lab tests for collecting these data.

Frank: And what do epidemiologists do with their data?

Alice: For starters, they want to predict how fast it will spread in a given population, like in a given country or among students of our university after we re-open.

Frank: Then tell me: Will I get infected in the first week of classes?

Alice: Did your grandpa ever tell you whether you will hit a deer in any given week?

Frank: Stupid question; of course not! He told me though that there is a high likelihood that I will eventually hit one, especially if I don't drive extra carefully around dusk.

Alice: Right. Scientists would not be able to predict when any particular driver would hit a deer. But with good data on density of deer populations and driving habits, they might be able to roughly predict the total number of such accidents in a given area per week.

Similarly, epidemiologists will not be able to predict who, in particular, will catch the disease at what time. As you had mentioned earlier, every single transmission depends on a lot accidental factors. But with good data, epidemiologists may be able to roughly predict how many people in a given population will become infected with Covid-19 during a given week.

Bob: When I read about this stuff it always says that there is some model that predicts such a number. What do they mean by "model"?

Cindy: This sounds like "model airplane". But that would be a toy, not something scientific.

Frank: We use them in engineering, Cindy. You can actually learn a lot about real airplanes from playing with toy models. For example, which wing shapes will give enough aerodynamic lift and a stable flight. When a model airplane crashes, it is not nearly as big a deal as when the real thing does. But before you build the real thing, you need to do a lot of computer simulations.

Alice: Exactly. What we call models in epidemiology are actually computer simulations. In a sense, we let the infection run its course inside the computer and observe what happens.

Cindy: And no real people get hurt by the outbreak when it's all on the computer! I like that.

Bob: I read that there are many different such models and they all predict different numbers.

Frank: So it seems that these models are all wrong.

Alice: There are two main reasons why different models give somewhat different predictions.

The first is that any model is a simplified version of the real world. This is true for epidemiological models as much as for model airplanes. When we construct a model, we make decisions about which aspects of the real world to put into our model and which to ignore. This is like building different models of real airplanes: Some are smaller and inexpensive, others are bigger, more realistic, more complicated, and more expensive. Some will fly better than others. By playing with all of these models, one would get a pretty good idea how the real thing flies.

Similarly, epidemiological models differ in how closely they match the real world. We learn only gradually which aspects of Covid-19 transmission make the biggest difference to the predicted spread. Therefore, we always will have some discrepancies between predictions of models that take into account different aspects of the real-world situation. But if most of our models predict the same general pattern, we can be confident in this prediction.

The second issue is that all models rely on data. With a new disease like Covid-19, it takes some time before we will have enough reliable data for more precise modeling.

Cindy: So with last month's data, you would get a prediction that is different from the one when you use the most recent numbers?

Alice: A slightly different one, usually. And the second prediction will likely be more accurate as it will be based on more and better data.

Frank: Still, what is all this modeling good for if it's not going to be accurate anyways? Why not just wait and see what actually will happen?

Alice: That's an important question. The spread of Covid-19 not only depends on what the virus does to us, but also on what we do in order to prevent its transmission. Whether or not we will be under lockdown, to what extent we practice social distancing, how many of us will wear masks. These human responses to the pandemic matter a lot.

Bob: Would they be among the aspects of the real world that one needs to put in the model to get accurate predictions?

Alice: Yes. They are actually the most important aspects.

Cindy: But how do we know how many people will wear masks and practice social distancing?

Alice: We don't, and this is why epidemiologists explore What-If scenarios. Run one simulation assuming that very few people will wear masks and practice social distancing, and run another one where most people do.

They can compare the predictions and see how many new infections will likely be avoided by adopting these preventive or—as they are often called in epidemiology—control measures.

Then epidemiologists recommend the ones that work best.

Bob: I see. They could then tell people how many new infections and deaths from the disease will likely be avoided by wearing masks, social distancing, and frequent hand-washing.

Alice: Exactly. This is what epidemiologists can do for us.

Frank: That's what I thought. Those guys will make us put on masks. In a free country, nobody should be forced to wear them.

Alice: Did your grandpa *force* you to slow down around dusk?

Frank: No. He just told me about the likelihood of that expensive trip to the body shop. I made the calculation and my own decision.

Alice: So he gave you the *information* that allowed you to make a wise decision. Similarly, the job of scientists is only to supply the information that we all need to "make the calculation", as you put it, and decide wisely.

Cindy: But don't we wear masks to protect others? And put others in danger by not wearing them? So how can we then leave it to each of us to "make the calculation" and decide individually?

Alice: Very important point, Cindy! The only effective way of protecting any one person is by limiting the spread in the population, by protecting everybody. And this is possible only if all of us contribute.

Some decisions have to be made collectively. Even in a free country, we cannot each decide separately whether we want to drive on the right side of the road, as we do in the U.S., or on the left, as they do in Britain.

Bob: So who should make the decisions?

Alice: Local, state, and federal authorities can mandate some preventive measures. Scientists do not make these decisions; their role is only to provide the information that is needed for deciding wisely.

But various mandates and recommendations set only boundaries for what is and what is not permissible. In many situations, each of us needs to decide what to do. The choices we make will have consequences for all of us. We need to think through these consequences if we want to avoid the worst scenarios.

My goal is to help you understand the science. Making wise decisions is then up to each of us.

Bob: Sounds good. I have so many questions. Shall we take a short break now and then continue our discussion?

Cindy: Yes, let's do this.

Frank: Fine with me.

Alice: See you all in a few!

Endnotes

[3] The story of this book is fictional and none of the characters is based on any real person. Ohio University `https://www.ohio.edu/` is the academic home of the author. It did in fact announce in June 2020 plans to re-open for on-site classes in Fall Semester 2020.

[4] A bobcat is the mascot of Ohio University, and its students often informally call themselves "bobcats". OU, as Ohio University is commonly abbreviated, does not offer a formal degree in epidemiology, but many graduate students work on various aspects of the subject under the guidance of faculty from several departments.

[5] Distrust of science and scientists is widespread in the U.S. and has been a major factor in impeding an effective response to the

pandemic. See, for example, the interview [1] given by Dr. Anthoni Fauci, the leading expert in the U.S. on infectious diseases.

References

[1] Howard J, Stracqualursi V. Fauci warns of 'anti-science bias' being a problem in US. CNN Politics 2020 Jun 18 [cited 2020 Dec 6]. Available from: https://edition.cnn.com/2020/06/18/politics/anthony-fauci-coronavirus-anti-science-bias/index.html

Chapter 3

How dangerous is COVID-19? And what do the numbers really mean?

Alice, Bob, Cindy, and Frank continue their discussion on June 29, 2020. In total, 10,226,574 Covid-19 infections and 517,350 deaths from the disease have been reported worldwide [1]. In the U.S., there has been a 79% increase in new reported infections over the last 2 weeks.[6]

Alice: So what would you all like to talk about?

Cindy: Will it be really safe to come back to campus in the fall? With so many students around? And many of them will party a lot; I think this is really dangerous.

Frank: Come on, Cindy! College students are young and healthy and have little to fear from coronavirus. We need to get a real education with real classes. We cannot put our lives on hold because of a few infections going around.

Cindy: But we may infect others who are more vulnerable. And the numbers of infections are going up so much right now! I've read that in the U.S., there has been a more than 100% increase in new cases over the last 2 weeks.

Bob: I've also read about the increase over the last 2 weeks, but that it was around 80%.

Cindy: But even if it's 80%, that's still so scary!

Bob: Maybe Alice can explain to us which number is the correct one. Either way, it's a huge increase.

But I have another question: I've read that the actual numbers of infections may be even much higher. Can you tell us about this, Alice?

Frank: Yeah, right. Nobody really knows how many people got infected. The numbers in the media are only the numbers of those who tested positive. There has been a lot more testing lately, and the more people we test, the more new infections we will see. So all this so-called increase is just caused by more testing.

Bob: I'm not sure whether that's all there is to it. Last week I was talking with some friends from Arizona and Florida. The daily numbers of infections in their states had been going up a lot, and I thought that was a very bad sign. But one of my friends told me that the reported numbers of deaths from Covid-19 were staying pretty flat in Arizona, and the guy from Florida told me that they were even trending downward in his state. If the numbers of deaths keep going down, perhaps new cases aren't really increasing after all.

Alice: We will need to carefully look at these data one-by-one. Let me start with—

Cindy: But if there really are many more new infections? Then we will soon have many more people dying from Covid-19. This would be so horrible. We cannot let this happen. Perhaps we need another lockdown?

Bob: No way, Cindy! Not another lockdown! People also died unnecessarily because they postponed doctor's visits during the lockdown.

And all these lockdowns did terrible damage to people's lives. My mom works in human resources for a large company. When they were forced to lay off people, she wasn't making the decisions, but she was the one who needed to call them in and tell them. Single mothers who lost their only source of income, people a few years from retirement who had been putting their hearts into their jobs for decades, you name it. And together with their jobs, they lost the health insurance that came with it. In the middle of a pandemic!

On those days when she needed to break the news to people, sometimes to a dozen people, mom came home and didn't say a word. Just went to her room and stayed there for hours. I'd never seen her like this before. I wanted to talk with her and give her some comfort, but dad told me not to disturb her. I really didn't know what to do.

Frank: At least your mom still does have a job, Bob. Mine lost hers.

Cindy: I feel so sorry for your mom!

Frank: Thank you, Cindy! If business keeps picking up again, they might re-hire mom. But not if someone slaps another lockdown or something on us.

So tell us, Alice: What were all these lockdowns for? Was it right to do so much damage to people's jobs? Is it right to restrict people's freedom and require them to wear masks?

Alice: I will be able to answer your first question. Science can explain how things work. My goal here is to share with you these explanations and show you how some control measures, also called preventive measures, can prevent new infections, hospitalizations, and deaths. Such control measures include social distancing, wearing masks, closure of selected businesses, and lockdowns of entire regions.

But science cannot all by itself answer ethical questions about what's right and what's wrong. Each of us needs to form our own opinions on these. I don't want to force my opinions about right or wrong upon you. But I can help you understand what's at stake.

All control measures have certain costs. For social distancing and wearing masks, the costs are relatively minor inconveniences. But full lockdowns have terrible economic costs. Epidemiologists can predict how many lives will be saved by control measures, and economists can predict the economic impact. But neither epidemiologists nor economists can answer the question how many jobs are worth preserving at the cost of cutting short one human life.

Cindy: This is such a terrible question. I don't even want to think about it.

Alice: Nobody wants to think of such a frightening choice. But if we close our eyes and just blindly follow our gut instincts, reality may catch up and present us with an answer that nobody would have chosen. If we want to make rational decisions, we need to clearly understand the tradeoffs.

Bob: Could we perhaps get by with only wearing masks and social distancing? Without closing businesses? Then we might not need to make such dreadful choices.

Cindy: Shouldn't we also isolate infected people and quarantine others whom they could have infected?

Alice: These are good questions. We'll need to first talk in some detail about how these preventive measures work and how effective they are.

Frank: Well, I think we should just let the infection spread through the population as quickly as possible, until we get herd immunity. They say that when 60% of all people have become infected, the pandemic will be over.

Alice: There are a lot of misunderstandings about herd immunity. We should talk some time about how, exactly, it works. One little-known fact is that even if the so-called herd-immunity threshold is 60% and no preventive measures are taken, a much larger percentage of people may experience infection, even more than 90%.

The strategy of ending the Covid-19 outbreak by achieving herd immunity has actually been tried in two European countries.

The U.K. quickly abandoned it when the numbers of infections and deaths went up too fast. They currently have one of the highest numbers of deaths per million of people in Europe and are still struggling to get the outbreak under control.[7]

Sweden is still following this strategy. They are trying to achieve herd immunity while slowing down the spread with relatively mild restrictions. In particular, the Swedes did not close schools. But they are still very far from achieving herd immunity, and have already many more deaths per million people than the U.S.[8]

Cindy: This is terrible! I cannot imagine how many more people would die until this herd immunity is achieved.

Frank: I don't believe that the Covid-19 pandemic will be as deadly as they say. A few years ago, there was a big panic about the swine flu. And then it turned out to be no more deadly than the seasonal flu. Why scare people unnecessarily?

Alice: The CDC, our Centers for Disease Control and Prevention, estimated that the swine flu pandemic in 2009–2010 may have claimed between 150 thousand and 575 thousand lives worldwide [2]. These are horrible numbers. As of yesterday, already more than 517 thousand deaths from Covid-19 had been reported worldwide. Probably more than the total number for the swine flu, while the Covid-19 pandemic is still in its early stages.

For the U.S., the CDC estimated a total number of about 61 million cases and 12.5 thousand deaths from the swine flu. This would put the mortality—which we can think of as the percentage of infected people who died from the disease—at around 0.2%, about twice as high as for a typical seasonal flu. As of yesterday, the U.S. had already reported more than 129 thousand deaths[9] from Covid-19, about 10 times more than died from the swine flu in our country.

Frank: But are these really deaths from coronavirus? I've read that most people who die from it are over 80 years old or have some underlying condition, like diabetes or heart diseases. I think those should be counted as their causes of deaths, not the coronavirus infection.[10]

Alice: You mentioned some of the risk factors that make it more likely that a Covid-19 patient will require hospitalization or die from the disease. There are many more; you can find a detailed list at the CDC website. Let me put the URL into the chat [3].

Think about it this way: For example, hypertension is a condition that puts a person at increased risk of a heart attack. But many people with hypertension lead long and productive lives. If a person afflicted by it does suffer a heart attack and dies, the cause of death would still be the heart attack, not the hypertension. It's the same with Covid-19.

Frank: So what is the mortality from Covid-19?

Alice: While the pandemic is still ongoing, the actual mortality cannot be calculated, only estimated. Estimates that I have seen range from 0.66% to over 1%, but these numbers will likely change as we continue to learn more about the disease.[11] So Covid-19 appears to be at least 6–7 times more deadly than the seasonal flu, and it is much more contagious.[12]

Cindy: What if the mortality turns out to be somewhere between these numbers, let's say 0.8%?

Alice: Then even if herd immunity could be achieved with around 60% of all people becoming infected, more than 37 million people worldwide would die from Covid-19; as many as the entire population of Canada, or almost as many as the entire population of California. In the U.S., the death toll would be on the order of 1.6 million people, which is roughly the population of Philadelphia.

Cindy: This sounds so horrible! But you have been talking only about numbers. Each one of these deaths ends the life of a human being. A real person like us, with dreams, hopes, and plans for the future! I cannot even imagine what it's like to die all alone under a ventilator with no relatives and friends allowed to visit.

Alice: It's a slow and lonely death. My mother's family came from Eastern Europe. After World War II, many people there had tuberculosis, which is also a potentially deadly infection [4]. My great-grandmother worked as a nurse in a tuberculosis ward. They didn't have much protective equipment back then. No relatives and no members of the clergy were allowed to visit. Great-grandma told me about those night shifts alone with dying patients. She was often the last person they could talk with, and she would sit at their bedside and hold their hand.

Cindy: Wasn't she afraid of becoming infected?

Alice: I asked her about this. She simply replied: "How could I be afraid? These patients needed me."

Cindy: Is this why you decided to study epidemiology, Alice?

Alice: Great-grandma wanted me to become a doctor. But I was more interested in science and mathematics. Medicine is about curing people from diseases. Epidemiology is about preventing people from becoming infected in the first place. As an epidemiologist, I will be able to work with numbers and mathematical models and help prevent suffering and death.

Cindy: I'm so glad I met you Alice. So please tell me: How can I make sure I don't catch a single one of these coronaviruses?

Alice: First of all, don't panic. A single virus particle will not make you sick. It takes many of them, probably several hundreds, to cause an infection. Your innate immune system will easily be able to cope with a handful of virus particles.[13]

But you can become infected by inhaling a large number of viruses. Unfortunately, it's impossible to make 100% sure this will never happen. There are a lot of ways to greatly reduce this risk though. If you and others meticulously follow the recommendations of epidemiologists, you will not be totally safe, but reasonably safe.

Cindy: But if I do get infected?

Alice: Then you need to isolate yourself as soon as you develop symptoms or test positive and stay in isolation as long as you are likely to remain infectious. This will typically take about 10 days, and will prevent the spread of the infection to others.

Most Covid-19 patients experience only mild flu-like symptoms, such a fever, cough, headache, and fatigue.[14] Many of them, perhaps one third of all who became infected, stay entirely asymptomatic. This is a big problem, as they may spread the infections to others without realizing that they pose a danger. A similar problem is that people tend to be most infectious right before the onset of symptoms.

Cindy: But what if I get so sick that I need to go to the hospital?

Alice: This is rather unlikely, but it may happen, even to young and healthy people. Patients with severe symptoms have described the experience as feeling like they would slowly drown for days in pain that felt like having glass in their lungs. On the more optimistic side, as we continue to learn more about Covid-19, hospitals are getting more successful at treating it, and some medications that help in improving people's recovery are becoming available.[15] But I am not a specialist in medicine and cannot tell you more about symptoms and treatments than you probably already know.

Cindy: Yes, I'm reading a lot about this. But if I need treatment, all hospitals will be full, and they cannot admit me?

Alice: This is a big concern. It happened in northern Italy in March. Covid-19 cases were suddenly increasing so fast that they run out of everything: Hospital beds, ventilators, protective equipment, and medical staff to care for all patients with severe symptoms. Some Covid-19 patients had to be put in makeshift beds outside of hospitals, nurses were totally exhausted from constantly working overtime, and many of them became infected.[16] One of the main reasons why most countries and most of our states imposed lockdowns was that they wanted to prevent a similar situation.

Cindy: Let's hope this won't happen here. But I have heard that even people who recover may still have problems several months later. Our neighbor down the street is a young guy, in his early 30s. But he caught coronavirus with severe symptoms. After a few days in the hospital, he recovered from the disease. Ever since then, for two months now, he has been in a mental fog, almost like people who have Alzheimer's disease. I'm friends with his sister, and she told me that he has forgotten how to say "toothbrush," and is still on leave of absence from his work, because he cannot concentrate on anything. And he had adopted such a cute puppy before he became sick. But he had to return it to the shelter, because he keeps forgetting to feed it and take it out for a walk.

Alice: Yes, being in such a mental fog even months after recovery from Covid-19 seems to happen quite frequently, even to young people. Also, a large proportion of Covid-19 survivors suffer persistent fatigue, breathing disorders, or cardiac problems for months after recovery.[17]

Bob: I always thought that even if I catch Covid-19, it would be over after a week or so. Being in a mental fog and unable to concentrate on anything for several months afterwards, that does sound frightening.

But we interrupted Alice when she was trying to tell us about the numbers. Are the actual numbers of infections really many times larger than the numbers of infections that the media report?

Frank: And different media outlets report different numbers for the same day. Are they just making these numbers up or what?

Alice: Good questions! When we want to interpret data, we need to first understand what the numbers really mean and how they were obtained.

Let me first talk about two kinds of numbers that get reported most often: The daily numbers of infections, or daily numbers of cases, and the cumulative numbers of infections, or cumulative numbers of cases.

Cindy: So there are different names for the same number? I find this so confusing.

Alice: You are not alone, Cindy! For example, the daily numbers of infections correspond to something that in the scientific literature is called incidence of the infection. Journalists who want to sound like experts sometimes mix them up with the prevalence of the infection, which would be the number of people who are currently infected and have not yet recovered.

Here I want to use a more intuitive terminology that directly shows what these numbers stand for. So I will talk about the daily numbers of reported new infections and the total numbers of reported infections up to a given day for a given country, state, or region.

Bob: Would "reported" mean the same as "confirmed"?

Alice: Yes. Most of the published statistics show the numbers of people for whom a Covid-19 infection has been confirmed by a test.[18] If such a test comes out positive—that is, shows presence of the virus—a new infection is recorded and reported to appropriate health authorities.

Bob: So, for people who get Covid-19 and never take a test, perhaps because they never develop symptoms, or perhaps because testing is not easily available, their infections will not show up in these statistics?

Alice: Correct. Many, probably most, actual infections never get reported. So the number of actual infections will be higher than the number of reported infections.

Bob: Sounds like there is no way of knowing the precise numbers of actual infections.

Alice: Right. We can only estimate them. Some studies indicate that, in the early stages of the pandemic, the actual numbers may have been approximately 10 times higher than the reported numbers. I think that now, as we are doing more testing, the ratio may be smaller than 10:1.[19]

Cindy: This sounds so scary! Even these reported numbers already look so terribly large.

Frank: So how can epidemiologists model the epidemic if they don't even know the actual numbers?

Alice: Very good question, Frank! Remember that all models are What-If scenarios that can give only reasonable estimates of future numbers, but never the exact numbers for any future day or week. For this purpose, it may be sufficient if we have a good estimate of the ratio between reported and actual infections.

Also, the purpose of each model is to answer a specific question. For example, if we are trying to estimate the required number of hospital beds, the model can use the number of reported cases, since Covid-19 hospitalizations are always reported.

Bob: But wouldn't this difference between the reported and actual numbers make it difficult to estimate the mortality?

Alice: Yes, it would. The only quantity we can reliably calculate is what's called the case-fatality rate or case-fatality ratio. It is the proportion of confirmed cases who die from the disease. But even this ratio cannot be precisely determined on a daily basis, as there is a time lag between the reporting of infections and of deaths. People don't die from Covid-19 right after symptoms start, but typically only after suffering for a couple of weeks.[20]

The case-fatality ratio also greatly differs between countries.[21] For example, as of yesterday, it was as high as 15.7% in Belgium. In the U.S. it was around 4.9%, in Norway it was 2.8%, in Israel it was 1.3%, and in Singapore it was only 0.06%. Some of these differences can be explained by how many people in these countries got tested and by the quality of their health care. But nobody quite understands why the differences are that large.

In the U.S., there are big differences in hospitalization and death rates between ethnic groups, with Native, African, and Hispanic Americans suffering a disproportionally larger share of severe and fatal infections.[22] These are also the groups of our citizens who more often lack access to high-quality health care.

There are also large differences between age groups. Older people are at the highest risk. But among the people whose deaths from Covid-19 were reported by the CDC last week, between 1 in 5 and 1 in 4 were under 65 years old.[23]

All this makes it very difficult to estimate the mortality of Covid-19. And it is not even clear whether a single percentage would be very meaningful for the entire world or even an entire country.[24]

Frank: OK. But let's get back to these reported numbers. Why do different sources give different numbers for the same day?

Alice: Let's look at two sources of data on Covid-19 infections. The World Health Organization, the WHO, reported a total number of 9,831,896 confirmed Covid-19 cases up until yesterday [5]. Another source, called Worldometer, reported a total of 10,226,574, also up until yesterday.

Frank: Looks to me like somebody is simply making up these numbers.

Alice: Neither of the sources I mentioned here makes anything up. To understand where these differences come from, let's think about the word "reported".

Cindy: Do you mean, somebody has to record the numbers of positive tests in a testing center and report the tally to an office before they are included in the statistic?

Alice: Exactly. The process actually involves reporting at several levels: Testing centers send their reports to an office at the county level, the counties send their reports to a statewide office, the states send their numbers to the CDC at the federal level. The WHO gets their data from the CDC, while some other sources include data directly from reports at earlier stages of this process. Worldometer cuts out the intermediate levels and reports the most up-to-date numbers. You can, for example, find the latest numbers for our county of Athens directly at this source right after they appear. Let me put the URL into the chat [1].

Sources like the Johns Hopkins Coronavirus Resource Center [6] and the New York Times [7] also cut out many of these intermediate levels. So the reporting by the WHO is probably the most reliable, but it lags about two days behind the reporting of Worldometer, which is the fastest. For example, Worldometer listed a big spike of 185,420 new cases reported on June 19, 2020 for the entire world. The WHO reported almost the same number, 184,172 new cases, two days later, on June 21. Speedier reporting may introduce some inaccuracies, but they appear to be fairly small.

Bob: But even with the speedy reporting by Worldometer, are these really the number of infections that occurred on that day? I think there would already be a time lag before the numbers get reported by the county.

Alice: Very important observation, Bob! Even with the fastest possible reporting, we get only the number of infections that occurred some time in the past, around a week earlier at best. It takes on average 5 days to develop symptoms of the disease after exposure to the virus. And it might take a couple of days after onset of symptoms before a person would decide to get tested, and then some more time until the test results come back from the lab and get included in the tally.

Cindy: So these reported numbers of daily infections give us, like, a snapshot of the recent past?

Alice: That's a very good way to put it, Cindy! Epidemiologists can then use models for estimating current and future numbers based on data that only tell us directly what happened last week or 10 days ago.

Bob: So that increase over the last 2 weeks that Cindy talked about earlier today would then really be an increase of now infections between, say, 3 weeks ago and 1 week ago. But was it really over 100% or closer to 80%?

Alice: This depends how we calculate the increase. If we compare the reported numbers of daily new infections for June 14 and June 28 from Worldometer, we get an increase of 101.09%, from 20,523 for June 14 to 41,269 for June 28 in the U.S. On the other hand, the 7-day moving averages were 22,449 for June 14 and 40,221 for June 28, which corresponds to an increase of 79.17%.

Frank: There you have it. Can't trust those numbers. They calculate something to make things look really bad, and then it turns out not to be so bad if they calculate it differently.

Bob: This may be like in economics. There are various indicators of how well the markets are doing, and we need to really understand what the numbers mean to make sense of them. I think that the 7-day moving average would be a more reliable indicator.

Cindy: What does "7-day moving average" mean? I'm so bad at math!

Bob: Maybe Alice can explain this to us. But I am wondering about this 10:1 ratio between actual and reported infections. How can anyone possibly estimate it if all the data are on reported infections?

Frank: I still think this so-called increase is just because of more testing. Especially since we don't know the actual numbers of infections. Can you tell us about this, Alice?

Cindy: But tests prevent new infections! How can they increase their numbers?

I'm so scared about catching coronavirus and perhaps infecting others. Please tell us, Alice, what can we do to keep us safe? Or at least reasonably safe, as you said.

Frank: Alice also told us not to panic. I still think we might just let the virus spread, at least among young and healthy people like college students, and go for herd immunity. But how come that more than 90% of people could become infected if herd immunity would require only 60%?

Alice: These are all very important questions.

Cindy: And I also wonder whether it is safe to touch anything these days or travel anywhere.

Frank: And I would want to talk about these damn masks. People shouldn't be forced to wear them.

Bob: I have a few more questions myself, but it's getting late. Should we schedule regular meetings with Alice and talk about these questions one-by-one?

Alice: I'll be happy to keep meeting with you. Some of these questions don't have very short answers. We will first need to discuss how, exactly, infections spread among people.

Cindy: Please keep meeting with us, Alice, and tell us exactly how to protect ourselves. But my schedule over the summer keeps changing from day to day.

Frank: Mine too. Let's exchange phone numbers and schedule on short notice as time permits.

Bob: Yes, let's do it this way.

Alice: I'm looking forward to meeting you all next time!

Endnotes

[6]   Throughout this book, numerals are used for all single-digit numbers that pertain to epidemiological data and models, characteristics of the infection, control measures under discussion, or

quantities that are used in calculations. In all other cases, the usual convention of writing single-digit numbers as words is followed.

7 A Wikipedia article [8] is a good starting point for reading more on the response to the pandemic in the U.K. Numbers of deaths per million in the U.K. and several other European countries for a day close to when this conversation took place can be found in the tables of Chapter 6.

8 Sweden never issued a nationwide stay-at-home order, as such measures are prohibited by the Swedish constitution. The country focused instead on selectively protecting especially vulnerable populations. A Wikipedia article [9] is a good starting point for reading more on the response to the pandemic in Sweden. The longer-term effectiveness of the response in the U.K. and Sweden to the Covid-19 pandemic are described in [10]. By September 6, 2020, Sweden had the ninth highest number of COVID-related deaths per capita in the world, at 57.3 per 100 thousand people, while the U.K. has the fifth highest, at 62.6 per 100 thousand people.

9 According to [1], the exact number was 129,391.

10 For example, a study of 5,700 Covid-19 patients admitted between March 1 and April 4 to a dozen hospitals in the New York City area [11] found that only 6% of them had no chronic conditions like hypertension, obesity, and diabetes. For a nontechnical description of this study, see [12].

11 Estimates of mortality, or more precisely, infection-fatality rates, during an ongoing pandemic necessarily keep changing as more data become available and treatment options improve. At the time of this conversation, Alice would have been familiar with an estimate of 1% given by Dr. Fauci, the leading expert on infectious disease in the U.S. in testimony to the U.S. congress in early March [13], an estimate of 0.66% for China calculated in the paper [14], and several significantly higher estimates like the ones quoted at [15]. A subsequent meta-analysis of the literature [16] that was posted on July 7 found estimates of the infection-fatality

rate that ranged from 0.53% to 0.82%, with a one-point estimate of 0.68%, but cautioned against over-interpreting these findings, as there are large heterogeneities between subpopulations and potential issues with underreporting.

[12] The most important measure of contagiousness of an infection is the basic reproduction number R_0; see Chapter 9 for details. For seasonal influenza, the value of R_0 varies from year to year. A review of research papers [17] found a mean value of $R_0 \approx 1.3$. The same paper quotes a slightly higher value of R_0 between 1.4 and 1.6 for the H1N1 "swine flu" of 2009, and an estimate of $R_0 \approx 2$ for the "Spanish flu" pandemic of 1918–1919 that claimed approximately 50 million lives. As will be discussed in Chapter 9, for Covid-19, the value of R_0 has been estimated to be between 2 and 3. This makes Covid-19 significantly more contagious than all known strains of the flu.

[13] Chapter 27 gives a brief explanation why multiple virus particles are required for causing an infection. The infectious dose—that is, the minimum number of viruses required to cause an infection—is difficult to estimate and appears to be unknown for SARS-Cov-2 at the time of this writing. Based on the similarity to the SARS virus, it has been hypothesized that the number would most likely be on the order of several hundreds [18].

[14] For a comprehensive list of Covid-19 symptoms, see [19].

[15] An up-to-date overview of treatment options for Covid-19, including experimental ones, can be found at [20].

[16] A Wikipedia article [21] gives many details on the Covid-19 outbreak in Northern Italy. A New York Times article [22] investigates the history of the response to the outbreak and reasons why it was insufficient to prevent the tragedy.

[17] Some examples of Covid-19 induced "brain fog" are described in detail in [23]. This article, as well as the studies [24] and [25] that demonstrate the high frequency of cardiological and other long-term complications came out only after the conversation took place. But as a student of epidemiology, Alice would have been familiar with anecdotal evidence at the time.

[18] Some published data sets also give numbers of suspected Covid-19 illnesses or cases where Covid-19 was the likely cause of death. This distinction is ignored in the text in an attempt to keep the main lines of argument as straightforward as possible.

[19] See Chapter 17 for a detailed discussion of this ratio.

[20] It also takes additional time before deaths from Covid 19 are reported. An approximate timeline for Covid-19 deaths is given in [26].

[21] The ratios that Alice quoted here were calculated based on cumulative data from [1] until June 28, 2020. Continuously updated current ratios can be found at [27].

[22] The CDC publishes detailed data on hospitalization rates by race and ethnicity at [28] and data on disparities in deaths from Covid-19 by race and ethnicity at [29].

[23] Based on data from [30] for the week ending June 27, 2020. The actual percentage of deaths reported for this week that involved patients under 65 years old was 22.3%.

[24] These complications are one reason why only the most cursory treatment of hospitalization and death rates has been included in this elementary text.

References

[1] Worldometers.info. Dover, Delaware, U.S.A. COVID-19 Coronavirus Pandemic. [cited 2020 Nov 12].
https://www.worldometers.info/coronavirus/

[2] Centers for Disease Control and Prevention. Influenza (Flu). 2009 H1N1 Pandemic (H1N1pdm09 virus). [cited 2020 Dec 23]. https://www.cdc.gov/flu/pandemic-resources/2009-h1n1-pandemic.html

[3] Centers for Disease Control and Prevention. Coronavirus Disease 2019 (COVID-19). People with Certain Medical Conditions. [cited 2020 Nov 29]. https://www.cdc.gov/coronavirus/2019-ncov/need-extra-precautions/people-with-medical-conditions.html

[4] Daniels M. Tuberculosis in Europe During and After the Second World War.—I Br Med J 1949 Nov 12 [cited 2020 Dec 6]; 2(4636):1065–1072. https://www.ncbi.nlm.nih.gov/pmc/articles/PMC2051747/
DOI: 10.1136/bmj.2.4636.1065

[5] World Health Organization. WHO Coronavirus Disease (COVID-19) Dashboard. [cited 2020 Nov 14]. https://covid19.who.int/

[6] Center for Systems Science and Engineering (CSSE) at Johns Hopkins University (JHU). Johns Hopkins University of Medicine. Coronavirus Resource Center. COVID-19 Dashboard. [cited 2020 Nov 14]. https://coronavirus.jhu.edu/map.html

[7] The New York Times. Coronavirus World Map: Tracking the Global Outbreak. [cited 2020 Nov 14]. https://www.nytimes.com/interactive/2020/world/coronavirus-maps.html

[8] Wikipedia: The free encyclopedia. Wikimedia Foundation, Inc. COVID-19 pandemic in the United Kingdom. [cited 2020 Dec 6]. https://en.wikipedia.org/wiki/COVID-19_pandemic_in_the_United_Kingdom

[9] Wikipedia: The free encyclopedia. Wikimedia Foundation, Inc. COVID-19 pandemic in Sweden. [cited 2020 Dec 6]. https://en.wikipedia.org/wiki/COVID-19_pandemic_in_Sweden

[10] Fottrell Q. Sweden embraced herd immunity, while the U.K. abandoned the idea—so why do they both have high COVID-19 fatality rates? MarketWatch 2020 Sep 6. [cited 2020 Dec 6]. https://www.marketwatch.com/story/uk-abandoned-herd-immunity-while-sweden-embraced-it-how-possible-is-it-to-achieve-herd-immunity-without-a-vaccine-2020-08-26

[11] Richardson S, Hirsch JS, Narasimhan M, Crawford JM, McGinn T, Davidson KW. Presenting characteristics, comorbidities, and outcomes among 5700 patients hospitalized with COVID-19 in the New York City area. JAMA, 2020 Apr 22 [cited 2020 Dec 6]; 323(20):2052–2059. https://jamanetwork.com/journals/jama/fullarticle/2765184 DOI:10.1001/jama.2020.6775

[12] Rabin RC. Nearly all patients hospitalized with Covid-19 had

chronic health issues, study finds. The New York Times. 2020 April 23. [updated 2020 Jul 22; cited 2020 Nov 29]. https://www.nytimes.com/2020/04/23/health/ coronavirus-patients-risk.html

[13] User Clip: Dr. Anthony Fauci addresses COVID-19 mortality rate. C-Span 2020 Mar 11. [cited 2020 Dec 6]. https://www.c-span.org/video/?c4860450/user-clip-dr-anthony-fauci-addresses-covid-19-mortality-rate

[14] Verity R, Okell L, Dorigatti I, Winskill P, Whittaker C, Imai N, et al. Estimates of the severity of coronavirus disease 2019: A model-based analysis. Lancet Infect Dis. 2020 Mar 30 [cited 2020 Dec 6]; 20(6):669–677. https://www.thelancet.com/journals/laninf/article/PIIS1473-3099(20)30243-7/fulltext DOI: 10.1016/S1473-3099(20)30243-7

[15] Worldometers.info. Dover, Delaware, U.S.A. COVID-19 Coronavirus Pandemic. Coronavirus (COVID-19) Mortality Rate. [cited 2020 Dec 6]. https://www.worldometers.info/coronavirus/coronavirus-death-rate/

[16] Meyerowitz-Katz G and Merone L. A systematic review and meta-analysis of published research data on COVID-19 infection-fatality rates. Int J Infect Dis. 2020 Dec [cited 2020 Dec 28];101:138–148. https://www.sciencedirect.com/science/article/pii/S1201971220321809 DOI: 10.1016/j.ijid.2020.09.1464 Preprint version MedRxiv 2020 2020 Jul 7. [cited 2020 Dec 29]. https://www.medrxiv.org/content/10.1101/2020.05.03.20089854v4 DOI: 10.1101/2020.05.03.20089854

[17] Coburn BJ, Wagner BG, Blower S. Modeling influenza epidemics and pandemics: Insights into the future of swine flu (H1N1). BMC Med. 2009 Jun 22 [cited 2020 Dec 6]; 7:30. https://bmcmedicine.biomedcentral.com/articles/10.1186/1741-7015-7-30 DOI: 10.1186/1741-7015-7-30

[18] Mandavilli A. It's Not Whether You Were Exposed to the Virus. It's How Much. The New York Times 2020 May 29. [cited 2020 Dec 6]. https://www.nytimes.com/2020/05/29/health/coronavirus-transmission-dose.html

[19] Centers for Disease Control and Prevention. Coronavirus Disease 2019 (COVID-19). Symptoms of Coronavirus. [cited 2020 Dec 6]. https://www.cdc.gov/coronavirus/2019-ncov/symptoms-testing/symptoms.html

[20] Harvard Medical School. Harvard Health Publishing. Treatments for COVID-19: What helps, what doesn't, and what's in the pipeline. 2020 Mar. [updated 2020 Nov 23; cited 2020 Dec 6]. https://www.health.harvard.edu/diseases-and-conditions/treatments-for-covid-19

[21] Wikipedia: The free encyclopedia. Wikimedia Foundation, Inc. COVID-19 pandemic in Italy. [cited 2020 Dec 6]. https://en.wikipedia.org/wiki/COVID-19_pandemic_in_Italy

[22] Horowitz J, Buciarelli F. The lost days that made Bergamo a tragedy. The New York Times. 2020 Nov 29. [Updated 2020 Dec 6; cited 2020 Dec 6]. https://www.nytimes.com/2020/11/29/world/europe/coronavirus-bergamo-italy.html

[23] Belluck P. 'I feel like I have dementia': Brain fog plagues Covid survivors. The New York Times. 2020 Oct 11 [updated 2020 Oct 14; cited 2020 Nov 10]. https://www.nytimes.com/2020/10/11/health/covid-survivors.html

[24] Puntmann VO, Carerj ML, Wieters I, Fahim M, Arendt C, Hoffmann J, et al. Outcomes of Cardiovascular Magnetic Resonance Imaging in Patients Recently Recovered From Coronavirus Disease 2019 (COVID-19). JAMA Cardiol. 2020 Jul 27, 2020 [cited 2020 Nov 11]; 5(11):1265–1273. https://jamanetwork.com/journals/jamacardiology/fullarticle/2768916 DOI:10.1001/jamacardio.2020.3557

[25] Garrigues E, Janvier P, Kherabi Y, Le Bot A, Hamon A, Gouze H, et al. Post-discharge persistent symptoms and health-related quality of life after hospitalization for COVID-19. J Infect. 2020 Aug 25 [cited 2020 Nov 11]; 81(6): e4–e6. https://www.ncbi.nlm.nih.gov/pmc/articles/PMC7445491/ DOI: 10.1016/j.jinf.2020.08.029

[26] Moser W, Kelly C. To understand the US pandemic, we need hospitalization data — and we almost have it. The Atlantic Monthly Group. The COVID Tracking Project. 2020

Jul 4. [cited Nov 29]. https://covidtracking.com/blog/hospitalization-data

[27] Johns Hopkins University of Medicine. Coronavirus Resource Center. Maps and Trends. Mortality analyses. [cited 2020 Dec 6]. https://coronavirus.jhu.edu/data/mortality

[28] Centers for Disease Control and Prevention. Coronavirus Disease 2019 (COVID-19). COVIDView. A Weekly Surveillance Summary of U.S. COVID-19 Activity. [cited 2020 Dec 6]. https://www.cdc.gov/coronavirus/2019-ncov/covid-data/covidview/index.html#hospitalizations

[29] Centers for Disease Control and Prevention. National Center for Health Statsitics. COVID-19 data from NCHS. COVID-19 death data and resources. Health disparities: Race and Hispanic origin; provisional death counts for coronavirus disease 2019 (COVID-19). [cited 2020 Dec 6]. https://www.cdc.gov/nchs/nvss/vsrr/covid19/health_disparities.htm

[30] Centers for Disease Control and Prevention. National Center for Health Statistics. COVID-19 data from NCHS. COVID-19 death data and resources. Weekly updates by select demographic and geographic characteristics. [cited 2020 Nov 14]. https://www.cdc.gov/nchs/nvss/vsrr/covid_weekly/index.htm

Chapter 4

How does the spread of COVID-19 depend on our contacts?

Alice, Bob, Cindy, and Frank meet on July 3, 2020. Over the preceding week, on average 184,617 new Covid-19 infections per day have been reported worldwide, a 13% increase over the previous week [1]. In the U.S., the corresponding increase has been 39%. The Fourth of July national holiday is coming up in the U.S., and there is concern that with people gathering for the celebrations, many more of them will become infected.

Cindy: My aunt wants to have all the family over so that we can celebrate the Fourth of July. I don't know whether that's reasonable. I really want to be with my aunt and my little nephews. But I'm so scared of catching coronavirus and then perhaps infecting others. Please tell me, Alice, should I go?

Alice: That's a difficult question. Family gatherings involve many contacts with a lot of people. Some activities, like having dinner in the house, are a lot more dangerous than others, like having a barbecue outside.

Cindy: Could we then all get together if we only have the barbecue outside? Will this keep everybody safe?

Alice: Every family gathering is different. A lot would depend on how many people are expected to attend, how big the backyard is, and how conscientious all people who attend will be about taking precautions.

You said, "keep everybody safe". This is very important. Infections spread in groups of people, and each person in the group is only as safe as the entire group. It is not possible to completely eliminate all risk, but I can help you understand a few general principles that will allow us to make good decisions about reducing this risk in many different situations.

First we will need to talk about how exposure to the infection leads to infectiousness after some time, how contacts lead to transmissions, and how Covid-19 spreads among groups of people along chains of transmissions. Let's make this our goal for today. When we have a clear picture of how this can happen, then we will discuss in more detail how to protect ourselves.

Cindy: *(Sigh)* OK, I'll be patient. But let's talk about this soon.[25]

Alice: A new Covid-19 infection is caused by transmission of virus particles from an infectious person to another person. Let's say from Ingham, who is infectious, to Sue. It can happen when Ingham and Sue are in close contact.

If Sue is susceptible to contracting Covid-19, and if sufficiently many virus particles are transmitted to her from Ingham, she will become infected.

Frank: Simply put: Sue will then catch coronavirus from Ingham.

Alice: Right. But it takes some time for the virus to multiply in Sue's body before she will shed virus particles that may infect others. This time is called the latency period. Its length differs from person to person. On average, it may last about 3 days.[26]

Epidemiologists say that a person in the latency period is in the exposed state and refer to the moment of transmission as the time of exposure. In my example, Sue was exposed to Covid-19 at the time of her contact with Ingham. At the end of the latency period, Sue will become infectious. Both exposed and infectious people are considered infected.

Cindy: Is the latency period the same as the incubation period?

Alice: No. The terms often get mixed up, but technically the incubation period lasts from the moment of exposure to the onset of symptoms. In Covid-19 infections, the incubation period also varies from person to person, from 2 to 14 days. In rare cases, it may be even shorter or longer. On average, it appears to be about 5 days.[27]

Bob: So, is the incubation period for Covid-19 then approximately 2 days longer than the latency period?

Alice: Yes, this is what the data show. It is a big problem. People infected with Covid-19 can already infect others before they develop any symptoms and become aware that they pose a danger. And many of them, somewhere around one third, or 33% of all cases,[28] never show any symptoms at all. But these asymptomatic cases can still infect others.

Typically, people recover from Covid-19 within 2 weeks, but in severe cases it may take much longer. After recovery, they are immune from becoming reinfected, at least for some time.[29] So they are no longer susceptible. Most importantly, they are no longer infectious. When a person is no longer susceptible or infected, epidemiologists call that person removed.

Frank: Removed? Sounds like the person has died from the disease.

Alice: Yes, people who died from the disease are also in the removed state. But fortunately, most of the time a person becomes removed by recovery from Covid-19 with immunity.

Bob: Lots of terminology here. Let me see whether I got this straight.

I will talk about Sue, as in your example.

At any given time, Sue will be in exactly one of the following states:[30] susceptible, exposed, infectious, or removed. Sue starts out susceptible but can become exposed as a result of a transmission. She will become infectious after about 3 days. She may or may not develop symptoms. If she does, as in my picture, this would happen a couple of days after she becomes infectious. After about 2 weeks after exposure, she will be in the removed state, which means that she can no longer become infected or infect others.

Let me try to draw a picture and share my screen with you:

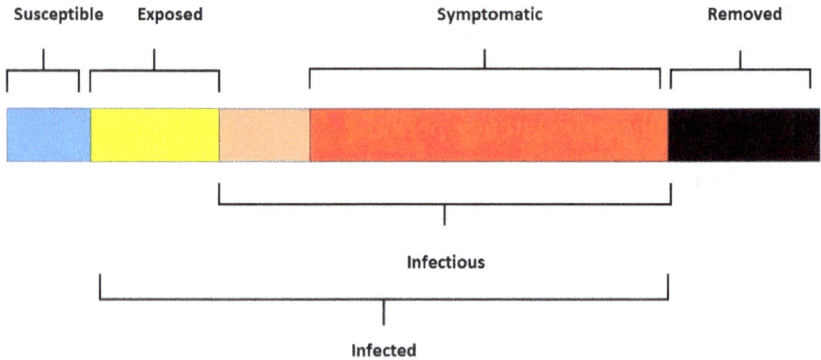

Fig. 4.1   Progression of a person through the states that were discussed above.

Alice: Thank you, Bob! This nicely sums it up for us.

We need to keep in mind though that not everybody with Covid-19 becomes symptomatic and that the times until onset of infectiousness and recovery that you mentioned differ from person to person.

Cindy: Aw, poor Sue! Hopefully she didn't suffer too much and quickly recovered!

Alice: Let's wish Sue well. Unfortunately, many Covid-19 patients are not that lucky.

Now let's discuss in more detail when a transmission of the virus between two people can occur. This requires a contact between them.

Frank: Wait a sec! Aren't they telling us that we can catch the virus if we get closer than six feet of somebody not wearing a mask? Even if we don't touch that person?

Alice: Very good point, Frank! The word "contact" in this context does not mean actual physical contact. It means any interaction that *could* lead to transmission of sufficiently many virus particles for causing a new infection. Like getting within six feet of each other without wearing masks. Or even being in the same poorly ventilated room for an extended period of time when wearing masks and keeping a distance of more than six feet.

Cindy: But can't the disease also be transmitted when Ingham touches an elevator button and Sue touches it some time later? Even if they are not in that elevator the same time? I am so worried about touching anything these days!

Alice: Yes, this may be possible. We would then say that they had an indirect contact.

Cindy: So the contacts in our previous examples would be called direct contacts?

Alice: Right.

Bob: But then each of us makes hundreds of contacts each day; basically anytime we do anything!

Frank: And no transmissions happen during most of them. So why is everyone freaking out?

Alice: Important points, Bob and Frank! Most contacts don't lead to new infections. So we should not panic about every single contact.

But there are many, many contacts during the day. Even though in each one of them a transmission is very unlikely, these chances, or probabilities of transmission, add up over time to a real danger that one of them may lead to a new infection.

To really understand what is going on, we need to think about populations. That's what epidemiologists call groups of people who share some specified space for some time. Like the people who live in Ohio, or all people who go to the same party.

Let me share my screen and show you pictures of a population of 50 people. Think of them as all people in a small residential neighborhood.

The members of this population are represented as little dots. The contacts they have over a short time interval, perhaps lasting 15 minutes, are represented as line segments. Please keep in mind that over the course of an entire day, there would be many more contacts:

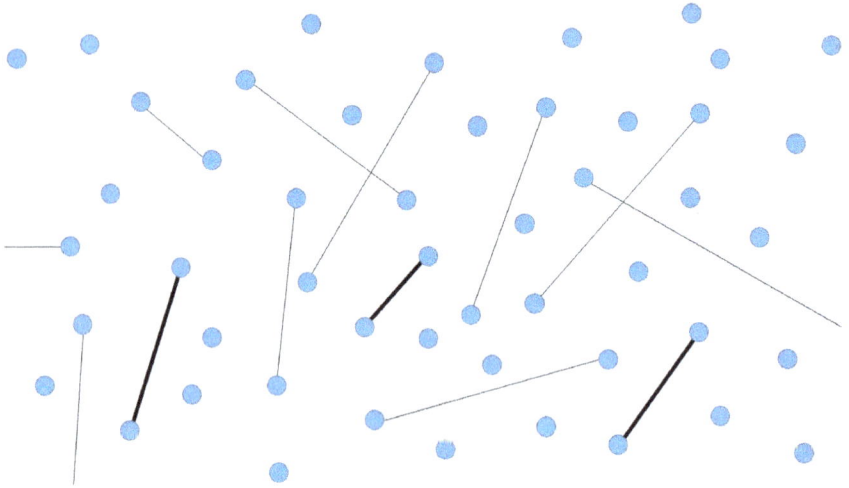

Fig. 4.2   Contacts in a small population over a short time interval.

Bob: Why are some lines only drawn to the margin? And why do some dots overlap the margin?

Alice: Here most of the contacts occur within this group of people, but some contacts are with people outside of this population. They are represented by lines drawn only up to the margin.

For some people it may not be entirely clear whether they belong to the population. Think of students who live in the neighborhood during vacation but are away during much of the academic year. I have drawn them here as little dots that overlap the margin. Let me count them in and draw their dots entirely inside the margin in my next pictures.

I have used the color blue to indicate that a person is susceptible.

What do you think? How many of these contacts will lead to transmissions of Covid-19?

Frank: None, because all contacts are between two susceptible persons.

Cindy: But the contacts with people outside the picture? Could they lead to transmissions? We don't know from Alice's picture whether the person on the other end of the line is infectious.

Alice: Very important points, Frank and Cindy! Contacts between two susceptible people will not lead to transmission. My picture shows that this would be the case for the contacts within this population, but does not give this information for the contacts with people outside of it.

In real life, we usually don't know whether or not the other person is infectious. Due to the time lag between the end of the latency period and the onset of symptoms, we may not even know whether we ourselves are infectious and pose a danger to others.

Bob: Why did you draw thicker lines for three of the contacts in your picture (Fig. 4.2)?

Alice: Not all contacts are equal. When two people touch the same elevator button, they technically speaking have a contact. It is then possible that a transmission of enough virus particles will occur. But it is very, very unlikely. Similarly, when we quickly pass a person almost shoulder-to-shoulder in a corridor, transmission is possible. But it is very unlikely, as we would be close only for a second or so.

Most of our contacts are of low intensity in this sense. I have drawn them here with thin lines.

But there are also contacts that are much more intense. Think about kissing, hugging, or talking for 15 minutes while standing close to each other and not wearing masks. Or when we spend an hour together in the same poorly ventilated room, even sitting more than six feet apart. Here I have drawn three high-intensity contacts with thick lines.

High-intensity contacts have a large probability of being what is called effective. An effective contact is one that would lead to a transmission of sufficiently many virus particles to cause a new infection *if* one of these people is infectious and the other is susceptible.

Bob: But in your picture, they will not lead to transmissions, because each is between two susceptible people.

Alice: Right.

Cindy: How about when we talk with a friend for half an hour while wearing masks and sitting six feet apart, would this be a high-intensity or a low-intensity contact?

Alice: Good question, Cindy! It depends where you talk. Outdoors, the contact would be low-intensity; in a poorly ventilated room it may be high-intensity.

The distinction between low-intensity and high-intensity contacts is not clear-cut. In reality, there is a sliding scale of chances of transmission for hundreds of different kinds of contacts. Here I'm sorting contacts into two types only because this will help us visualize how Covid-19 infections spread and how we can prevent them from spreading.[31] My pictures are models; greatly simplified representations of a complex real world.

Now let us take a look at the contacts during the next short time interval:

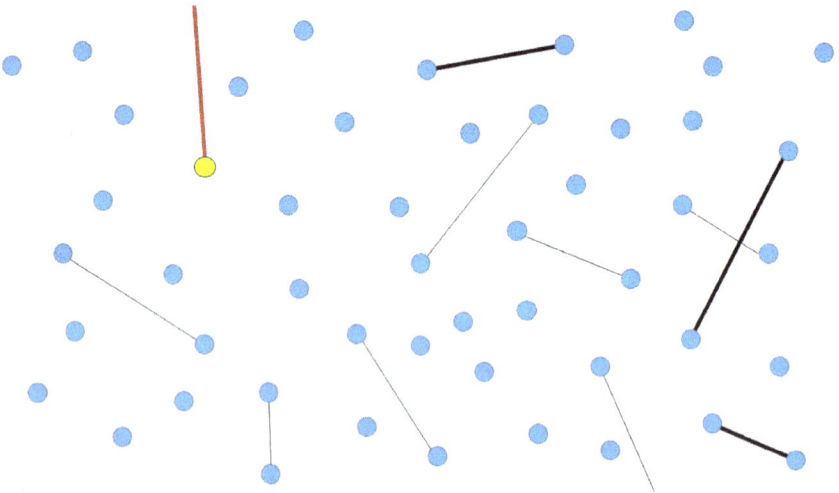

Fig. 4.3   Ingham becomes infected.

Here one person, let's call him Ingham again, had an effective high-intensity contact with someone from outside the population.

This contact led to a transmission, and now Ingham is in the exposed state, which is shown in yellow.

Epidemiologists often call the first infected person in a population the index case. The index case could only have become infected through contact with somebody from outside the population. Perhaps Ingham had a couple of beers in a crowded bar outside of the neighborhood.

Next let's look at the contacts during a short time interval the next day:

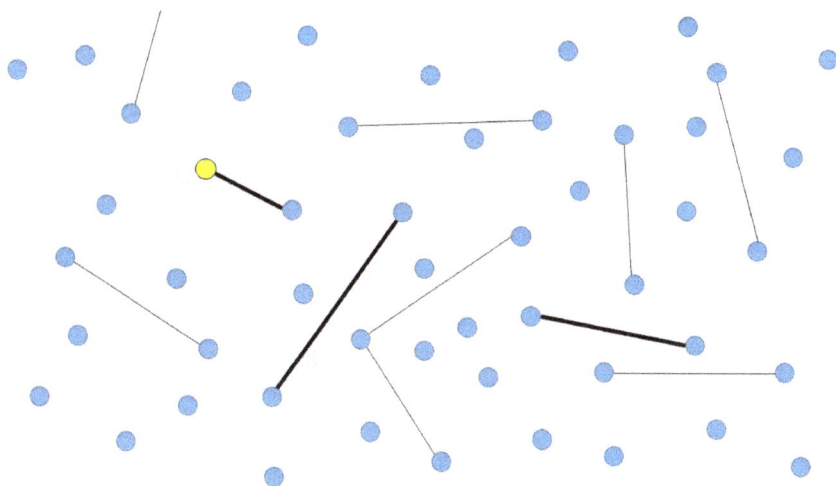

Fig. 4.4   The contacts during a time interval when Ingham is in the exposed state.

Ingham had a contact with another member of our population, even a high-intensity and quite likely effective contact. But this contact did not lead to a transmission and new infection, because he was still in the latency period and unable to infect others.

Let's fast-forward a couple of days to a time when Ingham has become infectious. Right now, I'll not make the distinction between asymptomatic and symptomatic infections and use bright red for showing infectious states:

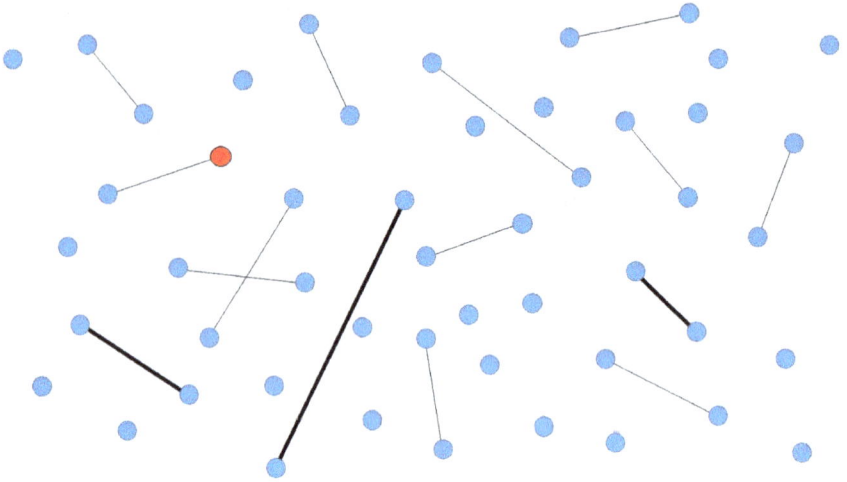

Fig. 4.5   Ingham has become infectious; shown in red.

Alice: Here Ingham had only a low-intensity contact that would be unlikely to lead to a new infection. I've assumed it did not.

Let's fast-forward to another short time interval:

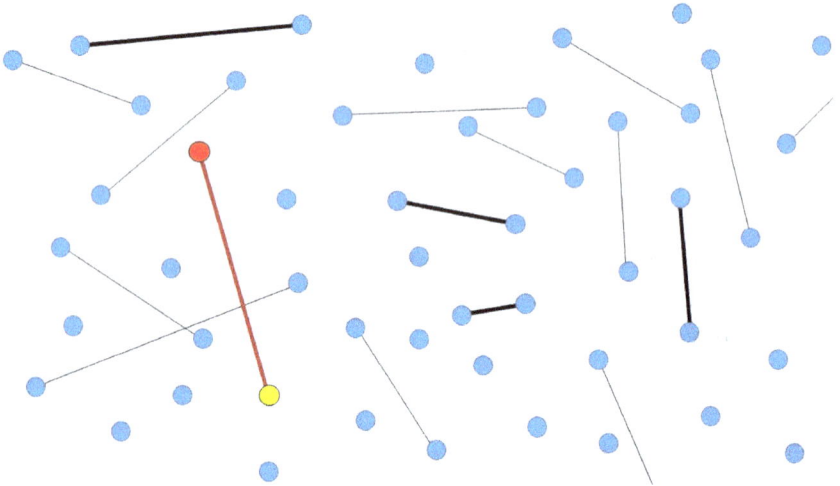

Fig. 4.6   Ingham infects Sue.

Here Ingham had a high-intensity effective contact with another person. Let's call her again Sue. The contact led to a new transmission, and Sue is now in the exposed state.

We can think of Ingham and Sue as siblings living in the same household where they would have many high-intensity contacts.

Let's fast-forward again:

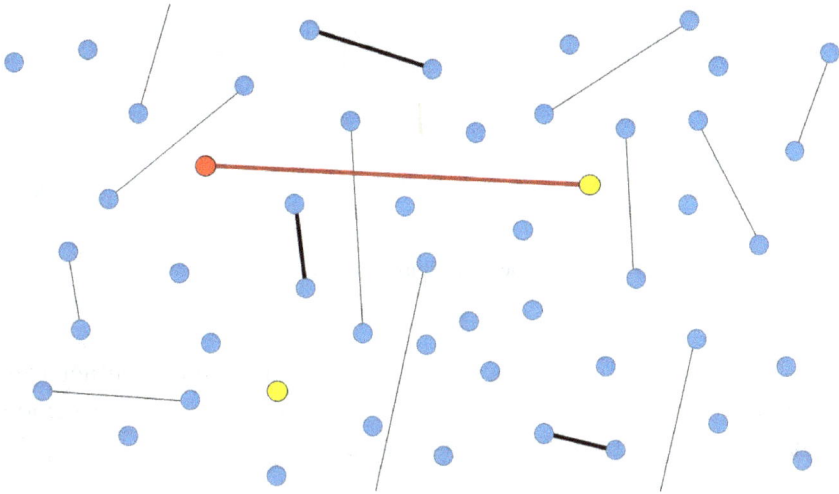

Fig. 4.7   Ingham infects Emily.

Here Ingham had a high-intensity effective contact with a second person. Let's call her Emily. She may be Ingham's girlfriend. Ingham has now caused two new infections.

Let's fast-forward again, to a time when both Sue and Emily will have become infectious. Then we have three infectious people in our population: Ingham, Sue, and Emily.

During this time interval, Ingham had a high-intensity contact and Sue's contact was low-intensity.

Bob: So Ingham would then cause yet another infection, but Sue would not?

Alice: Quite likely, but not necessarily:

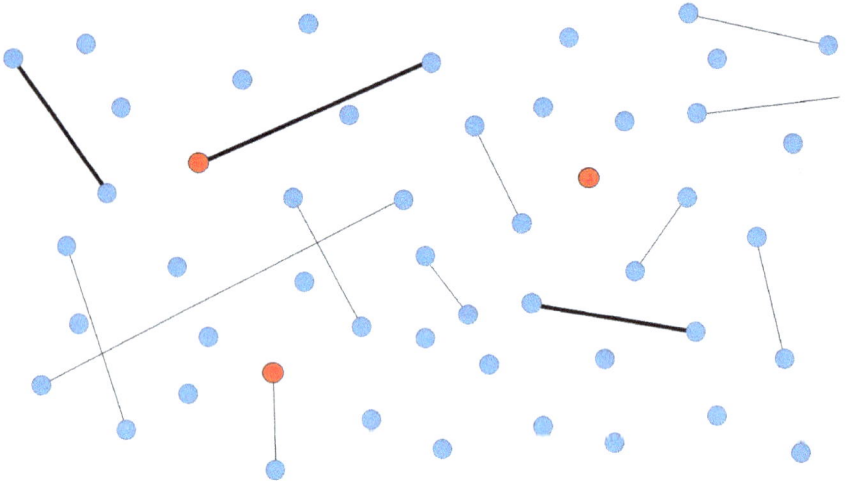

Fig. 4.8   Both Sue and Emily have become infectious.

Not all high-intensity contacts are effective. Ingham's contact certainly put the other person in danger. But in my example, I assumed that it caused no harm. Let's fast-forward again:

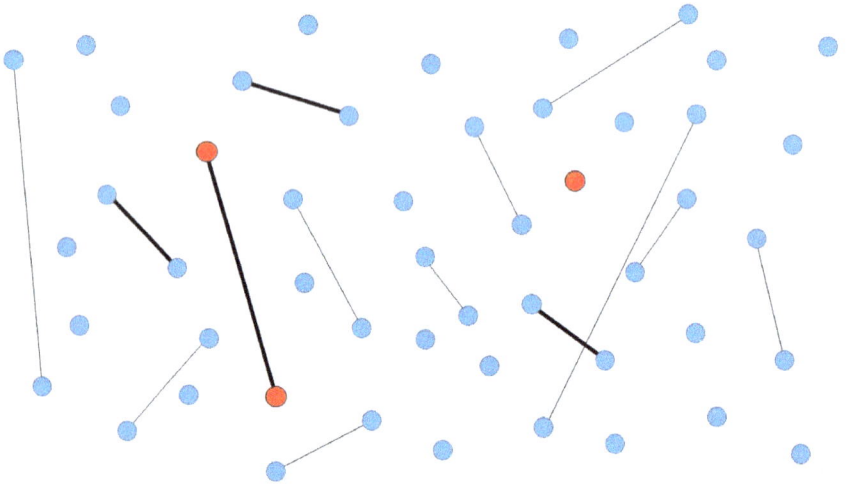

Fig. 4.9   Ingham and Sue have another contact.

We still have three infectious people in our population. Sue and Ingham have another high-intensity contact.

Cindy: This would happen a lot if they are siblings living together. But if both of them are already infected, it does not cause further harm.

Alice: Right. This is why I drew the line in black. No new infection was caused.

Let's fast-forward to a time around two weeks after Ingham got exposed:

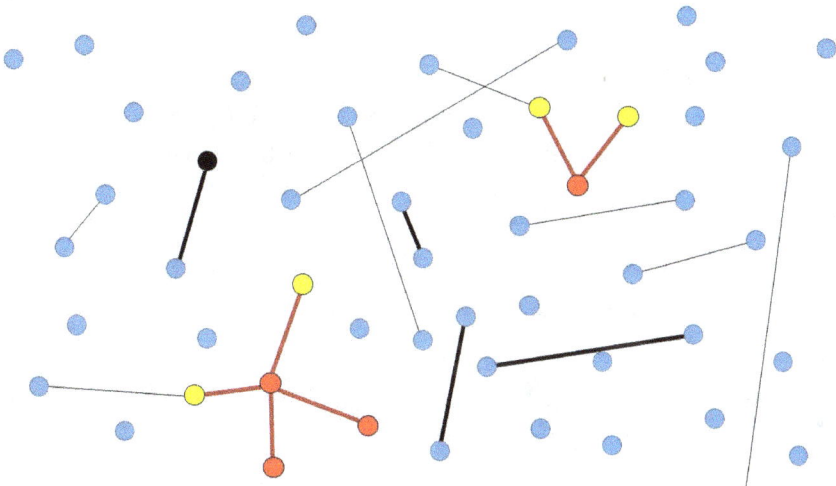

Fig. 4.10   Ingham recovered; Sue and Emily have caused new infections.

By now, Ingham has recovered with immunity. He can no longer infect other people, even through high-intensity contacts.

Emily has infected two members of her family, and Sue went to choir practice where she infected four other people, two of whom have already become infectious.

Frank: Come on, Alice! In your picture, Emily would infect the members of her family at the same time when Sue's choir was singing. How likely is that?

Alice: You are right, Frank, this is very unlikely. Here I have drawn all these contacts in the same picture so that it better illustrates an important point: Ingham has directly infected only two people: Sue and Emily. But both have become links in several chains of transmissions that were started by Ingham, the index case in our example.

Cindy: Can we also see from the picture how many people were directly infected by Sue and by Emily?

Bob: I don't think so. At least four by Sue and at least two by Emily. But neither Sue nor Emily has recovered yet, so they may cause even more infections.

Alice: Right. A person may infect others at any time between becoming infectious and becoming removed. We can count the total number of infections that are directly caused by a given person only after this person has reached the removed state.

Bob: So what would happen in the long run?

Alice: Let me show you a possible scenario:

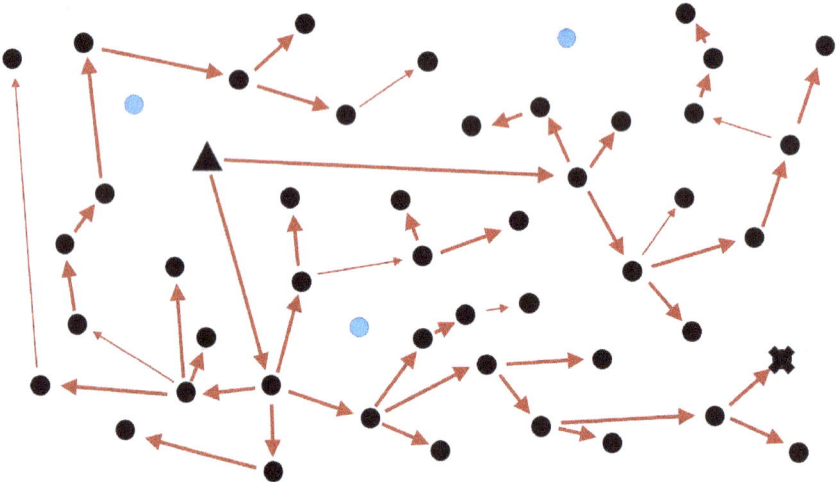

Fig. 4.11   The outbreak has run its course.

Instead of a snapshot in time, I've shown all those effective contacts within the population that over the course of the outbreak have led to new infections.

I've marked Ingham, our index case, with a triangle rather than a circular disk and the transmissions with arrows rather than lines, and have used thick arrows when the transmission occurred through a high-intensity contact and thin arrows when it occurred through a low-intensity contact.

We can see that the index case was the only one infected by somebody from outside this population. For each other person who experienced infection, there is a chain of transmissions from the index case.

Cindy: Wow! So this single index case caused so many infections! Only 3 people in this population never got infected!

Frank: I think this picture is nonsense. In a real population, it would certainly be a smaller percentage of people who caught coronavirus at some time.

Alice: This is a good question. In my picture, 47 out of the 50 people, or 94% of the population, experienced infection at some time during the outbreak. Unfortunately, this may be a quite realistic percentage for Covid-19 if no preventive measures whatsoever are taken. We may discuss some other time why things may get that bad.[32]

Bob: Why did you cross out one disk in your population?

Alice: To indicate that one person in my example has died from Covid-19. All the others have recovered, most after experiencing only mild symptoms or no symptoms at all, some after suffering a lot, and a few may have recovered, but still experience long-term effects.

Cindy: This is terrible! Ingham has caused so much suffering and even one death.

Alice: This is a very important observation, Cindy. Ingham may not have experienced any symptoms himself. But Ingham's one contact with somebody from outside the population has also led to infections in 46 other people, and even to one death. It takes only one index case to start a large outbreak in a population.

This is the most important lesson that we can learn from this picture: One person's careless behavior may cause suffering or even death of many others. And conversely, when we behave in a careful way, we may protect both ourselves, and many, many others.

Cindy: If only he had not gone to that bar!

Alice: This would have prevented the transmission in the story as I have told it. But in a similar story, Ingham might have been infected by a colleague who works in the same office.

Bob: You certainly couldn't blame Ingham in that case.

Alice: We need to be careful with using the word "blame". Let me give you an example of what might have happened in the chain of transmissions that led to the death in my picture.

Ingham contracts Covid-19 in a bar. Sue gets infected while watching TV together with her brother. At choir practice, Kathy catches the infection from Sue. Kathy and her neighbor Hannah share rides to work, and Hannah gets infected during the ride share. Then Hannah infects her 10-year old son Ethan during dinner, who in turn infects his friend Pablo during soccer practice. At home, Pablo gives hugs to his mom and grandma and infects both. Grandma dies.

Cindy: This is so terribly, terribly sad! It makes me cry. We cannot blame little Pablo; we cannot even tell him that he was the one who infected grandma. Never, ever!

Alice: And we cannot blame Ethan for getting close to Pablo when they played. Soccer is a contact sport after all.

Bob: Neither should we blame Hannah, Kathy, or Sue. They were just making normal contacts as we all do.

Frank: Let's not blame Ingahm either, even if he caught it in a bar. Perhaps he had a rough day and wanted a cold one. And he may not have known that it was dangerous.

Alice: I agree. Careless behavior during the Covid-19 epidemic is often being compared to reckless driving. Going to a party while having symptoms of Covid-19 would certainly be every bit as irresponsible as drunk driving.

But none of the people in my example did anything nearly as reckless. All contacts in this chain of transmissions were normal interactions of considerate people. And yet the chain led to the death of one person.

Frank: Glad you see it this way. So nothing can be done. We just need to let the pandemic run its course.

Cindy: But then so many people will suffer and die! Look at all the black dots in Alice's picture! As she said, 94% of all people may eventually become infected.

I think we should avoid all contacts while Covid-19 goes around.

Alice: Would you want Pablo not to get close to his grandma? This would make her feel lonely. Would you want Hannah to not talk with her son over dinner?

Cindy: No, of course not! I was thinking only that we should avoid all contacts outside of our homes.

Bob: That's impossible. People need to go to work. Most jobs require contacts with other people.

Alice: Right. Some contacts as necessary, even outside of our homes. But we do not need to cut all contacts. Pablo's grandma might be still with us if any one of the contacts in my example had not occurred. Cutting unnecessary contacts will go some way towards protecting ourselves and many other people.

Frank: Perhaps, but let's not overdo it. Some people would want to keep Ethan and Pablo indoors all the time. But healthy boys need exercise and need to play with their friends. When I was 10, me and our neighbor's kids were running around outside all the time and playing together. It often got pretty rough. Now we are all healthy adults, and some of my friends already have kids themselves. Do we want these kids to grow up being glued all day to their computer screens, or what?

Bob: I played tennis, which seems safer than soccer. But Sue and Hannah need to go to work. They could perhaps go in separate cars, but would that help all that much? With the economy in shambles, they may need to save some money. Sharing rides protects the environment and cuts in half the probability that either of them would get into a car accident.

Alice: Good points, Frank and Bob. We need to think about risks in ways we are not accustomed to.

We would like to eliminate all risks, but this is not possible. With Covid-19, we need to weigh one risk against another. Like the risk of kids spreading the disease against the risk of stunting their development when we keep them isolated at home too much. The risk of Hannah and Sue contracting Covid-19 during the ride share versus doubling the risk of getting into a car accident when they take separate cars.

And when we evaluate these risks, we need to think not only about the people directly involved in the contact, but also about people who may suffer further down a chain of transmissions. Ingham, Emily, Sue, Hannah, Ethan, and Pablo may be young and healthy and have little to fear from a Covid-19 infection. But this was not true for Pablo's grandma.

Cindy: So we should cut the most risky contacts.

Alice: This would be a good strategy.

Cindy: Then Ingham should not have gone to that bar. This was the most risky and unnecessary contact.

Alice: How about Sue's choir practice? She infected four people.

Cindy: But singing in a choir is a good thing! How can this be risky?

Alice: Actually, singing in a choir is as risky as going to a bar. We cannot base our judgement of the risk that a certain activity poses on the value we see in it.

Cindy: Will you tell us which activities are too risky, Alice?

Alice: Yes and no. I can explain to you what makes certain contacts very risky and why. We will then see why singing in a choir, going to crowded bars, and attending large parties are among the most risky ones.

But I cannot give you a definite list. There are too many human activities, and each of them can be done in a number of different ways. When we understand some basic principles, each of us will be able to assess risk on a case-by-case basis.

Bob: Sounds like in your example Ingham should not have gone to that bar and Sue's choir should have canceled practice, but the other contacts were acceptable.

Alice: This would have worked in the example. But in real life things are more complicated. Ingham and Sue might not have known at the time that what they were doing was dangerous. This is what we can do here: We can talk about what makes an activity dangerous so that we all can make informed decisions.

Let's look at the picture again:

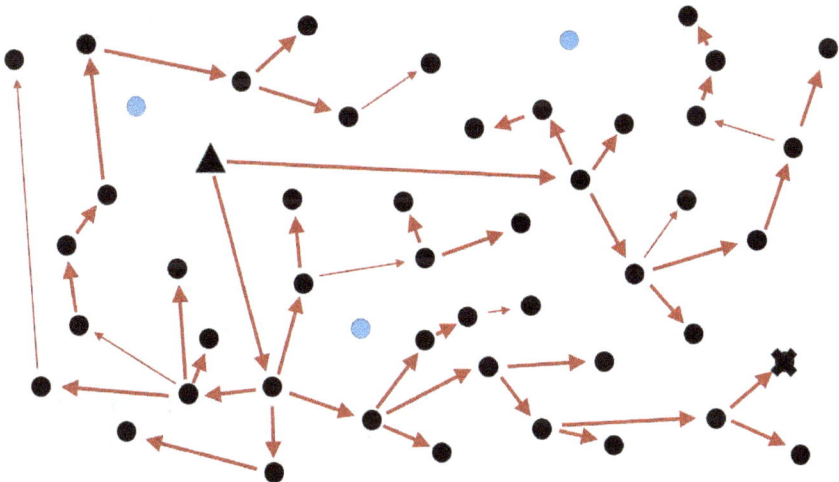

Fig. 4.12   The outbreak has run its course.

As you can see, all contacts in this particular chain of transmission were high-intensity ones, and so were most of the contacts that led to new infections of anybody in this population. They are represented here as thick arrows, and they are the contacts that pose the highest risk. Some transmissions also occurred during low-intensity contacts, but very few of them. Despite the fact that most of our contacts are of low intensity.

Cindy: Are you saying, Alice, that if we just cut out all of our high-intensity contacts, new infections could not spread very far?

Alice: In theory this would work.

Bob: But in practice it would not. Some of our necessary contacts are of high intensity.

Alice: Right. We cannot cut all of these contacts. But we often can turn them into low-intensity contacts.

For example, Sue and Hannah might wear masks while sharing their ride to work. Ingham and Sue would not need to give up on watching their favorite TV shows together, but they do not need to sit on the same couch.

Ingham could protect himself and all others by having his drinks in the patio, and Sue's choir might be able to practice in somebody's backyard standing far enough apart.

Bob: So, when we cut out the unnecessary contacts and turn the necessary ones that are normally high-intensity into low-intensity contacts, would we then be able to control the spread of Covid-19?

Alice: Yes, quite likely. At least with enough testing, contact tracing, and quarantining. We should talk about all these preventive measures in some detail in later chats.

As I said, in reality there is no clear-cut distinction between high-intensity and low-intensity contacts. I classified contacts into these two categories only so that we can better understand what is going on. Instead of saying "turn our high-intensity contacts into low-intensity ones", it would be more accurate to say "turn our contacts into lower-intensity ones". But I like Bob's phrase better than mine, because it gives us a good intuition about what we need to do.

Frank: I might agree with Bob, but only up to a point. I don't know how to say this in mixed company, but we all have certain human needs. For very intense contacts, if you want to call them this way.

Alice: We are among adults, Frank. We can discuss some time how to keep ourselves and our partners safe without giving up intimacy and sex. Today we have covered enough material.

Cindy: There were so many new technical terms and facts. Will we need all of them later?

Alice: Yes. Let me briefly list them for easier reference:

- Epidemiology studies the spread of infections in populations.
- At any given time, each member of the population is in one of the following states: susceptible, exposed, infectious, or removed. Both exposed and infectious persons are considered infected. The removed state signifies that the person can neither become infected nor infect others.
- New infections are caused by transmission of sufficient numbers of virus particles through an effective contact between an infectious and a susceptible person. High-intensity contacts are much more likely to be effective than low-intensity contacts. While most of our contacts are low-intensity, most transmissions of Covid-19 occur during high-intensity contacts.
- A newly exposed person first goes through a latency period before becoming infectious. In Covid-19 infections, the latency period is usually about 2 days shorter than the incubation period, which lasts from exposure to the onset of symptoms. A significant proportion of Covid-19 cases remain entirely asymptomatic while able to infect others.
- Infections spread within a population via chains of transmissions whose links are effective contacts. Even a single infectious person, called an index case, can start sufficiently many such chains so that a large proportion of the population will experience infection at some time. Regardless of whether or not the index is at high risk for developing complications from

Covid-19, other people further down these chains of transmissions may greatly suffer or even die.

- We cannot eliminate all risk. But we can mitigate the spread of Covid-19 by limiting our contacts to the necessary ones and turning as many of those of high intensity into low-intensity contacts as possible.

Endnotes

[25] The material in this book is organized so that basic concepts of epidemiology are discussed first. For greater transparency, each chapter focuses on a single concept or a few related ones. For this reason, detailed coverage of specific control measures such as social distancing or quarantining close contacts of confirmed cases starts only in Chapter 12. While the discussions in these chapters rely to some extent on the material on reproduction numbers that is covered in Chapters 9 through 11, the dependence is not very heavy. Readers who wish to do so will be able to follow most of the discussions on control measures if they choose to skip ahead.

[26] He et al. reported in [2] that infectiousness usually starts 2–3 days before onset of symptoms with significant variability from person to person. Assuming a median incubation period of a little more than 5 days, this implies an estimate of around 3 days for the latency period.

[27] In [3], the median length of the incubation period has been estimated at 5.1 days. Actual incubation periods vary from person to person.

[28] The proportion of asymptotic cases is very difficult to estimate, as such cases are hard to detect. Estimates in the literature vary. Alice's number of 33% was reported in a study based on over 60,000 randomly selected persons [4, 5]. This study is described in some detail in Chapter 17.

[29] Duration of infectiousness differs between individuals, but in most cases does not appear to extend for a longer time period than 8 days after onset of symptoms, which roughly corresponds to 2 weeks after exposure. At the time this conversation took

place, there were no definitely confirmed cases of re-infection with Covid-19. While such cases have subsequently been documented [6–8], they remain rare. Recent studies [9, 10] suggest that the immune response against Covid-19 would typically last at least 5 or 6 months, and might last significantly longer.

[30] In epidemiological modeling, the sets of individuals who at a given time are in the susceptible, exposed, infectious, or removed states are called compartments.

[31] Some epidemiological models do classify contacts into high-intensity and low-intensity ones, but most don't. Here the distinction is made from the outset, as it naturally leads to intuitive descriptions of how important control measures like social distancing and wearing masks contribute to limiting the spread of Covid-19.

[32] See Chapter 26.

References

[1] Worldometers.info. Dover, Delaware, U.S.A. COVID-19 Coronavirus Pandemic. [cited 2020 Dec 29]. https://www.worldometers.info/coronavirus/

[2] He X, Lau EH, Wu P, Deng X, Wang J, Hao X, et al. Temporal dynamics in viral shedding and transmissibility of COVID-19. Nat Med. 2020 Apr 15 [cited 2020 Dec 29]; 26:672–675. https://www.nature.com/articles/s41591-020-0869-5 DOI:10.1038/s41591-020-0869-5

[3] Lauer SA, Grantz KH, Bi Q, Jones FK, Zheng Q, Meredith HR, et al. The incubation period of coronavirus disease 2019 (COVID-19) from publicly reported confirmed cases: estimation and application. Ann Intern Med. 2020 May 5 [cited 2020 Dec 29];172(9):577–582. https://pubmed.ncbi.nlm.nih.gov/32150748/ DOI: 10.7326/M20-0504

[4] Spanish Ministry of Health. Estudio ENE-COVID19: Segunda ronda estudio nacional de sero-epidemiología de la infección por SARS-COV-2 en España. Preliminary report 2020 Jun 3. [cited

2020 Dec 29]. `https://www.mscbs.gob.es/gabinetePrensa/`
`notaPrensa/pdf/04.06040620180155399.pdf`

[5] Pérez P. España sigue sin inmunidad frente al coronavirus. El Mundo. Salud. 2020 Jun 4. [cited 2020 Dec 29]. `https://www.elmundo.es/ciencia-y-salud/salud/` `2020/06/04/5ed8e530fdddffda998b4675.html`

[6] To KK, Hung IF, Ip JD, Chu AW, Chan WM, et al. COVID-19 re-infection by a phylogenetically distinct SARS-coronavirus-2 strain confirmed by whole genome sequencing. Clin Infect Dis. 2020 Aug 25. [cited 2020 Dec 29]. `https://www.ncbi.nlm.nih.` `gov/pmc/articles/PMC7499500/` DOI: 10.1093/cid/ciaa1275

[7] Van Elslande J, Vermeersch P, Vandervoort K, Wawina-Bokalanga T, Vanmechelen B, et al. Symptomatic SARS-CoV-2 reinfection by a phylogenetically distinct strain. Clin Infect Dis. 2020 Sept 5. [cited 2020 Dec 29].
`https://academic.oup.com/cid/advance-article/doi/10.` `1093/cid/ciaa1330/5901661` DOI:10.1093/cid/ciaa1330

[8] Prado-Vivar B, Becerra-Wong M, Guadalupe JJ, Marquez S, Gutierrez B, Rojas-Silva P, et al. COVID-19 re-infection by a phylogenetically distinct SARS-CoV-2 variant, first confirmed event in South America. SSRN 2020 Sept 8. [cited 2020 Dec 29]. `https://papers.ssrn.com/sol3/papers.cfm?abstract_` `id=3686174` DOI: 10.2139/ssrn.3686174

[9] Wajnberg A, Amanat F, Firpo A, Altman DR, Bailey MJ, Mansour M. Robust neutralizing antibodies to SARS-CoV-2 infection persist for months. Science 2020 Dec 4; 370(6521):1227–1230. `https://science.sciencemag.org/` `content/370/6521/1227.full` DOI: 10.1126/science.abd7728

[10] Dan JM, Mateus J, Kato Y, Hastie KM, Faliti CE, Ramirez SI, et al. Immunological memory to SARS-CoV-2 assessed for greater than six months after infection. bioRxiv 2020 Dec 18. [cited 2020 Dec 29]. `https://www.biorxiv.org/content/10.` `1101/2020.11.15.383323v2` DOI: 10.1101/2020.11.15.383323

Chapter 5

Have travel restrictions helped?

Alice, Bob, Cindy, and Frank meet on July 8, 2020. Over 3 million Covid-19 infections have been reported in the U.S. The latest U.S. jobs report showed an unemployment rate of 11.1% for June; down from 14.7% in April, but still nearly three times as high as the rate of 3.5% for February [1].

Bob: Over 3 million people have been infected with Covid-19 in the U.S., and millions have lost their jobs because of the restrictions. In late March and early April, we had over 6 million initial jobless claims per week, and even now there are still more than 1.4 million each week [2]. Every day, more than 200 thousand people are losing their jobs! And three months ago, it was close to 1 million people each day.

I wonder whether all this could have been prevented by blocking the virus from coming to our country.

Frank: The U.S. did impose a travel ban on China, where Covid-19 infections started. I have heard that it saved hundreds of thousands of lives.

Bob: I have read the same. But the infection started spreading here anyway. So I am wondering how much the travel ban really helped. Would it have been more effective if it had been imposed earlier or had been stricter? Can you tell us, Alice?

Alice: When there is an outbreak of a disease in another country, it seems very natural to impose travel restrictions. But many people don't quite understand what they can and what they cannot achieve. Let's discuss today in some detail how they actually work.

Let me share my screen and show you some pictures. We will consider What-If scenarios where there is an outbreak in a neighboring country that has not yet spread to our country. Our country is shown on the left, the other country on the right in my pictures. The colors of the dots in my pictures indicate disease states: blue for susceptible, yellow for exposed, salmon pink for asymptomatic infectious, bright red for symptomatic infectious, and black for removed. The vertical line represents the border. In my first picture, I drew a thin line to suggest that people can move rather freely between the two countries:

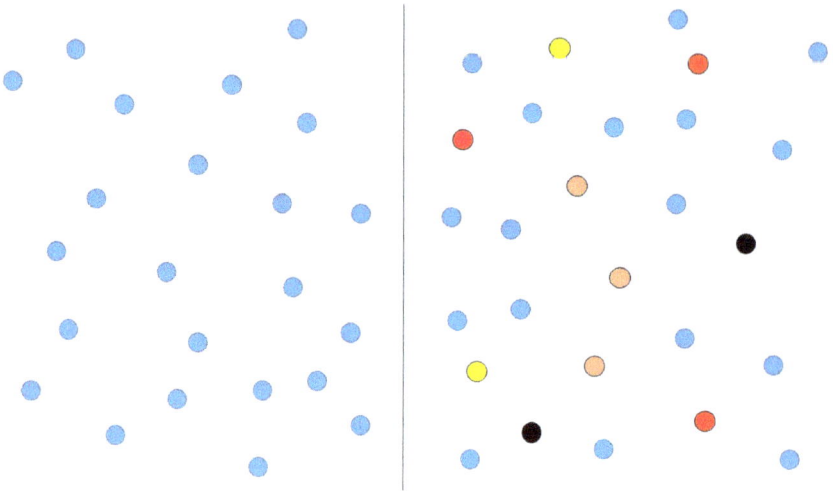

Fig. 5.1   People can move freely between the two countries.

In today's world, all countries are neighbors in a sense. You can think about the country on the left as the U.S., the country on the right as China, and the border as airports. But I want to keep the discussion more general.

So some people will travel, as shown in the next picture. Most travelers from the neighboring country will be disease-free and pose no danger to us. But some of them will arrive with Covid-19 infections. I have shown only those in the picture so as not to crowd it with too many arrows. Also, travelers from our country will go to a place where they can be exposed to Covid-19 infections:

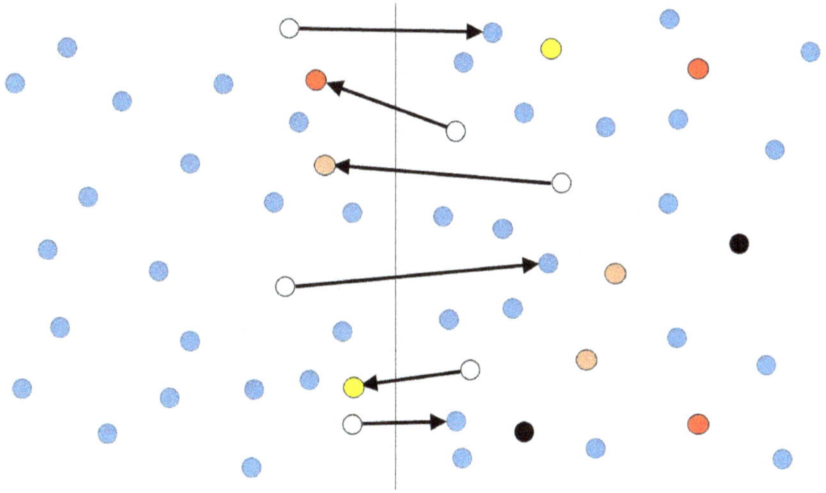

Fig. 5.2 Examples of travel without restrictions.

In my next picture I show how over the next week the infection might have spread further:

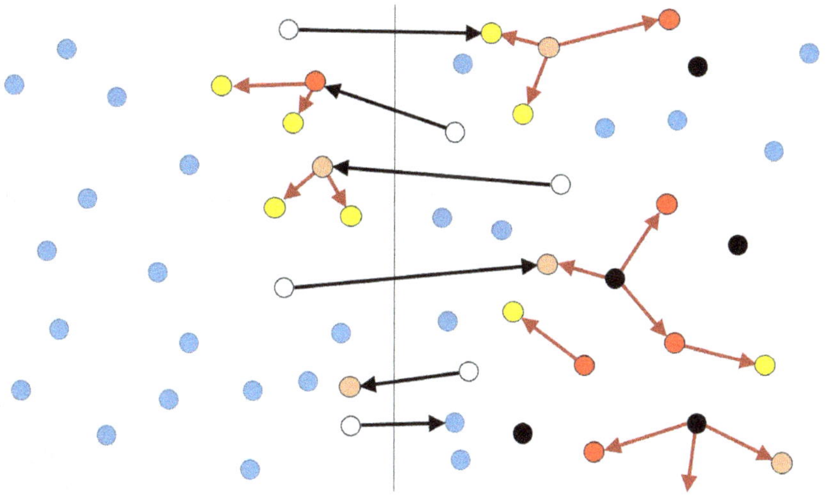

Fig. 5.3 Possible effects of unrestricted travel a week later.

Some of our travelers have been exposed. And travelers who arrived in our country already infected may have caused new infections.

There are many different types of travel restrictions. The least disruptive ones are travel advisories that do not prevent, but try to dissuade our citizens from visiting another country.

Let's see what might happen if we combine travel advisories with screening travelers for symptoms at the border and preventing those who have a fever from entering:

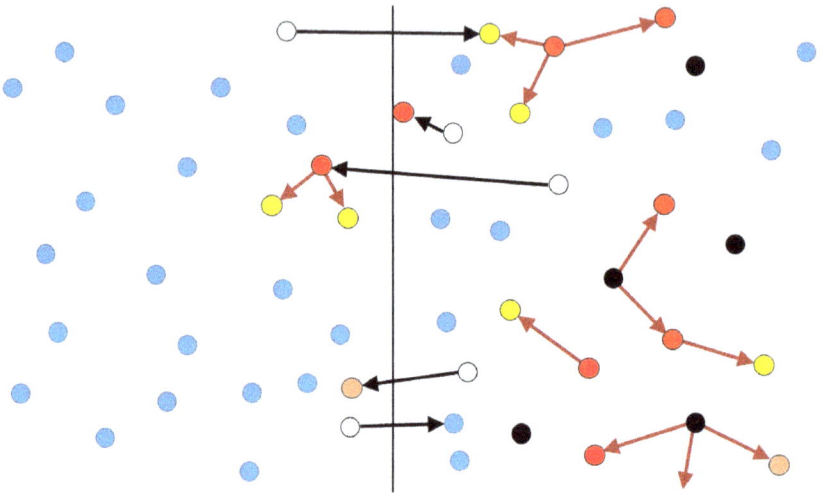

Fig. 5.4   Possible effects of travel advisory and screening for symptoms at ports of entry.

Note the bright red dot that got stuck right at the border. It represents the symptomatic case of our previous picture, who was not allowed to enter our country. Also, one of our travelers canceled the trip.

Bob: This has prevented some infections of our people, but not all of them.

Alice: Right. The asymptomatic case, shown in salmon color in my second picture (Fig. 5.2), could still enter, and so could the one that was merely exposed at the time and has by now also become infectious.

Cindy: Later on, this case may cause infections that start chains of transmissions. And the traveler from our country who caught Covid-19 abroad could start such chains after returning.

Alice: Yes. These restrictions will delay the eventual spread of the infection in our country a little, but they cannot prevent it from happening.

Frank: But the U.S. travel ban on China was much stricter than that!

Alice: True. Most, but not all, flights between the countries were canceled, and most, but not all, people were prevented from traveling between the two countries.[33]

Under this type of travel ban, some people will still travel, and with the sheer volume of regular international travel, especially between large countries as the U.S. and China, eventually somebody will bring the infection to our country:

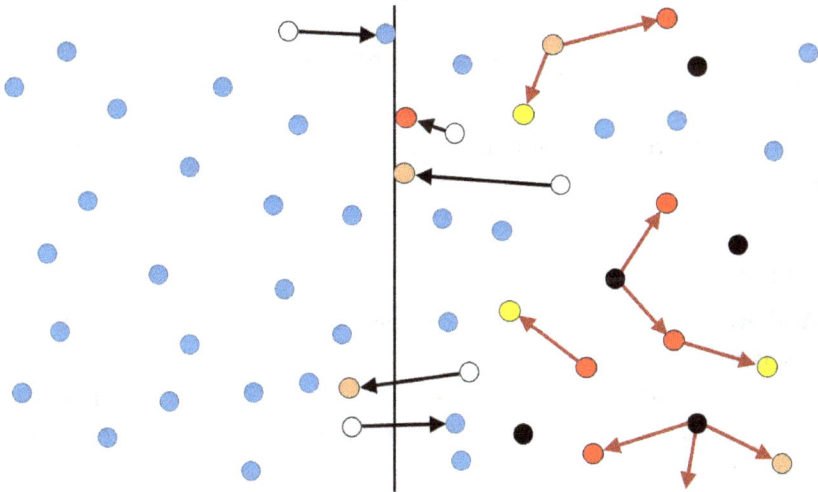

Fig. 5.5 Possible effects of a more restrictive travel ban.

In my picture, the infected visitor has not yet started chains of transmissions, but is likely to do so soon. We can see that this travel ban might have delayed the spread in our country, by a couple of weeks perhaps, but could not have prevented it.

Only a total travel ban could in theory prevent the infection from entering our country. As in the next picture:

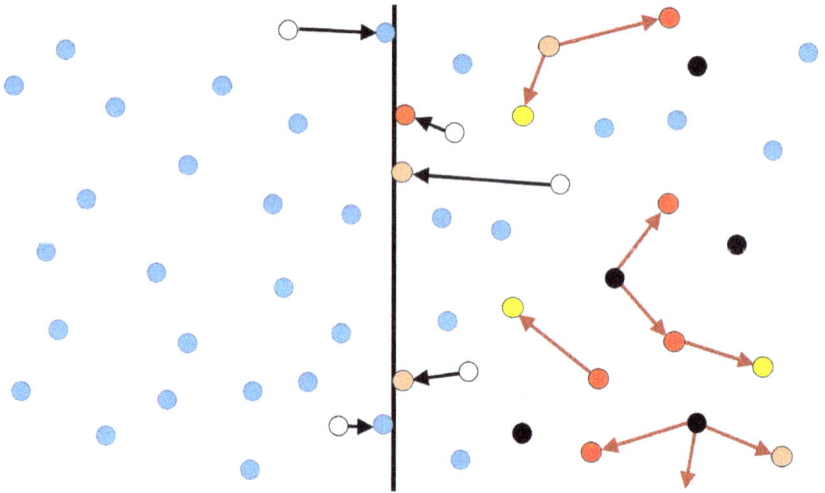

Fig. 5.6   Possible effects of a total travel ban between two countries.

Bob: In theory, but not in practice. In our global economy, goods and services have to move between countries. Some people need to travel in order to deliver them.

Alice: Right.

And even if it were possible to completely seal off one border, it would not completely prevent infections from entering our country. There are around 200 countries in the world, and people travel between all of them. So somebody will eventually bring the infection from another country.

Something like this seems to have happened after travel between the U.S. and China was greatly restricted. We saw a large outbreak in New York and neighboring states in the second half of March and in April. Genetic sequencing has shown that it was most likely started by visitors who brought in the virus from Europe some time in late February or early March.[34]

In my next picture, the red arrow at the bottom left shows an infection that somebody might have brought from a third country:

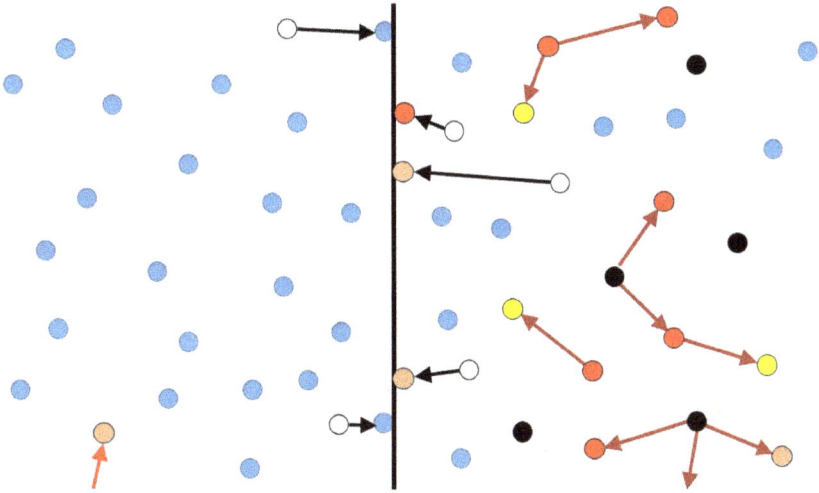

Fig. 5.7   Infections can still enter after completely sealing off one border.

Frank: But the U.S. also imposed a travel ban on visitors from many European countries.

Alice: Yes, on March 13. It came way too late and most likely had no significant effect on the spread of Covid-19 infections in the U.S.

Only by totally sealing off all of its borders, a country could in theory prevent all infected individuals from entering it.

Bob: Perhaps a country on remote islands, like New Zealand, could do this, but not the U.S.

Alice: Yes, it would be nearly impossible in a country like the U.S. New Zealand and Australia did in fact impose travel bans of this type, and they contributed to their success in limiting the spread of Covid-19.

Let me show you a picture of how such a travel ban might work if it could be imposed:

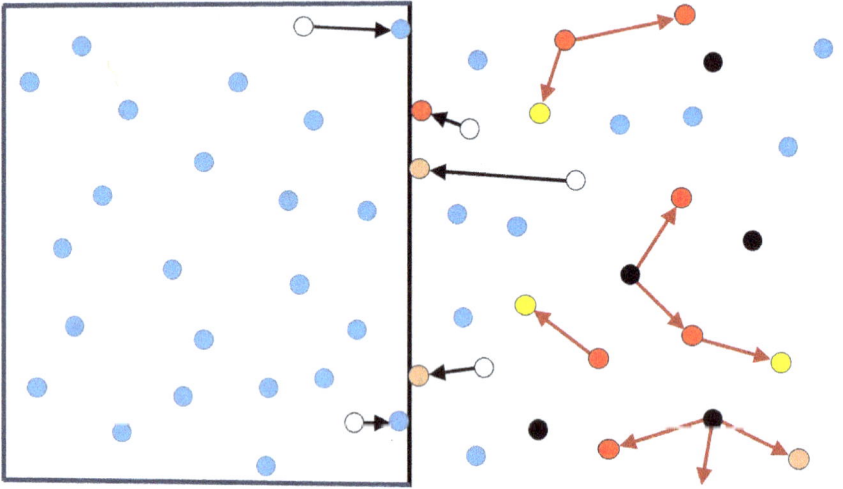

Fig. 5.8   A possible scenario when all borders are completely sealed.

But even if it could be done, by the time the borders were sealed, one or more infected individuals might already have entered:

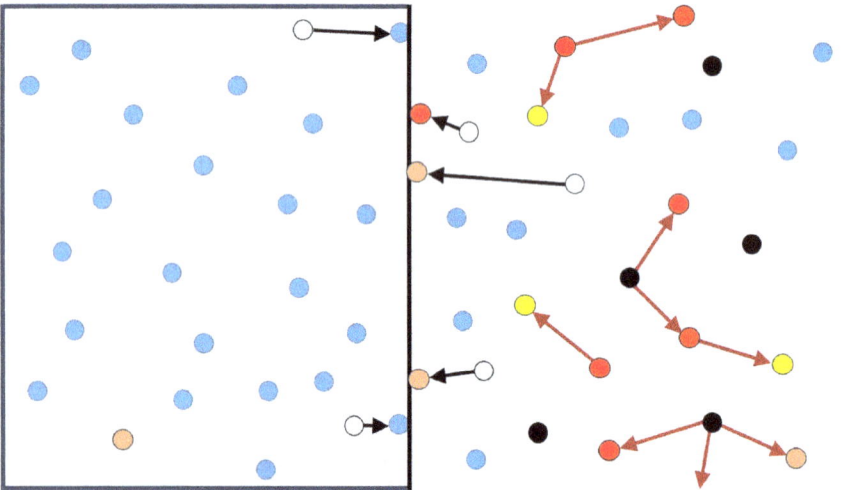

Fig. 5.9   Another possible scenario when all borders are completely sealed.

Cindy: The infected person in this picture would likely start chains of transmission, and the infection would then spread inside our country as much as in the other scenarios!

Alice: Yes. It takes only one index case to start an outbreak. And when no control measures beside the travel ban are put in place, our models predict that the number of people who will eventually become infected does not depend much on how many infections are brought in from abroad.[35]

A scenario like in the last picture did occur in the U.S. We now know that by January 31, when the U.S. imposed a partial travel ban on China, infections were already spreading inside our country. The first documented transmission inside the U.S. happened some time in late January, and it is likely that unconfirmed transmissions occurred even earlier.[36]

Bob: It almost looks to me now that travel restrictions and travel bans have no effect whatsoever.

Alice: They certainly are much less effective than most people believe them to be. If a travel ban gives people a false sense of security that the virus will not get into their country, it will have no effect and down the road the outbreak will be as large as without any travel restrictions.

But they have their uses. While they will generally not prevent an outbreak in a given country, they may slow down its onset. We can see this when we compare my earlier pictures with the later ones. With travel restrictions, fewer infectious people will enter, and many of these few may still not be infectious at the time. It takes only one index case to start a large outbreak. But if it is started by more people, it will grow faster.

With some travel restrictions in place, a country may have a couple more weeks to prepare for what's almost certainly to come. Ramp up the production of ventilators and personal protective equipment, like face masks. And, most importantly, warn its people of the dangers ahead, and explain to them how to best protect themselves and others. If the additional preparation time is used in this way, the outbreak can be kept small. I did not see much evidence of such steps being taken in the U.S. in February [3].

There is a second scenario where travel restrictions may help. Suppose a country has already brought its outbreak under control. Then the numbers of transmissions inside their population will be low. With control measures like social distancing, extensive testing, and contact tracing, they may be able to keep them at bay. We should talk about these preventive measures in detail some other time.

But in this situation, when the outbreak is still large elsewhere and many visitors arrive from abroad, the new infections brought in by these visitors could be a substantial fraction of all cases. They would also be difficult to detect by contact tracing. Therefore, it would make sense to limit the numbers of these visitors from regions where Covid-19 is still rampant. In such a situation, even partial travel restrictions can help. That's why the European Union, where there are currently relatively few new infections, still does not admit visitors from the U.S. and most other countries.[37]

Endnotes

[33] For a description of the U.S. travel ban on China, see for example, [4]. The order temporarily barred most foreign nationals who had traveled in China within the last 14 days. U.S. citizens, permanent residents, and their immediate families where still allowed to enter the U.S. even on direct flights from China, but faced screening at select ports of entry and were required to undertake 14 days of self-screening to ensure they didn't pose a health risk.

[34] This was confirmed by comparing genomes of different strains of the virus. See, for example, [5].

[35] See, for example, [6] for a description of such a model and for an explanation why the final size of an outbreak does not significantly depend on the number of initially infected individuals as long as this number is relatively small.

[36] Patient 1—a woman in her 60s—returned from China in mid-

January, 2020. One week later, she was hospitalized with pneumonia and tested positive for SARS-CoV-2. Her husband (Patient 2) did not travel but had frequent close contact with his wife. He was admitted 8 days later and tested positive for SARS-CoV-2 [7].

[37] A comparison of daily new infections in the U.S. and selected European countries will be discussed in Chapter 6. At the time of this conversation, restrictions on travel to countries in the EU had been lifted only for residents of the 27 members of the EU itself, the Schengen-associated nations of Iceland, Liechtenstein, Norway, and Switzerland, as well as residents of the following countries: Algeria, Australia, Canada, Georgia, Japan, Montenegro, Morocco, New Zealand, Rwanda, Serbia, South Korea, Thailand, Tunisia, Uruguay [8].

References

[1] Trading Economics. United States unemployment rate. [cited 2020 Nov 19]. https://tradingeconomics.com/united-states/unemployment-rate

[2] Macrotrends LLC. Initial jobless claims historical chart. [cited 2020 Nov 20]. https://www.macrotrends.net/1365/jobless-claims-historical-chart

[3] Leonhardt D, Leatherby L. The unique U.S. failure to control the virus. The New York Times 2020 Aug 6. [updated 2020 Aug 8; cited 2020 Dec 8]. https://www.nytimes.com/2020/08/06/us/coronavirus-us.html

[4] Reichmann D. US declares public health emergency from coronavirus. The Boston Globe 2020 Feb 1, 2020. [cited 2020 Dec 8]. https://www.bostonglobe.com/news/nation/2020/01/31/declares-public-health-emergency-from-coronavirus/9WMXL38AdA08GJworROtII/story.html

[5] Zimmer C. Most New York coronavirus cases came from Europe, genomes show. The New York Times 2020 Apr 8. [cited 2020 Dec 8]. https://www.nytimes.com/2020/04/08/science/new-york-coronavirus-cases-europe-genomes.html

[6] Just W, Callender H, LaMar MD. Exploring Erdős-Rényi random graphs with IONTW. QUBES. Community. Groups. Exploring Transmission of Infectious Diseases on Networks with NetLogo. 2015 May 9. [cited 2020 Dec 31]. https://qubeshub. org/community/groups/iontw/iontwmodules

[7] Ghinai I, McPherson TD, Hunter JC, Kirking HL, Christiansen D, Joshi K, et al. First known person-to-person transmission of severe acute respiratory syndrome coronavirus 2 (SARS-CoV-2) in the USA. Lancet 2020 Apr 4. [cited 2020 Dec 29]; 395(10230), 1137–1144. https://www.thelancet. com/journals/lancet/article/PIIS0140-6736(20)30607-3/fulltext DOI: 10.1016/S0140-6736(20)30607-3

[8] European Council/Council of the European Union. Press release. Council agrees to start lifting travel restrictions for residents of some third countries. 2020 Jun 30. [cited 2020 Nov 22]. https://www.consilium.europa.eu/en/press/press-releases/2020/06/30/council-agrees-to-start-lifting-travel-restrictions-for-residents-of-some-third-countries/

Chapter 6

How can we compare numbers of infections in different countries?

Alice, Bob, Cindy, and Frank continue their meeting on July 8, 2020. A week earlier, on July 1, the European Union had lifted cross-border travel restrictions for residents of its member states and 18 other countries.[37]

Bob: Speaking of travel: It's summer, time for a vacation. I was planning on going to Spain and hoping that they would lift their travel restrictions. They did last week, for visitors from 44 different countries, but not from the U.S. There are just a few countries that we can visit right now as tourists. Perhaps I could go to Jamaica, which re-opened its borders on June 15 [1].

Frank: Good for you. I'm just hoping people will stay put over the summer and do home improvements. A friend of mine has a construction business. We do everything: decks, siding, masonry. We serve customers within 75 miles. Reasonable rates. I'll put the contact in the chat, in case you need something.

It's hard work, long hours in the heat when there's a job, weekends and all. But I don't mind. Now that mom is unemployed, she needs every penny that I can bring home.

Cindy: I'd be happy to help you out, Frank. I'll share your contact with the neighbors on our street.

Frank: Thank you, Cindy. We do solid work. I can send you references.

Cindy: But about your trip, Bob: I don't know whether it would be safe to go on a vacation this summer. Especially to a foreign country. I would be so scared of catching coronavirus over there and bringing it back home.

Bob: Don't worry too much, Cindy. Some places are harder hit by Covid-19 than others. I would need to compare how bad it is in different countries and then go to a place where there are few infections.

Cindy: But how can we compare the numbers of infections in different countries? How would we know which countries are safer to visit than others? Perhaps Alice can tell us.

Alice: It's not too difficult. We can compare the numbers that are available online. But we will need to carefully think about what these numbers really mean and how they relate to our questions.

Bob: I think we can use the Worldometer web site that you told us about. Let me share the link in the chat [2].

Alice: Thank you, Bob. Let's look at the data for yesterday:

#	Country, Other	Total Cases	New Cases	Total Deaths	New Deaths	Total Recovered	Active Cases	Serious, Critical	Tot Cases/ 1M pop	Deaths/ 1M pop	Total Tests	Tests/ 1M pop	Population
	World	11,942,330	+208,301	545,678	+5,504	6,844,977	4,551,675	58,195	1,532	70.0			
1	USA	3,097,084	+55,442	133,972	+993	1,354,863	1,608,249	15,371	9,356	405	38,801,591	117,211	331,039,330
2	Brazil	1,674,655	+48,584	66,868	+1,312	1,072,229	535,558	8,318	7,878	315	4,316,284	20,304	212,587,032
3	India	743,481	+23,135	20,653	+479	457,058	265,770	8,944	539	15	10,211,092	7,398	1,380,233,788
4	Russia	694,230	+6,368	10,494	+198	463,880	219,856	2,300	4,757	72	21,537,771	147,584	145,935,812
5	Peru	309,278	+3,575	10,952	+180	200,938	97,388	1,265	9,378	332	1,821,328	55,227	32,978,661
6	Chile	301,019	+2,462	6,434	+50	268,245	26,340	2,060	15,744	337	1,210,326	63,305	19,119,079
7	Spain	299,210	+341	28,392	+4	N/A	N/A	617	6,400	607	5,734,599	122,652	46,755,169
8	UK	286,349	+581	44,391	+155	N/A	N/A	209	4,218	654	10,777,399	158,741	67,892,858
9	Mexico	261,750	+4,902	31,119	+480	159,657	70,974	378	2,030	241	641,142	4,972	128,955,195
10	Iran	245,688	+2,637	11,931	+200	207,000	26,757	3,270	2,925	142	1,846,793	21,983	84,009,505
11	Italy	241,956	+137	34,899	+30	192,815	14,242	70	4,002	577	5,703,673	94,338	60,459,826
12	Pakistan	234,509	+2,691	4,839	+77	134,957	94,713	2,306	1,061	22	1,445,153	6,541	220,943,702
13	Saudi Arabia	217,108	+3,392	2,017	+49	154,839	60,252	2,268	6,235	58	2,018,657	57,972	34,821,448

Fig. 6.1 Data from Worldometer.info [2] for July 7, ordered by total number of reported infections per country.

Worldometer constantly updates their data and for different countries they show up at different times. But when we look at the data for yesterday, we get numbers for each country for a full day.

Bob: So from these numbers we can answer a question like this one: "Where has the Covid-19 outbreak been the worst so far?"

Cindy: That would be in the U.S. The website shows 3,097,084 total reported infections in our country. Over three million!

The country with the second highest total is Brazil, with 1,674,655 total reported infections, or a little more than half of the number for the U.S.

Frank: Your comparison is unfair to the U.S., Cindy.

Cindy: Why would this be unfair? The number of total reported infections is higher in the U.S. than anywhere else in the world. This is simply a fact.

Frank: Yes, but the U.S. is also one of the largest countries in the world, and larger countries will have higher numbers of infections than smaller ones, even if the outbreak in both countries has been equally bad.

Bob: I can see that. So how can we then compare the numbers of infections in different countries with different population sizes?

Frank: Simple. Let's divide the numbers of reported cases for each country by its population in millions. This would give us a fair comparison.

Alice: Scientists call this scaling the data by population size. Frank is right, when we want to meaningfully compare numbers for different countries, we first need to scale them by population size.

Bob: But for that we would need to look up the population sizes somewhere and calculate these fractions.

Cindy: Wait! I think the Worldometer site already shows all these numbers.

Alice: Yes it does. And a lot of other useful numbers as well. That's what I like about this site.

Cindy: The website shows that the U.S. has a population of a little over 331 million people, while Brazil has about 212 and a half million people. In the column "Tot Cases/1M pop" it then gives a total number of 9,356 cases per million for the U.S. and 7,878 cases per million for Brazil.

So, after scaling for population size, the total reported infections are still higher in the U.S.

Frank: Things may change if cases in Brazil rise faster than in the U.S. And who knows how accurate these numbers really are? Perhaps Brazil reports fewer cases than the U.S., but in reality has more undetected ones?

Alice: Even the reported numbers for Brazil are horribly high. This worries me a lot, especially since I'm half Brazilian. My official first name is Aline, but most people don't know how to pronounce it right, and I go by Alice. My father's family is from Salvador in the province of Bahia, and I have many relatives there. This is such a wonderful place. The food is incredible, so delicious! And their carnival celebrations may be the largest in the world, like a giant block party spread out 15 miles. I can't even imagine what will happen over there if Covid-19 is still around during next carnival in February.

Frank: I didn't want to hurt your feelings, Aline. I didn't know your dad was from Brazil.

Alice: No offence taken, Frank. And you are right: There are a lot of problems with the response to Covid-19 in Brazil. Some are very similar to the ones we have in the U.S.[38]

Other problems are different in our two countries. For example, Brazil has been conducting very few tests; only about 10% as many as the U.S. did per million people. This is also shown in the Worldometer table. It wouldn't surprise me if the proportion of undetected cases were a lot higher in Brazil than in the U.S.

Bob: And the total number of 9,356 reported cases per million in the U.S. is not the highest in the world. We can see right from this chart that it is much higher in Chile, where it shows 15,744.

Chile has a population of only a little more than 19 million people. If we were only comparing the number of roughly 300 thousand total reported infections in Chile with the over 3 million reported in the U.S., we would get a totally misleading picture.

Alice: I agree. Isolated numbers quoted out of context can give misleading impressions. If we want to really make sense of any kind of data, we need to put them into the proper context.

Frank: So did Chile report the highest number of total Covid-19 infections per million of any country so far?

Cindy: Let me try toggling here at Tot Cases/1M and see what will happen:

All Europe North America Asia South America Africa Oceania													
#	Country, Other ↓↑	Total Cases ↓↑	New Cases ↓↑	Total Deaths ↓↑	New Deaths ↓↑	Total Recovered ↓↑	Active Cases ↓↑	Serious, Critical ↓↑	Tot Cases/ 1M pop ↓	Deaths/ 1M pop ↓↑	Total Tests ↓↑	Tests/ 1M pop ↓↑	Population ↓↑
1	Qatar	100,945	+600	134	+1	94,903	5,908	154	35,952	48	390,997	139,254	2,807,805
2	San Marino	698		42		656	0		20,571	1,238	5,729	168,838	33,932
3	Bahrain	30,321	+500	98		25,570	4,653	60	17,817	58	621,362	365,122	1,701,793
4	French Guiana	5,178	+124	21	+1	2,119	3,038	30	17,332	70	8,707	29,145	298,748
5	Chile	301,019	+2,462	6,434	+50	268,245	26,340	2,060	15,744	337	1,210,326	63,305	19,119,079
6	Vatican City	12				12	0		14,981				801
7	Kuwait	51,245	+601	377	+4	41,515	9,353	159	11,997	88	413,530	96,812	4,271,479
8	Andorra	855		52		800	3		11,065	673	3,750	48,532	77,268
9	Armenia	29,285	+349	503	+12	16,907	11,875	10	9,882	170	125,088	42,212	2,963,359
10	Mayotte	2,688	+9	34		2,446	208	3	9,851	125	8,800	32,249	272,877
11	Oman	48,997	+1,262	244	+6	31,000	17,773	127	9,593	44	217,194	42,522	5,107,767
12	Peru	309,278	+3,575	10,952	+180	200,938	97,388	1,265	9,378	332	1,821,328	55,227	32,978,661
13	USA	3,097,084	+55,442	133,972	+993	1,354,863	1,608,249	15,371	9,356	405	38,801,591	117,211	331,039,330
14	Panama	40,291	+957	799	+29	18,726	20,766	160	9,336	185	150,542	34,882	4,315,710

Fig. 6.2 Worldometer data for July 7, ordered by total number of reported infections per 1 million people in each country.

Alice: Not Chile. That country would be Qatar, with 35,952 total reported infections per million.

Bob: It seems Qatar did a terrible job at controlling the spread of Covid-19.

Alice: Qatar is a relatively small country, with less than 1% of the population of the U.S. For countries of such small size, the number of cases per million may strongly depend on a few large local clusters. This may give us a misleading picture of how well the country did overall in terms of getting the spread under control. There are also a few other small countries ahead of Chile, like the tiny city-state of San Marino.

The U.S. is number 13 on that list. This shows that we have had so far more reported cases per million than any large country with the exceptions of Chile, Peru, and Brazil.

Bob: What, exactly, do you mean by "large country", Alice?

Alice: Excellent question, Bob! Expressions like "large country" are imprecise. If we want to use them in science, we need to specify a cutoff. But this would be to some extent an arbitrary decision.

Bob: Can we set the cutoff here at a population of 10 million people?

Alice: We can go with this one and see where it leads us.

Let's now take a closer look at the situation across the Atlantic by clicking on "Europe":

	Country, Other ↓↑	Total Cases ↓↑	New Cases ↓↑	Total Deaths ↓↑	New Deaths ↓↑	Total Recovered ↓↑	Active Cases ↓↑	Serious, Critical ↓↑	Tot Cases/ 1M pop ↓F	Deaths/ 1M pop ↓↑	Total Tests ↓↑	Tests/ 1M pop ↓↑	Population ↓↑
1	San Marino	698		42		656	0		20,571	1,238	5,729	168,838	33,932
2	Vatican City	12				12	0		14,981				801
3	Andorra	855		52		800	3		11,065	673	3,750	48,532	77,268
4	Luxembourg	4,603	+61	110		4,056	437	3	7,352	176	237,755	379,729	626,117
5	Sweden	73,556	+271	5,470		N/A	N/A	103	7,282	542	520,208	51,503	10,100,443
6	Belarus	64,003	+199	436	+7	51,902	11,665	89	6,773	46	1,074,240	113,685	9,449,255
7	Spain	299,210	+341	28,392	+4	N/A	N/A	617	6,400	607	5,734,599	122,652	46,755,169
8	Iceland	1,873	+7	10		1,847	16		5,488	29	91,350	267,666	341,284
9	Belgium	62,058	+42	9,774	+3	17,122	35,162	27	5,354	843	1,313,064	113,287	11,590,614
10	Gibraltar	179				176	3		5,313		14,934	443,264	33,691
11	Ireland	25,538	+7	1,742	+1	23,364	432	12	5,171	353	473,974	95,972	4,938,681
12	Russia	694,230	+6,368	10,494	+198	463,880	219,856	2,300	4,757	72	21,537,771	147,584	145,935,812
13	Moldova	18,141	+235	603	+11	11,241	6,297	391	4,497	149	101,180	25,083	4,033,748
14	Portugal	44,416	+287	1,629	+9	29,445	13,342	76	4,356	160	1,271,425	124,698	10,196,020
15	UK	286,349	+581	44,391	+155	N/A	N/A	209	4,218	654	10,777,399	158,741	67,892,858
16	Italy	241,956	+137	34,899	+30	192,815	14,242	70	4,002	577	5,703,673	94,338	60,459,826

Fig. 6.3   Worldometer data for July 7, ordered by total number of reported infections per 1 million people in each European country.

Sweden would then have the highest number among large European countries, with 7,282 total cases per million people. Belarus has almost the same population as Sweden and would be next if we had set our cutoff for the population of a large country just a little lower than 10 million.

Bob: Now I can see what you meant when you said that setting a cutoff would be an arbitrary decision.

Next would be Spain with 6,400 total cases per million people. That looks pretty bad. Maybe it wouldn't be such a good idea to travel to Spain this summer.

Frank: They won't let you in anyway. Supposedly because there are many more infections here than in Spain.

But I wonder how they came up with this idea. The number for Spain is about two thirds of the one for the U.S. Definitely lower, but in the same ballpark. So why do the Europeans claim that the pandemic in the U.S. is *much worse* than over there? Sounds totally over-the-top to me.

Alice: They are making a different comparison than we have been discussing so far.

Bob's question was "Where has the Covid-19 outbreak been the worst so far?"

Bob: Right.

Alice: And for answering it we compared the total numbers of reported infections per million people. But such comparisons don't answer Cindy's question which countries might be safer to visit right now. This would be a question about the current situation, about where the pandemic is worse right now.

Cindy: Yes, this was my question.

I'm too scared to travel anywhere, and we can't visit Europe anyway. But if I think about it as one of those What-If scenarios, I would not want to get infected and then bring the virus back home. If I meet people who have recovered a long time ago, this shouldn't do any harm. But I don't want to be around people who are still infectious.

Would their number be the number of those "Active cases" in the table?

Alice: Almost. The numbers in this column are estimates of the reported cases that are still infectious. In each country, they are only a fraction of the actual numbers of infectious people at the current time. But if these fractions don't differ too much between countries, the numbers of active cases can be used for comparing the current situation in different countries.

Let's look at the first table again:

#	Country, Other	Total Cases	New Cases	Total Deaths	New Deaths	Total Recovered	Active Cases	Serious, Critical	Tot Cases/ 1M pop	Deaths/ 1M pop	Total Tests	Tests/ 1M pop	Population
	World	11,942,330	+208,301	545,678	+5,504	6,844,977	4,551,675	58,195	1,532	70.0			
1	USA	3,097,084	+55,442	133,972	+993	1,354,863	1,608,249	15,371	9,356	405	38,801,591	117,211	331,039,330
2	Brazil	1,674,655	+48,584	66,868	+1,312	1,072,229	535,558	8,318	7,878	315	4,316,284	20,304	212,587,032
3	India	743,481	+23,135	20,653	+479	457,058	265,770	8,944	539	15	10,211,092	7,398	1,380,233,788
4	Russia	694,230	+6,368	10,494	+198	463,880	219,856	2,300	4,757	72	21,537,771	147,584	145,935,812
5	Peru	309,278	+3,575	10,952	+180	200,938	97,388	1,265	9,378	332	1,821,328	55,227	32,978,661
6	Chile	301,019	+2,462	6,434	+50	268,245	26,340	2,060	15,744	337	1,210,326	63,305	19,119,079
7	Spain	299,210	+341	28,392	+4	N/A	N/A	617	6,400	607	5,734,599	122,652	46,755,169
8	UK	286,349	+581	44,391	+155	N/A	N/A	209	4,218	654	10,777,399	158,741	67,892,858
9	Mexico	261,750	+4,902	31,119	+480	159,657	70,974	378	2,030	241	641,142	4,972	128,955,195
10	Iran	245,688	+2,637	11,931	+200	207,000	26,757	3,270	2,925	142	1,846,793	21,983	84,009,505
11	Italy	241,956	+137	34,899	+30	192,815	14,242	70	4,002	577	5,703,675	94,338	60,459,826
12	Pakistan	234,509	+2,691	4,839	+77	134,957	94,713	2,306	1,061	22	1,445,153	6,541	220,943,702
13	Saudi Arabia	217,108	+3,392	2,017	+49	154,839	60,252	2,268	6,235	58	2,018,657	57,972	34,821,448

Fig. 6.4   Worldometer data for July 7, ordered by total number of reported infections per country.

Frank: The website doesn't give these numbers for Spain.

Alice: No, it doesn't. Such problems of missing data often occur in large data sets. Scientists then need to find a workaround.

Cindy: Could we compare these numbers for the U.S. and Italy instead? I mean, as a workaround?

Alice: Good idea, Cindy. The outbreaks in Italy and Spain followed similar patterns and we have the relevant data for Italy. They have had about 4,000 total reported cases per million so far.

Frank: Also in the same ballpark as the number of roughly 9,000 for the U.S., I'd say.

Alice: Epidemiologists estimate that currently about 1.6 million of the total reported cases in the U.S. are still active. This is the majority of all reported cases in our country.

For Italy, roughly 14 thousand of the total reported cases are still active. This is only a small fraction of the total for Italy.

Cindy: Wouldn't we still need to scale these numbers by population size before we making comparison?

Alice: Right. The website did not do this for us, so we need to do the calculations ourselves. After dividing by population size, I got

4,858 active cases per million for the U.S. and 236 per million for Italy. Would these numbers still be in the same ballpark?

Frank: No. So I guess it would be safe to travel to Italy.

Alice: Much safer than traveling to another place in the U.S.

Bob: Tourists from the U.S. are not permitted entry into the European Union right now. They shouldn't do this to us. But when we compare the numbers as we just discussed, I can see where they are coming from. They are afraid that we may be infected with Covid-19 and start new chains of transmissions in Europe.

Frank: So how about Spain? They didn't report their number of active cases, so how could we get an idea about their current situation?

Bob: Could we compare the numbers of reported daily infections for the U.S. and Spain? I meant to say: First scale them by population size and then compare?

Alice: Yes. These scaled numbers will give us a reasonable comparison of the current likelihood of becoming infected.

The table only shows us data for new reported infections for one day. In general, we need to be careful about drawing conclusions based on reported numbers for a single day. But as long as we only want to know whether the numbers are in the same ballpark, we can use these data.

Bob: So, for the U.S., 55,442 newly reported infections for July 7 would translate into $55,442/331$, or approximately 167 reported new infections per million people on that day.

Cindy: And for Spain, the number 341 of new reported infections for July 7 would translate into $341/46.8$, or approximately 7 reported new infections per million people on that day.

Frank: Not in the same ballpark, not even close.

Bob: If only they would let me travel to Spain!

Endnotes

[38] The most striking similarity between Brazil and the U.S. was that the presidents of both countries had been downplaying the threat of Covid-19. For details about the stance of Brazil's president, Jair Bolsonaro, see, for example [3]. The U.S. president Donald Trump explicitly admitted that he was intentionally downplaying the pandemic [4].

References

[1] The Office of the Prime Minister, Jamaica. PM Announces Phased Reopening of Jamaica's Borders with Strict Protocols 2020 Jun 1. [cited 2021 Jan 2]. `https://opm.gov.jm/news/pm-announces-phased-reopening-of-jamaicas-borders-with-strict-protocols/`

[2] Worldometers.info. Dover, Delaware, U.S.A. COVID-19 Coronavirus Pandemic. [cited 2020 Jul 8]. `https://www.worldometers.info/coronavirus/`

[3] Phillips T. Jair Bolsonaro claims Brazilians 'never catch anything' as Covid-19 cases rise. The Guardian 2020 March 26. [cited 2020 Dec 29]. `https://www.theguardian.com/global-development/2020/mar/27/jair-bolsonaro-claims-brazilians-never-catch-anything-as-covid-19-cases-rise`

[4] Woodward B. Rage. New York: Simon and Schuster; 2020. 480p.

Chapter 7

Why are trend curves useful and what do they show?

Alice, Bob, Cindy, and Frank meet on July 9, 2020. The numbers of daily reported Covid-19 cases have been trending downwards in many countries. Between June 8 and July 8, the 7-day moving average decreased from 648 to 309 in Canada, from 170 to 59 in the Netherlands, and from 6 to 4 in Thailand. In the U.S., daily reported infections are trending upwards. Over the same time interval, their 7-day moving averages increased from 21,927 to 55,530 [1].

Bob: Thank you, Alice, for meeting with us again today. Yesterday, we discussed some things that we need to keep in mind when making sense of published data: scaling by population size and using the numbers that are most relevant for a particular question.

Can we continue this discussion today and talk more about making sense of data?

Cindy: This would be good. I've read in the news that cases are trending downward in many countries, but sharply trending upward in the U.S. What do they mean by this? And what are these trend curves and 7-day moving averages that the press writes about?

I've also read that many people may have become infected over the Fourth of July weekend when people got together and celebrated the holiday. This sounds so scary!

Frank: Don't get scared by everything you read in the news!

Even the New York Times reported the opposite: For July 3, their graph shows 57,153 new Covid-19 cases in the U.S., for July 4, only 50,005, and for July 5 only 44,763 [2]. These numbers went down over the weekend, not up.

Bob: So it seems that there was a downward trend over the weekend. But then numbers went up again. And Alice had mention yesterday that we need to be careful about drawing conclusions based on reported numbers for just one day. I don't know what to make of it.

Alice: Yes, comparisons of reported numbers of infections on two or three consecutive days may give us a misleading picture.

Bob: Why?

Alice: Let me share my screen and put up a chart of daily reported new infections in the U.S. up to July 6:

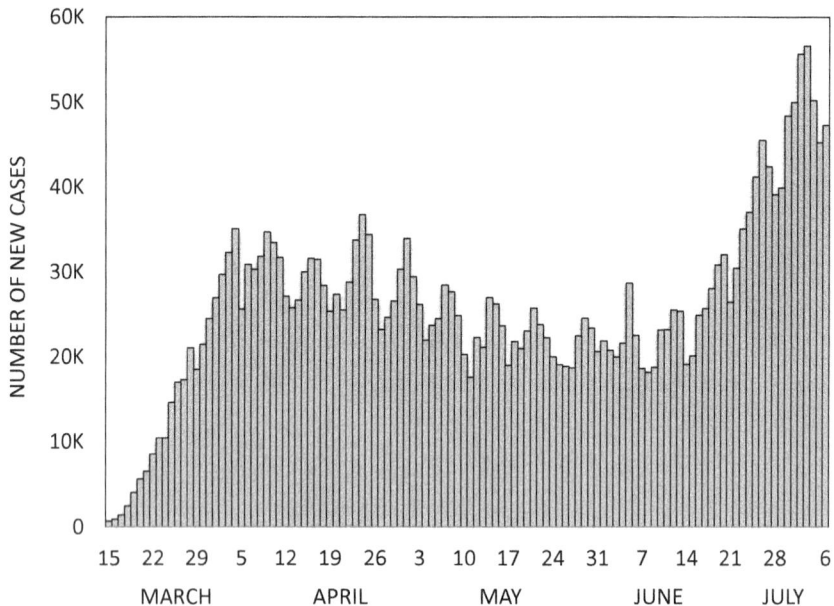

Fig. 7.1   Daily reported new Covid-19 infections in the U.S. up to July 6. The charts in this chapter are based on data from the New York Times [3].

Cindy: The numbers jump up and down from day to day. This is so confusing.

Bob: There seems to be some regular pattern though to these ups and downs.

Alice: Yes, there is. What do you think is the reason for this pattern?

Frank: Must be that they tend to be higher on certain days of the week.

Alice: Let's mark Fridays on the horizontal axis of our chart and make the bars for Fridays darker:

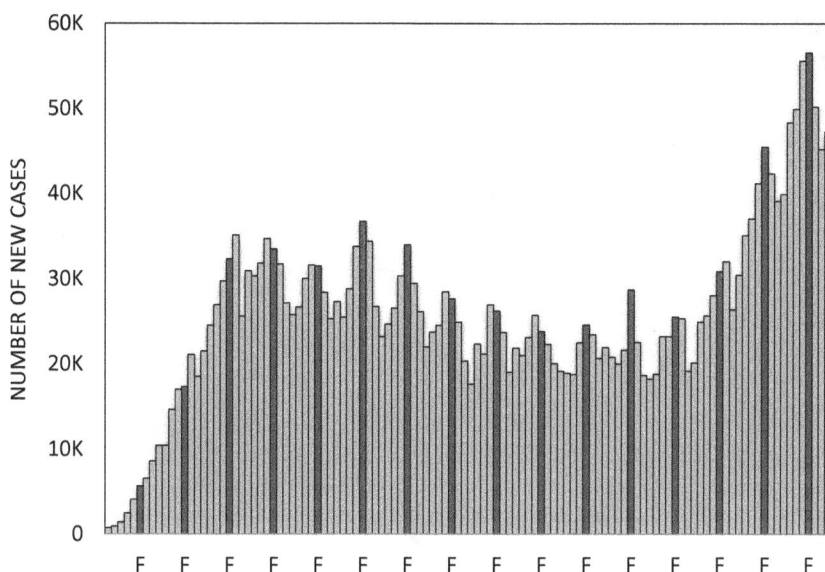

Fig. 7.2   Chart for the same data with Fridays marked.

Frank: Exactly what I thought. The numbers are higher at the end of the week, usually highest on Fridays, and lower early in the week.

Bob: That's probably because of delays in reporting. Many offices would not process data on weekends. And some may put out reports only at the end of the week.

Cindy: It would explain Frank's observation about the Fourth of July weekend. July 3 was a Friday, where one would typically see a very high number of reported cases. Then the numbers were lower for the next few days when not many reports came in.

Alice: Right. Also, remember that it takes some time after a transmission for the newly infected person to get tested and then for the results to be reported to the data bases. As you had mentioned, many new infections may have occurred over the Fourth of July weekend, and that worries me. But these cases would not yet have shown up in the charts even by today, July 9.

Frank: I see. We may get a wrong idea about the overall trend when we compare the data for a Friday with the data for a Saturday or Sunday.

How about comparing the data for two consecutive Fridays or two consecutive Mondays?

Alice: That's a better method. But not all Mondays are equal. July 6 was the Monday after Independence Day, and reporting might have even been slower than after a more typical weekend.

Let me show you a better method:

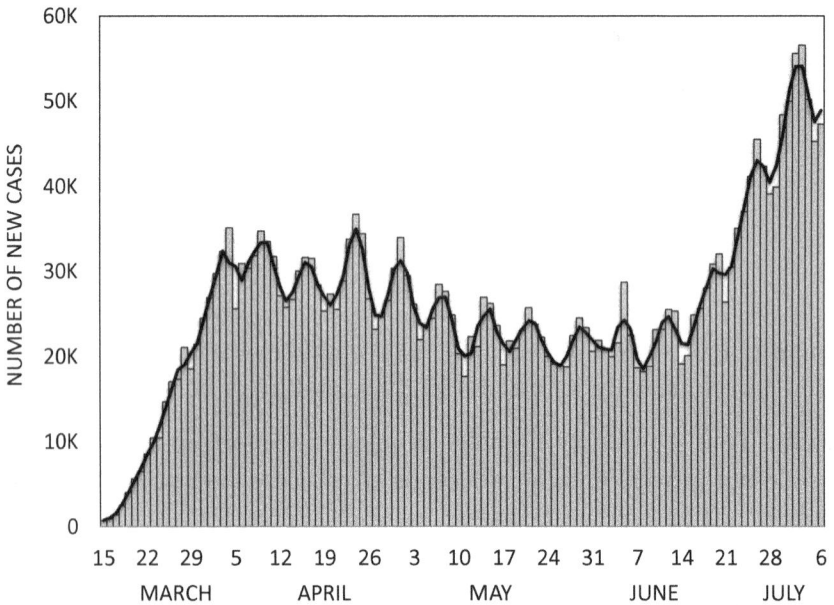

Fig. 7.3   The same data with a trend curve based on 3-day moving averages.

To get a clear visual picture of trends, we need to average data over several days and then plot these so-called moving averages on a curve. Such curves are sometimes called trend curves. For data on new infections, they are also called epidemic curves.

Bob: Over how many days should we average?

Alice: That depends on whether we want to visualize only long-term trends, or also short-term ups and downs. In the third chart (Fig. 7.3), I have added a trend curve based on 3-day moving averages to my first chart (Fig. 7.1).

Cindy: The curve shows all the ups and downs over the course of each week. Is this what you meant by short-term trends, Alice?

Alice: Yes. The longer-term trends are still obscured by this pattern.

Let's instead add a trend curve based on 5-day moving averages:

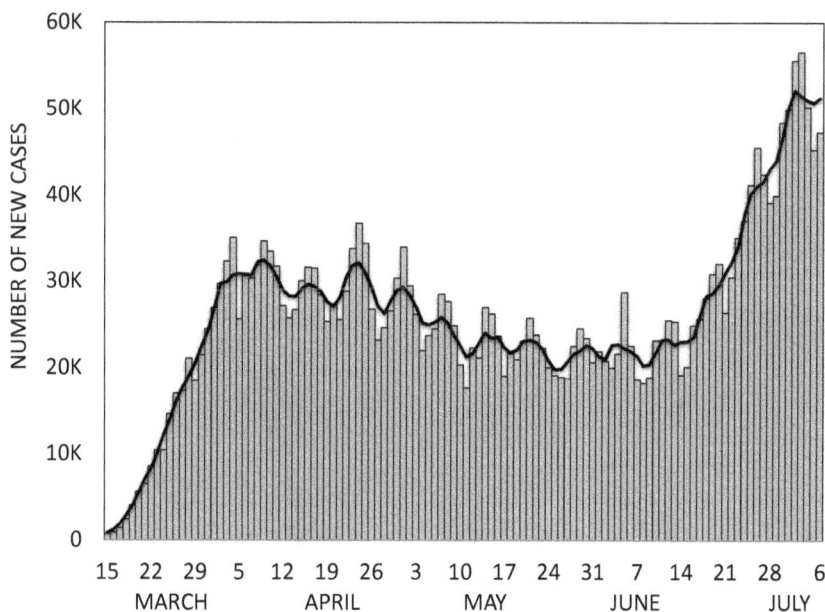

Fig. 7.4 The same data with a trend curve based on 5-day moving averages.

Bob: Now the longer-term trends become more visible. But we also clearly see the shorter-term fluctuations over the course of each week.

Cindy: I still find the many ups and downs of the curve confusing.

Alice: So let us try 7-day moving averages:

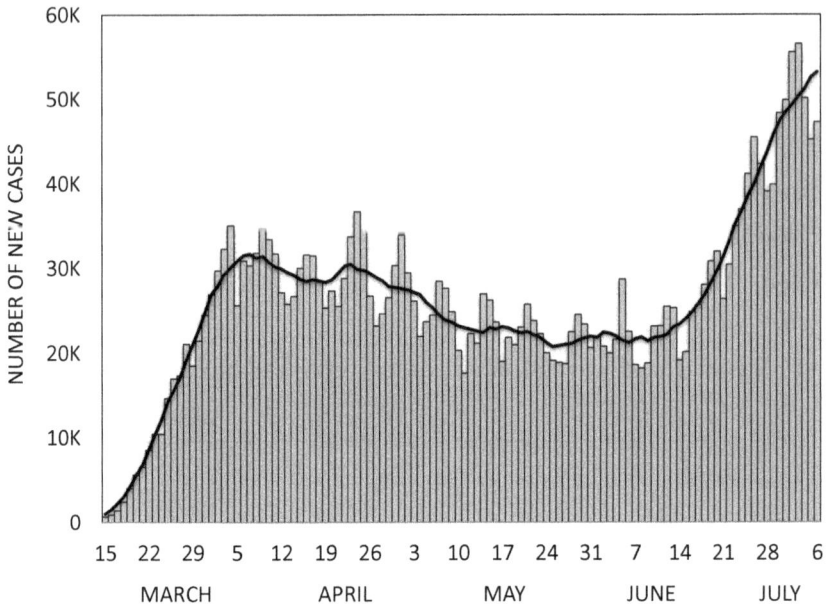

Fig. 7.5   The same data with a trend curve based on 7-day moving averages.

Now we can clearly see from this picture that there was a steep upward trend in the second half of March, a moderate downward trend in May, followed by a fairly steep upward trend that started mid-June.

Bob: Neat! I have one more question though: Should these 7-day moving averages be calculated for the given day, the 3 days before, and the 3 days after, or for the given day and the six days immediately preceding it?

Alice: Good question! Both methods are fine. Here I used your first idea. It often gives a trend curve that fits the data more snugly.

But we can use it only for historical data, that is, when we already know the numbers for the next 3 days after the last day on the chart. My charts display the data up to July 6, and as we talk here on the evening of July 9, we already know them for the next 3 days. But when we want to detect the current trend and don't know the future numbers yet, we need to use the second method.

References

[1] Worldometers.info. Dover, Delaware, U.S.A. COVID-19 Coronavirus Pandemic. [cited 2020 Nov 21]. https://www.worldometers.info/coronavirus/

[2] The New York Times. Covid in the U.S.: Latest map and case count. [cited 2020 Sep 22]. https://www.nytimes.com/interactive/2020/us/coronavirus-us-cases.html

[3] Github Inc. nytimes/covid-19-data. [cited 2020 Sep 22]. https://github.com/nytimes/covid-19-data

Chapter 8

Does the United States do enough testing?

Alice, Bob, Cindy, and Frank continue their discussion on July 9, 2020. More and more people are being tested for Covid-19 all over the world. Over the preceding month, the number of tests performed has increased by 59% in Turkey, 60% in Senegal, 87% in the U.S., and 119% in India.[39]

Cindy: I have read that the U.S. is not doing enough testing for Covid-19.

Frank: Nonsense. The U.S. has done way more testing than any other country on earth.

Bob: You cannot both be right, Cindy and Frank.

Alice: Actually, Frank's claim doesn't necessarily contradict what Cindy has read.

Bob: How could that be? Let's just look at the data and see who is right.

Alice: Let's do that. If we want to understand what is really going on, we need to look at the data. We can use the ones for yesterday from Worldometer (Fig. 8.1). I'll put the URL in the chat so that we all can access it: `https://www.worldometers.info/coronavirus/`

Frank: The data shows what I told you: The U.S. has conducted 39,479,437 tests up to now.

Nearly 40 million tests! No other country comes even close.

Cindy: No other country in the part of the chart that we see here. That's true. But how about the countries the countries further down the list? Some of them may have done more testing than the U.S.

| All | Europe | North America | Asia | South America | Africa | Oceania | | | | | | | |

#	Country, Other	Total Cases	New Cases	Total Deaths	New Deaths	Total Recovered	Active Cases	Serious, Critical	Tot Cases/ 1M pop	Deaths/ 1M pop	Total Tests	Tests/ 1M pop	Population
	World	12,156,029	+213,681	551,197	+5,507	7,025,772	4,579,060	58,325	1,560	70.7			
1	USA	3,158,932	+61,848	134,862	+890	1,392,679	1,631,391	15,457	9,542	407	39,479,437	119,257	331,044,624
2	Brazil	1,716,196	+41,541	68,055	+1,187	1,117,922	530,219	8,318	8,073	320	4,359,978	20,509	212,591,154
3	India	769,052	+25,571	21,144	+491	476,554	271,354	8,944	557	15	10,473,771	7,588	1,380,270,828
4	Russia	700,792	+6,562	10,667	+173	472,511	271,614	2,300	4,802	73	21,790,705	149,317	145,935,982
5	Peru	312,911	+3,633	11,133	+181	204,748	97,030	1,265	9,488	338	1,842,316	55,862	32,979,917
6	Chile	303,083	+2,064	6,573	+139	271,703	24,807	2,053	15,852	344	1,220,790	63,850	19,119,526
7	Spain	299,593	+383	28,396	+4	N/A	N/A	617	6,408	607	5,734,599	122,652	46,755,218
8	UK	286,979	+630	44,517	+126	N/A	N/A	197	4,227	656	11,041,203	162,625	67,893,830
9	Mexico	268,008	+6,258	32,014	+895	163,646	72,348	378	2,078	248	668,537	5,184	128,958,893
10	Iran	248,379	+2,691	12,084	+153	209,463	26,832	3,309	2,956	144	1,872,391	22,287	84,012,442
11	Italy	242,149	+193	34,914	+15	193,640	13,595	71	4,005	577	5,754,116	95,173	60,459,584
12	Pakistan	237,489	+2,980	4,922	+83	140,965	91,602	2,236	1,075	22	1,467,104	6,640	220,955,441
13	South Africa	224,665	+8,810	3,602	+100	106,842	114,221	539	3,787	61	1,944,399	32,777	59,322,322
14	Saudi Arabia	220,144	+3,036	2,059	+42	158,050	60,035	2,263	6,322	59	2,071,823	59,496	34,822,930
15	Turkey	208,938	+1,041	5,282	+22	187,511	16,145	1,172	2,477	63	3,782,520	44,840	84,356,463
16	Germany	198,765	+410	9,115	+12	182,700	6,950	292	2,372	109	6,376,054	76,096	83,790,088

Fig. 8.1   Data from Worldometer.info [1] for July 8, ordered by total number of reported cases per country [1].

Let me toggle the column "Total Tests" so that the countries will be ordered by the number of tests they have done:

| All | Europe | North America | Asia | South America | Africa | Oceania | | | | | | | |

#	Country, Other	Total Cases	New Cases	Total Deaths	New Deaths	Total Recovered	Active Cases	Serious, Critical	Tot Cases/ 1M pop	Deaths/ 1M pop	Total Tests	Tests/ 1M pop	Population
1	China	83,572	+7	4,634		78,548	390	5	58	3	90,410,000	62,814	1,439,323,776
2	USA	3,158,932	+61,848	134,862	+890	1,392,679	1,631,391	15,457	9,542	407	39,479,437	119,257	331,044,624
3	Russia	700,792	+6,562	10,667	+173	472,511	217,614	2,300	4,802	73	21,790,705	149,317	145,935,982
4	UK	286,979	+630	44,517	+126	N/A	N/A	197	4,227	656	11,041,203	162,625	67,893,830
5	India	769,052	+25,571	21,144	+491	476,554	271,354	8,944	557	15	10,473,771	7,588	1,380,270,828
6	Germany	198,765	+410	9,115	+12	182,700	6,950	292	2,372	109	6,376,054	76,096	83,790,088
7	Italy	242,149	+193	34,914	+15	193,640	13,595	71	4,005	577	5,754,116	95,173	60,459,584
8	Spain	299,593	+383	28,396	+4	N/A	N/A	617	6,408	607	5,734,599	122,652	46,755,218
9	Brazil	1,716,196	+41,541	68,055	+1,187	1,117,922	530,219	8,318	8,073	320	4,359,978	20,509	212,591,154
10	Turkey	208,938	+1,041	5,282	+22	187,511	16,145	1,172	2,477	63	3,782,520	44,840	84,356,463
11	UAE	53,045	+445	327	+1	42,282	10,436	1	5,362	33	3,720,000	376,038	9,892,612
12	Canada	106,434	+267	8,737	+26	70,247	27,450	2,151	2,820	231	3,055,341	80,939	37,748,830
13	Australia	8,886	+131	106		7,487	1,293	8	348	4	2,853,342	111,872	25,505,429
14	Saudi Arabia	220,144	+3,036	2,059	+42	158,050	60,035	2,263	6,322	59	2,071,823	59,496	34,822,930
15	South Africa	224,665	+8,810	3,602	+100	106,842	114,221	539	3,787	61	1,944,399	32,777	59,322,322

Fig. 8.2   Data from Worldometer.info [1] for July 8, ordered by total number of reported cases per country [1].

Bob: Well, China performed 90,410,000 tests; over 90 million of them. More than twice the total number of tests for the U.S. But China is the only country ahead of the U.S. What Frank said isn't literally true, but not too far off the mark.

Frank: I still think that in all fairness one should say that the U.S. performed more tests than China. Their population is more than 4 times as large as ours.

And when you scale the data by population size, as Alice has shown us, you get roughly 63,000 tests per million people in China, and 119,000 tests per million people in our country. That's what the second last column of the table shows. Our number is almost twice as large as theirs.

Bob: That makes sense. When we compare numbers between countries, we should scale them by population size.

Cindy: But then we can see that the U.S. did fewer tests per million people than Russia, the U.K., and Spain. And a lot fewer than the United Arab Emirates, where they did about 376,000 tests per million people so far. More than 3 times as many as the U.S.!

Bob: I wonder though ... are so many tests as in the United Arab Emirates even needed?

I think it's only important that a country does enough testing to keep the spread of the pandemic under control. What's the point of being world champion in the number of tests if they are not necessary?

Cindy: But the more people we test, the earlier we will be able to detect infections and quarantine those who might infect others. More tests will prevent more infections!

Bob: Tests are expensive. If we spend more money on testing than we need to, we may not have enough funding for other pressing needs.

Frank: So how many tests are actually needed for limiting the numbers of new infections?

Cindy: Could we perhaps look at the numbers for other countries, like Germany? I read that they have been quite successful. The total number of reported infections is currently 2,372 per million people in Germany; the number 9,542 for the U.S. is about 4 times higher.

Frank: But Germany has so far only performed 76,096 total tests per million people; a lot fewer than the U.S. at 119,257 per million. Like Bob said: Giving too many tests may be unnecessary.

If Germany did enough tests to keep their infections under control, then we must have done more than enough.

Bob: It would seem so, but how did Germany keep their infections down with relatively few tests, while ours are rapidly increasing as we speak?

Alice: Good question, Bob!

The German strategy is actually quite similar to ours. Let's think about it as follows: Most tests are taken by people who either show symptoms or have recently been in close contact with an infected person.

Cindy: But we also regularly test medical personnel and other people at especially high risk. Do they also do this in Germany?

Alice: Yes, they do. I don't know what the exact numbers of tests used for this purpose are. It is difficult to find reliable data on this.

Cindy: Can we assume that after giving these regular tests to people at high risk, they had 50,000 of their 76,000 tests per million people left over, while we had 100,000 of our 119,000 tests left over? To keep the numbers simple?

Alice: We can do this for our discussion.

These "left over" tests, as Cindy called them, are very important for identifying infected people and quickly isolating or quarantining them before they can infect many others. I'd like us to discuss some other time in more detail how this works and how it helps.[40]

For now, we only need to know that a sufficient number of such tests is needed to detect whether somebody with symptoms really has Covid-19 and whether those who have been in close contact with a Covid-19 patient have been infected. If a sufficient proportion of infections are detected by testing people with symptoms and their close contacts, it will be possible to keep the spread of Covid-19 under control.

Bob: I think I know what you are trying to get at, Alice. So we would need a certain number of tests per infected person to test all close contacts. The more infected people there are, the more tests we will need to test all people with symptoms and their contacts. Can we then say that a certain number of tests per reported infection is needed for successfully preventing sufficiently many further transmissions?

Alice: That's exactly right! So the number of tests that a country needs to perform for keeping the spread of Covid-19 under control depends only in part on its population size. It depends more strongly on the number of infections in this country.

Let's go with Cindy's numbers of 50,000 per million in Germany and 100,000 per million in the U.S. of tests for people with symptoms and contacts of confirmed cases. How do they compare with the total number of infections in the two countries?

Bob: If we divide the 100,000 in the U.S. by the 9,542 total reported infections per million, we get about 10.5 tests per reported infection.

Cindy: And if we divide the 50,000 in Germany by the 2,372 thousand total reported infections per million, we get about 21 tests per reported infection.

Frank: It would follow that Germany did about 2 times more testing per reported infection than the U.S. Or conversely, that the U.S. did only 50% as much testing per reported case as Germany.

But all this was based on very rough estimates.

Cindy: So the U.S. is doing only 50% as much testing as is needed! But earlier today I read in the New York Times[41] that it's only 39%. We calculated a different number. But it's similar to theirs.

Alice: We need to be a little careful about drawing conclusions. As Frank had mentioned, our calculations were based on very rough estimates. Also, we did not compare these ratios for all tests, only for the test that may not have been used for regular testing of certain groups of people.

Bob: And we don't know whether Germany did only as many tests as were necessary. Pretty cool though that we got a number that's close to the one in the New York Times!

Alice: I would have expected that the results of our calculations were probably a little off, but would be in the same ballpark as the actual percentage of needed tests.

The estimates published by the New York Times rely on much more detailed data than we had looked at and are based on recommendations by the Harvard Global Health Institute[42] rather than comparisons with another country. Also, they compare these recommendations with current testing volume instead of the total number of tests since the start of the pandemic.

Cindy: But this sounds so complicated! Thank you, Alice, for explaining it in a simpler way.

Bob: I can see now how Frank and Cindy could both be right with their takes on the number of tests in the U.S. Each of them was talking about something different. Our total number of tests is very impressive. But it may still not be nearly as large as it needs to be when our numbers of infections are so high.

Endnotes

[39] Based on data from [2] for June 8, 2020 and July 8, 2020.

[40] A detailed discussion about how testing fits into the overall strategy for limiting the spread of Covid-19 will be presented in Chapters 15, 16, and 19.

[41] At [3], the New York Times was giving regular updates on the numbers of current tests in the U.S. and all states as a percentage of the target number of tests that would be needed for successful mitigation of Covid-19. An archived copy that is available for July 10, 2020 shows that they reported a percentage of 39% at the time of this conversation.

[42] See [4] for details. This website also gives information similar to [3] for a number of different countries.

References

[1] Worldometers.info. Dover, Delaware, U.S.A. COVID-19 Coronavirus Pandemic. [cited 2020 Jul 9]. https://www.worldometers.info/coronavirus/

[2] University of Oxford. Oxford Martin School. Our World in Data. Total COVID-19 tests. [cited 2020 Nov 22]. https://ourworldindata.org/grapher/full-list-total-tests-for-covid-19?time=2020-02-20..latest

[3] Collins K. Is Your State Doing Enough Coronavirus Testing? The New York Times 2020 Jul 10. [cited 2020 Jul 10]. https://web.archive.org/web/20200710171908/https://www.nytimes.com/interactive/2020/us/coronavirus-testing.html

[4] Brown School of Public Health. Pandemics Explained. July 6, 2020 | State Testing Targets. New Testing Targets: As COVID-19 outbreaks grow more severe, most U.S. states still fall far short on testing 2020 Jul 6. [cited 2020 Dec 30]. https://globalepidemics.org/july-6-2020-state-testing-targets/

Chapter 9

What is the basic reproduction number and what does it tell us?

Alice, Bob, Cindy, and Frank meet on July 13, 2020. In March, the world had seen a nearly exponential increase in the numbers of Covid-19 infections, hospitalizations, and deaths from the disease. The healthcare system in Northern Italy had become overwhelmed. Most states in the U.S. and most countries around the world imposed lockdowns[43] that severely restricted people's movements and imposed heavy burdens on the economy. These largely succeeded in avoiding breakdowns of national or regional health care systems.[44] After increasing nearly exponentially during the second half of March, the 7-day moving average of worldwide deaths peaked in mid-April at slightly more than 7,000 reported daily deaths and stayed between 4,200 and 5,200 over the two months that preceded this conversation [1].

Bob: I read that epidemiological models predict how the numbers of Covid-19 infections will change. You told us, Alice, that these models are computer simulations. Can you tell us more about how they work?

Cindy: This must be awfully complicated. I'm not good at math and know nothing about computer simulations.

Alice: I can show you some simple ones that require very little math. Even from the simplest models we can learn a lot about how infections spread and how this can be prevented.

Cindy: Keep it as easy as possible, please!

Alice: Let's discuss today the simplest of all epidemiological models. It only uses only the basic reproduction number R_0.

Bob: I've heard a lot about R_0. What is it?

Alice: Let's think about the number of other people that an infectious person will infect before recovering. This number will differ from case to case. In the example that we studied when discussing contacts, our index case Ingham had transmitted the infection to 2 people while he was infected, to Sue and Emily. Before they recovered, Sue had infected 4, and Emily had infected 3 other people.

Cindy: Yes, I remember this from the last picture you showed us back then. So could we then say that Ingham, Emily, and Sue infected on average 3 people each?

Alice: Right! The average number of other people that an infectious person will infect before reaching the removed state is called the reproduction number or the reproductive number. You may see both terms in articles on Covid-19.

This number is denoted by R and is key in epidemiological modeling. Epidemiologists are interested in R for much larger populations than just the three people in our example. But let's keep our examples small so that we can better understand the general principle.

Bob: I have seen the symbol R_t somewhere. Is this the same as R?

Alice: Yes. Reproduction numbers may change over time,[45] and this is emphasized by the subscript t. But I want to keep the notation simple and will use only R for now.

Close to the beginning of an outbreak, almost everyone[46] in the population is susceptible, and no preventive or control measures have been taken. Then this number R will be roughly constant and is denoted by R_0. It is called the basic reproduction number, the basic reproductive number, or the basic reproductive ratio.

Today we will discuss a model that assumes that R is equal to R_0 all the time.

Bob: Wouldn't such a model only tell us what happens when just a few people have already caught Covid-19 and there are no control measures, such as school closures or social distancing?

Alice: Very important point, Bob! Today's model would only work under these assumptions. For studying the effect of control measures, we need different models. We may talk about such models later.

From the model based on R_0, we will see how the weekly numbers of new infections might quickly become too large if no control measures were taken.

Frank: Seems though that people are unable to agree upon what "too large" would be. Who is going to tell?

Alice: There are some numbers that almost everybody would agree with. What if more Covid-19 patients would need hospitalization than hospital beds are available? Or if the numbers of patients who need ventilators were to exceed the available intensive care units?

Cindy: Then we would need to turn away patients who need hospital care. Or let people die who might be saved in an ICU. This would be so horrible! I cannot even imagine how the doctors would feel if they need to decide whom to care for and whom to let die!

Frank: We would be in deep trouble; I can see this. So tell us, Cindy: What are these numbers for Ohio? You study health care administration, don't you?

Cindy: I don't know offhand. Let me google the American Hospital Directory. It says here that in Ohio we have about 27,000 hospital beds [2]. But I think about two-thirds of those may be needed for patients with other illnesses. This would leave at most 9,000 beds for Covid-19 patients.

Alice: In reality, this number may be lower. The real bottleneck could be the number of available ICU beds rather than the total number of hospital beds,[47] or a shortage qualified medical personnel, especially if too many nurses and doctors become infected.

Let's assume that a typical Covid-19 patient will require hospitalization for 2 weeks on average. Then we could handle at most 4,500 new Covid-19 hospitalizations per week. Moreover, let's assume that roughly 10% of Covid-19 infections require hospitalization. Then we could cope with at most 45,000 new reported Covid-19 infections per week, or roughly 6,500 per day. This is very optimistic. The actual percentage of reported Covid-19 cases that required hospitalization has been higher.[48]

I want to be clear that the true number of weekly reported cases in Ohio that would already overwhelm our healthcare system in the early stages of the pandemic may be much smaller than 45,000. But I don't want to sound alarmist here. So let us go with an overestimate.

Bob: So you are saying that if we had 45,000 reported cases per week, we would definitely be in trouble. But we may run out of resources much sooner.

Alice: Exactly. Now let us think about a week when there were only 10 reported[49] infections in our state.

Frank: That's a ridiculously small number compared to your 45,000. At that point in time, there was nothing to worry about.

Alice: We will see.

For Covid-19, the average number R_0 of new infections caused by an infectious individual has been estimated as being between 2.5 and 3.[50] Let's assume in our discussions that $R_0 = 3$. This will keep our calculations simple.

The average time it takes for one person between becoming infected and infecting another is sometimes called the serial interval. For Covid-19 it has been estimated to be less than 1 week.[51] To keep the numbers simple, let us assume in our model that it is 1 week.

How many new infections would we then expect to see in Week 1?

Cindy: I'm not sure. Some people with Covid-19 may infect only 1 or 2 others, while some may infect 4 or 5. But I think when you say "expect", you mean "on average". This would be $R_0 = 3$, right?

Alice: Right.

Cindy: So in Week 1, we would see about $3 \times 10 = 30$. Is this what you mean?

Alice: Yes, Cindy. We cannot be sure of the exact number. But the individual differences will roughly average out. You said it right: "about 30".

Bob: By the same calculation, in Week 2 we would then see about $3 \times 30 = 90$ new infections.

Frank: And in Week 3 about $3 \times 90 = 270$ new ones. Still far from being a problem for the healthcare system.

Alice: Yes. Let me share my screen and show you the graph:

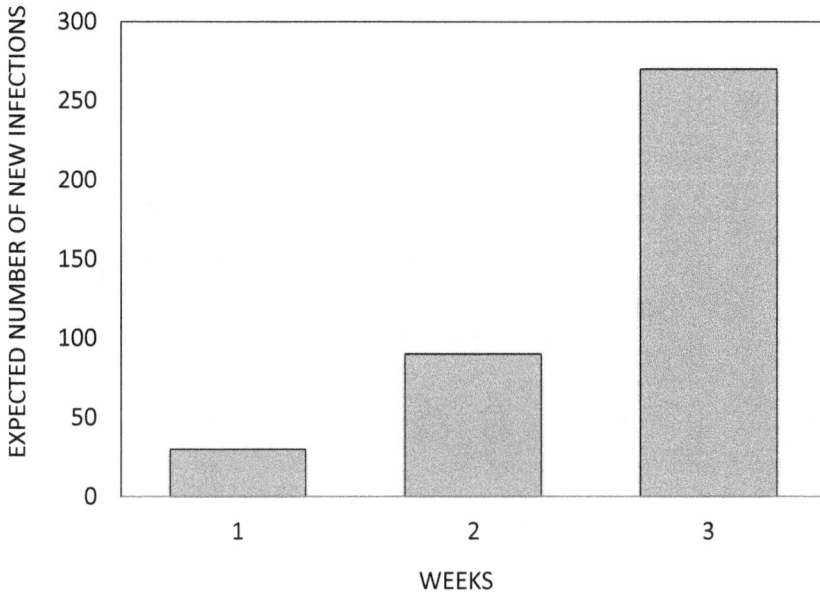

Fig. 9.1   Predicted new cases for weeks 1 to 3.

In a real epidemiological model, the calculations you did here would be done by a computer.

We would then predict about 810 new infections in Week 4, about 2,430 in Week 5, and about 7,290 in Week 6.

Cindy: These numbers are so much bigger!

Alice: Let me add them to my picture:

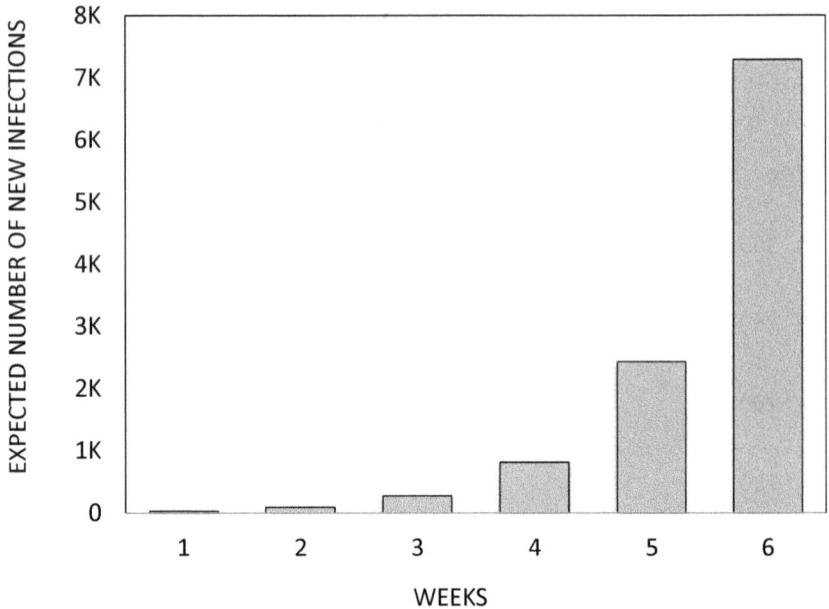

Fig. 9.2   Predicted new cases for weeks 1 to 6.

Bob: Yes, the numbers in Weeks 4 through 6 dwarf those in Weeks 1 through 3.

Frank: But even the number in Week 6 is only about 16% of your threshold of 45,000.

Bob: What does your computer show for the following weeks, Alice?

Alice: 21,870 new infections in Week 7, and 65,610 new infections in Week 8. Way above the threshold of 45,000.

This model predicts that, within less than two months, we would go from numbers that might appear miniscule and no cause for alarm to a situation where the disease would crush our healthcare system.

Let me show you the picture:

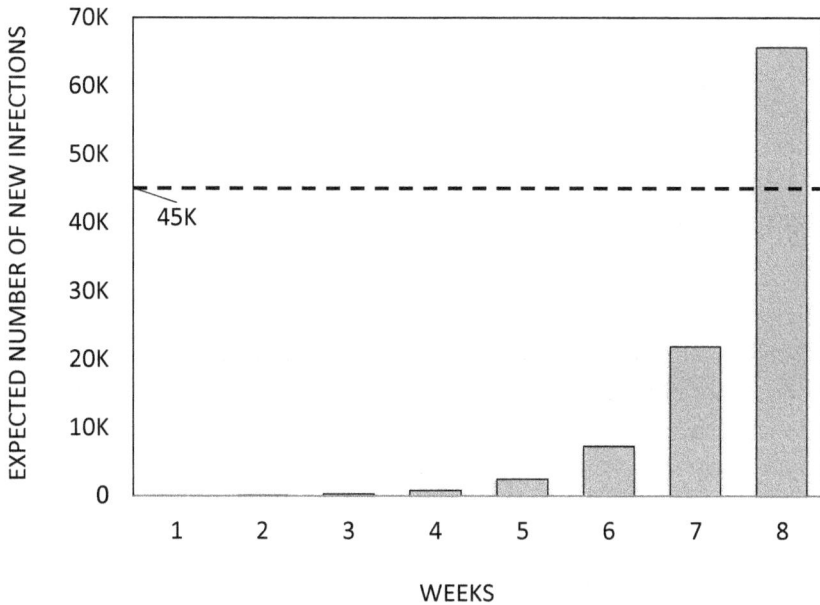

Fig. 9.3   Predicted new cases for weeks 1 to 8.

Bob: Do your graphs show the predicted numbers of actual cases or of reported cases?

Alice: We have been modeling here the increase of reported cases, because for these we can estimate hospitalization rates. The reproduction number predicts the growth of actual cases. But if we assume that a fixed proportion of all cases get reported, our model also also applies to the growth of reported cases.

Frank: Wait a minute! When was that week in Ohio when we had only reported 10 cases?

Alice: I used the number 10 only to make the calculations easy. It would have been early March. Between March 6 and March 13, the number was close[52] to 10.

Frank: Then in your model Covid-19 would have crushed our health care system by early May. But it didn't. In fact, even the total number of reported cases in Ohio went over 45,000 only on June 22, and the weekly numbers never got anywhere close [1].

So your model is wrong!

Alice: Good observations, Frank! But the model is not wrong, it actually did its job.

Frank: How can the model not be wrong if it predicts something so different from what actually happened?

Alice: Remember that our model is based on R_0 and works only before any control measures are taken. It is a What-If scenario that shows what is likely to happen if we don't do anything to limit the spread of the infection.

Starting on March 9, when Ohio had only 3 total reported cases, Governor Mike DeWine gradually imposed a series of restrictions.[53] Dr. Amy Acton, the Director of Ohio's Department of Health, then issued a stay-at-home order effective March 23.

After our state had implemented these drastic control measures, the assumptions of our model were no longer were satisfied. The data you described show that these measures did successfully prevent the dire predictions of our What-If model from becoming reality.

Cindy: So Dr. Acton and Governor DeWine knew about your model, and that's why they issued these orders?

Alice: More detailed and accurate models, but essentially models like the one we discussed. These models enabled them to enact an effective policy.

Bob: Well ... that's good.

But let's come back to our model. What would have happened in the long run without any control measures?

Alice: Good question! Our model actually gives a formula for the predicted number, which we will call $I(t)$, of new reported cases in week t:

$$I(t) = 10 \times 3^t.$$

Cindy: I remember seeing something like this is my math class! Is this, like, an exponential function?

Alice: Right! Every function of the form $f(t) = a \times b^t$ with $a > 0$ and $b > 1$ signifies exponential increase, also called exponential growth.

Bob: So, in our case we would have $a = 10$, which was the initial number of weekly reported infections, and $b = 3$, which was the basic reproduction number R_0.

Alice: Right! Eventually, the value of any exponential function $f(t) = a \times b^t$ with $a > 0$ and $b > 1$ will increase past any given threshold.

Frank: But this can't happen in the real world. For instance, we could never have more weekly infections in Ohio than there are people in our state.

Alice: Good observation! As I said, this model could work only near the very beginning of the outbreak. For later stages of the pandemic, we will need to work with more flexible models that do not assume that R is equal to R_0 all the time. We may discuss some of them later.

Even near the beginning of an outbreak, the actual increase would not be exactly exponential, only nearly exponential. Which means the model can give us only a good approximation, not the exact numbers. This is true of all models, by the way.

The most important property of a function $f(t)$ with exponential growth is this: For small t, we may get relatively small values and slow growth of $f(t)$, as we saw for the first few weeks in our model. But over time the function will grow much more rapidly. So if you draw its graph, it will bend upwards.

Bob: I see. In our example, small t would be the times near the beginning of the outbreak. That's why the numbers for the first few weeks in our model were so much dwarfed by later numbers!

Alice: Exactly! When some numbers grow exponentially, or nearly exponentially, we cannot expect them to stay small for long.

In early March, our reported numbers were still very small. Back then, many people believed that they posed no real danger. But they grew nearly exponentially, and our state took decisive action to avert looming disaster.

Cindy: I'm so glad that our hospitals did not become overwhelmed! But we talked about so much math today. It all went a little fast for me. Can you repeat the most important points?

Alice: Yes, let me summarize them:

- The reproduction number R, also called the reproductive number, is the average number of other people that an infectious person will infect before reaching the removed state. It is denoted by R.
- The reproduction number changes over time. Close to the beginning of a disease outbreak, when almost everyone in the population is susceptible and no preventive or control measures have been taken, the reproduction number R will be roughly constant and approximately equal to R_0.
- The constant R_0 is called the basic reproduction number or the basic reproductive number.
- For Covid-19, the value of R_0 has been estimated to be between 2 and 3.
- If no control measures are taken, mathematical models predict nearly exponential increase of numbers of new infections close to the beginning of the outbreak. Thus if no control measures are put in place, the numbers of new cases with severe symptoms may eventually overwhelm the capacity of the healthcare system.
- Exponential functions are functions of the form $f(t) = a \times b^t$. When both a and b are positive numbers, these functions increase exponentially. For small t, they may increase very slowly, but their graphs bend upwards and they will eventually cross any given threshold.

Endnotes

[43] For a list of countries and states in the U.S. that did not impose lockdowns, see [3].

[44] Not all lockdowns succeeded in preventing local healthcare systems from becoming overwhelmed. A tragic example occurred in April in the city of Guayaquil in Ecuador [4].

[45] Most importantly, reproduction numbers may decrease in response to control measures (see Chapter 11) and because at later stages of an outbreak, fewer people will be susceptible to infection (see Chapters 10 and 26).

[46] The official definition of R_0 requires that only the index case be infected. But for the time horizon discussed in this chapter, the depletion of susceptibles does not yet significantly alter the reproduction number.

[47] Data on current usage of ICU beds in Ohio by Covid-19 patients are published at [5].

[48] At the time of this conversation, the total hospitalization rate in Ohio had been higher 10% of all reported cases. In the early stages, it was significantly higher; currently it is below 10%. For details see [6]. The decrease in hospitalization rates over time is largely due to the fact that this rate is calculated as a percentage of reported cases and that with more widespread testing, a larger proportion of cases will be detected, while the proportion of patients who develop severe symptoms may remain unchanged. The threshold that Alice derived from her rough estimates would likely have been overly optimistic for the early stages of the pandemic that this discussion refers to. With current detection rates, the actual threshold would be somewhat higher. On November 24, 2020, the Ohio Department of Health [5] reported that 4,449 patients with Covid-19 were hospitalized and that the state was nearing the capacity of its healthcare system. Over the preceding week, there had been approximately 58,000 new Covid-19 infections in the state.

[49] The modeling in this chapter is based on reported cases. This allows for predicting future hospitalizations based on known fractions of hospitalizations relative to reported cases. While numbers of actual cases are likely much higher, under the simplifying assumption of a fixed detection rate, reported numbers would increase proportionally to actual numbers. The model then can give rough predictions for the increase of reported cases and required hospitalizations, even though the actual numbers remain

hidden. The assumption of a fixed detection rate might be approximately realistic for the short time horizon of the discussion in this chapter, but not adequate in the long run (see previous item).

50 The precise value of R_0 is difficult to estimate. It depends on how people behave under normal circumstances, which in turn depends on prevailing cultural norms. Thus R_0 will vary slightly between different countries and regions within countries. Also, as awareness of an ongoing pandemic already changes people's behavior and the reproduction number, estimates based on data from the earliest phases of the pandemic may give the most accurate picture. A meta-analysis of 12 published studies of data sets for December 2019 and January 2020, mostly from China, found that estimates of R_0 ranged from 1.4 to 6.49, with a mean of 3.28, and a median of 2.79 [7]. As the mean is strongly influenced by outliers, the median is presumably the more informative number. It falls into the range between 2.5 and 3 that is assumed throughout this text.

51 The serial interval of the Covid-19 pandemic is not a fixed quantity. Isolation and quarantining policies can significantly limit transmissions that occur relatively late after exposure, but are less effective in preventing transmissions that occur before the onset of symptoms. This would shorten the serial interval, as has been empirically observed. Analyzing publicly available data from China on 677 different pairs of infectors and infectees, researchers found that from January 9 to 22 of 2020, the serial interval averaged 7.8 days, whereas from January 30 to February 13, the average was 2.2 days, shortening by more than threefold over the 36-day period [8]. This study also cites several earlier papers that give estimates of the serial interval from 3.1 to 7.5 days. For example, in a paper that was submitted in February 2020, Nishiura et al. estimated a median of 4.6 days for the serial interval [9]. Alice puts the serial interval at exactly 7 days, which she admits to be an overestimate. However, the modeling in this chapter is for the early stages of an outbreak, before quarantine and isolation policies were in place. In this scenario, a 7-day serial interval may

not be very far off the mark. The assumption would no longer be accurate for the modeling at later stages when some control measures are in place, as is done in Chapters 11, 13, 23, and 24. However, in the interest of achieving greater transparency and simplifying the calculations, these subtleties are ignored in the text itself. The shortening of the serial interval will not alter the qualitative predictions of these models, only shorten the time spans over which the model predicts increases or decreases of new infections.

[52] On March 9, the first 3 cases of Covid-19 were confirmed in Ohio. By March 13, the total had reached 13. See [6].

[53] For more information on the time-line of restrictions in Ohio see [6] or [10].

References

[1] Worldometers.info. Dover, Delaware, U.S.A. COVID-19 Coronavirus Pandemic. [cited 2020 Sep 21].
https://www.worldometers.info/coronavirus/

[2] American Hospital Directory, Inc. Hospital Statistics by State. [cited 2020 Sep 21].
https://www.ahd.com/state_statistics.html

[3] Wikipedia: The free encyclopedia. Wikimedia Foundation, Inc. COVID-19 pandemic lockdowns. [cited 2020 Nov 24].
https://en.wikipedia.org/wiki/COVID-19_pandemic_lockdowns

[4] Cabrera JM, Kurmanaev A. Ecuador's death toll during outbreak is among the worst in the world. The New York Times 2020 Apr 23. [updated 2020 May 12; cited 2020 Nov 24]. https://www.nytimes.com/2020/04/23/world/americas/ecuador-deaths-coronavirus.html

[5] Ohio Department of Health. Coronavirus (COVID-19) Ohio Public Health Advisory System. [cited 2020 Sep 21]. Regionally available from:
https://coronavirus.ohio.gov/wps/portal/gov/covid-19/public-health-advisory-system/

[6] Wikipedia: The free encyclopedia. Wikimedia Foundation, Inc. COVID-19 pandemic in Ohio. [cited 2020 Sep 21]. https://en.wikipedia.org/wiki/COVID-19_pandemic_in_Ohio

[7] Liu Y, Gayle AA, Wilder-Smith A, Rocklöv J. The reproductive number of COVID-19 is higher compared to SARS coronavirus. J Travel Med. 2020 Mar 13 [cited 2020 Sep 21]; 27(2):taaa021 https://www.ncbi.nlm.nih.gov/pmc/articles/PMC7074654/ DOI: 10.1093/jtm/taaa021

[8] Ali ST, Wang L, Lau EHY, Xu XK, Du Z, Wu Y, et al. Serial interval of SARS-CoV-2 was shortened over time by nonpharmaceutical interventions. Science 2020 Aug 28 [cited 2020 Sep 21]; 369(6507):1106–1109. https://science.sciencemag.org/content/369/6507/1106.full DOI: 10.1126/science.abc9004

[9] Nishiura N, Linton NM, Akhmetzhanov AR. Serial interval of novel coronavirus (COVID-19) infections. Int J Infect Dis. 2020 Apr [cited 2020 Sep 21]; 93:284–286. https://www.sciencedirect.com/science/article/pii/S1201971220301193 DOI: 10.1016/j.ijid.2020.02.060

[10] Johns Hopkins University of Medicine. Coronavirus Resource Center. Critical Trends. Impact of opening and closing decisions by state. [cited 2020 Sep 21]. https://coronavirus.jhu.edu/data/state-timeline

Chapter 10

How are reproduction numbers related to our contacts?

Alice, Bob, Cindy, and Frank meet on July 16, 2020. They will talk about how reproduction numbers depend on our contacts. Reproduction numbers are key to epidemiological modeling. As the pandemic is spreading, scientists are trying to better understand it. By the end of June, over 23,000 research articles on Covid-19 had already become available [1], and the number keeps growing.

Bob: We talked about how Covid-19 is transmitted during contacts between two people. And we talked about reproduction numbers R. How are they related to our contacts?

Alice: Let's explore this today. Recall that each of us typically makes many, many contacts each day. Most of them are low-intensity, some are high-intensity. But transmissions of Covid-19 happen only during so-called effective contacts. High-intensity contacts have a much larger chance of being effective than low-intensity contacts.

Cindy: I remember! You told us that it takes many virus particles, probably at least hundreds, to cause a new infection[13] and that a contact will be effective if it is intense enough so that sufficiently many of them will be transmitted.

Frank: But only if one person is infectious and the other one is susceptible. Otherwise nothing will happen, even if the contact is very close.

Alice: Correct. A contact is considered effective when it would lead to a transmission of the infection *if* one of the individuals making this contact is infectious and the other susceptible. So not all effective contacts lead to new infections.

Only a small fraction of our contacts are effective. It appears that over the course of 10 days, which is the average duration of infectiousness[29] for Covid-19, a typical person would make effective contacts with about 3 other people.[50]

Bob: So, an infectious person would then infect on average 3 other people. Which means that $R = 3$, as I recall.

Frank: Hold on, Bob! Not all effective contacts of an infectious person lead to new infections. Only the ones with susceptible people do.

Bob: I was thinking about the start of an outbreak, when only the index case is infectious and all others are susceptible. The index case would then cause 3 new infections on average.

Alice: Excellent observations everyone! Bob has in fact given us here the official definition of the basic reproduction number R_0: It is the average number of new infections that a typical index case would cause in a large population that consists entirely of susceptible individuals.[54]

Cindy: Why does it say in this definition "typical" index case?

Alice: Some people make many more effective contacts than others. In very detailed epidemiological models, we need to take into account these individual differences, or heterogeneities, as they are called in the scientific literature.[55] Also, a given person is more likely to make effective contacts with friends and family members than with strangers. Such patterns of making contacts can be studied with fairly complicated models based on contact networks.[56] But here we will only cover the very simplest models that assume everybody is "typical" and everybody is equally likely to make contact with everybody else.[57]

Frank: But that's not the case, as you just admitted yourself!

Alice: A model is always a simplified version of reality. Some of its assumptions can only be rough approximations of reality. But simpler models are easier to understand and help us to see more clearly what is going on.

For now we only need to remember that our simplified estimate of $R_0 = 3$ translates into an assumption that people make on average effective contacts with 3 different individuals during the time when they are infectious. They may make multiple effective contacts with some of them during that time, especially with family members or close friends. Then only the first of these repeated contacts will lead to a transmission.

Frank: Alright. I can see what the deal is with this index case. But what about later on, when there are already other infected people and perhaps even some who have recovered with immunity?

Alice: Then some of the effective contacts of an infectious person would be with others who are no longer susceptible. This will make the reproduction number R smaller than R_0. For this reason, R will usually decrease over time, even if no control measures are put into place.

Bob: So could we then say that at any given time, the reproduction number R is the average number of *susceptible* individuals that a typical person makes effective contact with while being infectious?

Alice: This is a good way of thinking about R. It is not entirely accurate when there are multiple infectious individuals around, as they can make contact with the same susceptible person. But when the proportion of infectious people in the population is small enough, R will be approximately equal to the average that Bob has described.

Frank: Let's go back to R_0. The official definition talks only about one infectious person while everybody else is still susceptible. When we talked last time, we looked at a model where the numbers of infections were growing. But we assumed that the reproduction number R was equal to R_0 all the time. So we were fudging it, to say the least!

Alice: Whenever we build a model, we "fudge" a little by ignoring some aspects of the real world. This is perfectly okay if we keep in mind that predictions of models are only estimates of what is going to happen. Sometimes only rough estimates.

During the initial stages of an outbreak, only a very small fraction of all contacts will be between two people who are no longer susceptible.

For this reason, models that assume that R remains equal to R_0 over some time interval are reasonably accurate as long as the vast majority of people still remain susceptible.

Frank: I have another question: What if we don't do anything? Without any control measures, no social distancing, no masks, no lockdowns, none of this stuff, what percentage of people would catch coronavirus over time?

Alice: Very good question! It has an answer only if we assume that people who go through Covid-19 infections recover with permanent immunity and cannot be infected repeatedly. This may be too optimistic,[58] but let's make this assumption here.

Under this assumption, the percentage of the population who will experience infection at some time depends on R_0. It is called the final size of the outbreak.[59]

Bob: So what would the predicted final size be for $R_0 = 3$?

Alice: For a population of 50 individuals, the picture at the end of the pandemic would then look similar to this one:

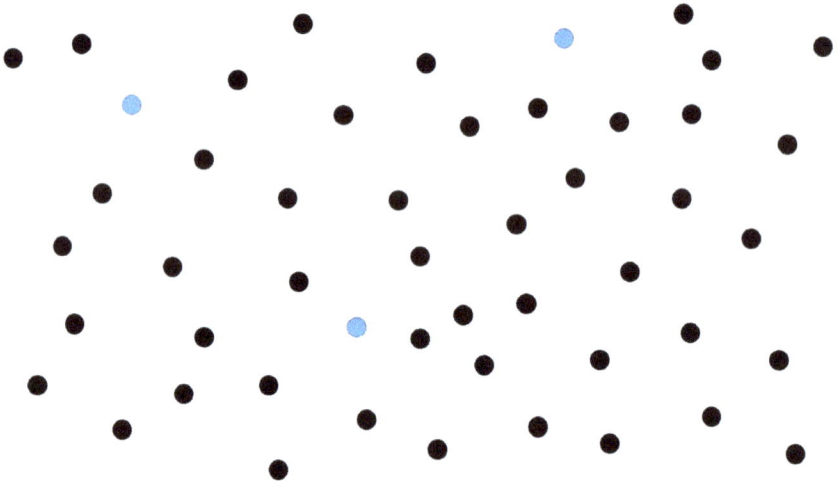

Fig. 10.1   Situation at the end of an outbreak without control measures when $R_0 = 3$.

The simplest models[60] give a final size of about 94% when $R_0 = 3$. Only 6% of the population will then escape infection and remain susceptible. The actual percentages may be a little different due to random effects, but might be close.

People who have experienced infection and are in the removed state are shown in black. People who have escaped infection and are still susceptible are shown in blue. It is the state of the population that we saw at the end of our discussion on contacts, but without the arrows.

Cindy: This looks so terrible! Almost everybody got infected.

Bob: Yes, Cindy, this looks terrible. But R_0 for Covid-19 may be a little smaller than 3, between 2.5 and 3. What would happen when R_0 were smaller?

Alice: Even for $R_0 = 2$, the models predict that the picture would look like this, with about 80% of individuals experiencing infection:

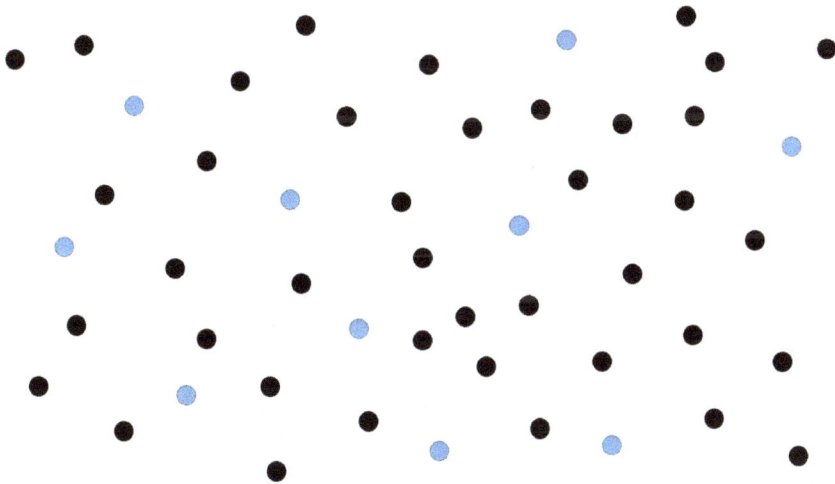

Fig. 10.2 Situation at the end of an outbreak without control measures when $R_0 = 2$.

Frank: Hold on! Don't they say in the media that the pandemic would be over when we reach what they call "herd immunity"? And that it would require somewhere between 60 and 70 percent of people having experienced infection? So how come you predict that for R_0 between 2 and 3, somewhere from 80% to 94% of all people would get infected at some point?

Alice: There are a lot of misunderstandings about herd immunity. Let's talk some other time about how it works and what it does to the spread of new infections.

Right now, I only want to show you how the final size of an outbreak without control measures depends on R_0. For $R_0 = 1.5$, the models predict that the picture would look like this, with about 58% of individuals experiencing infection:

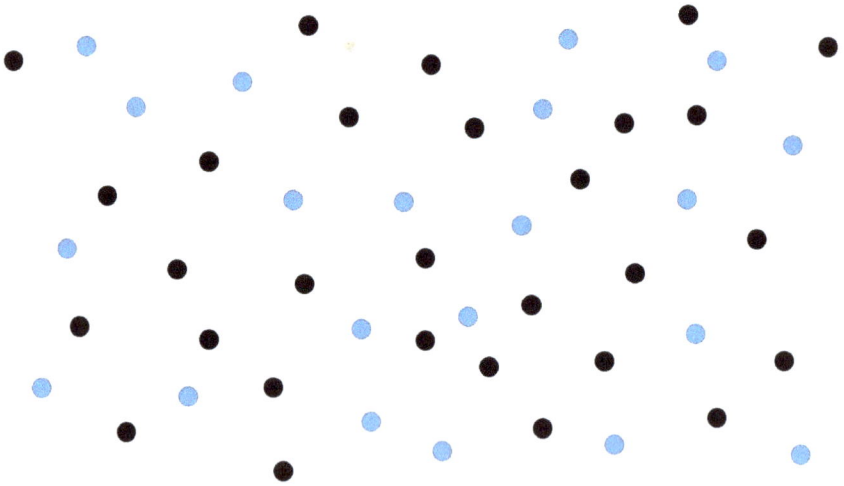

Fig. 10.3   Situation at the end of an outbreak without control measures when $R_0 = 1.5$.

Bob: Much better than for $R_0 = 3$, but still most people would get infected.

Alice: Yes. As long as $R_0 > 1$, always a significant percentage of the population would experience infection.

Frank: So what would the percentage be for $R_0 < 1$?

Alice: In this case, the models predict that in a large population, the percentage of people who will experience infection would be close to 0.

Let me show you some pictures that illustrate why. Instead of drawing lines for all contacts during short time intervals, we will only draw lines that show who infected whom. These transmission events will not necessarily occur in the order shown in our pictures, but we will get a better idea of what is going on when we focus on the entire time periods during which certain individuals remain infectious.[61] I will also talk more generally about R rather than R_0.

We will again look at a population of 50 individuals but will assume that initially 4 of them are infected, while all others are susceptible. Like this:

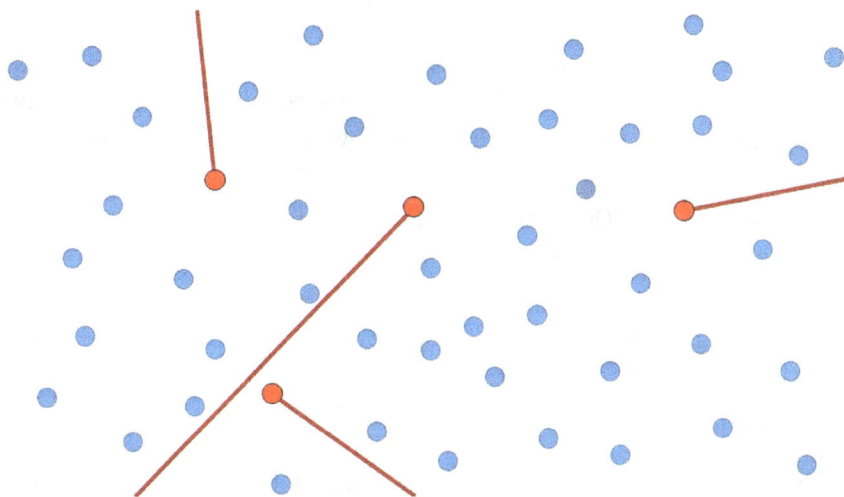

Fig. 10.4   Initially, 4 individuals got infected through contacts outside of the population.

We can think of those 4 infected individuals as index cases of 4 separate outbreaks. Let us assume $R = 0.75$ and look at a typical scenario for the new infections caused by those 4 index cases:

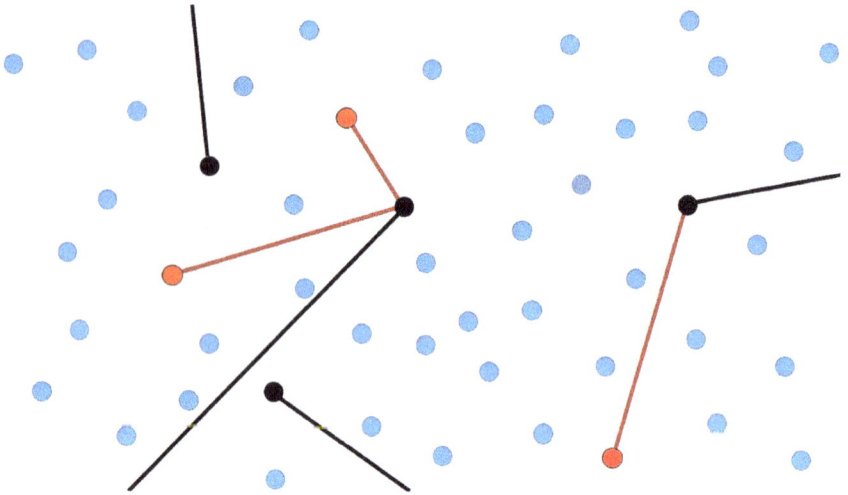

Fig. 10.5   New infections caused by the index cases.

We can see here that 1 of the index cases has caused 2 new infections, while 2 of them have caused none. The average—or, more precisely, the mean—number of infections caused by an index case is $\frac{2+1+0+0}{4} = 0.75 = R$.

In my next picture (Fig. 10.6), let us look at further infections caused by these 3 newly infected individuals.

I will assume that 2 of them cause 1 new infection each, while the third causes none. Then the mean number of infections caused by each of those 3 is $\frac{1+1+0}{3} \approx 0.67$.

Cindy: But this isn't equal to $R = 0.75$.

Alice: Not exactly equal, but close. Disease transmissions are random events, and we cannot expect to get the exact value of R_0 for the mean, only a value that is reasonably close.

Bob: And we could get the exact mean 0.75 if these three cases had caused a total of 2.25 new infections, which is impossible.

Alice: Right! Let's look at the picture:

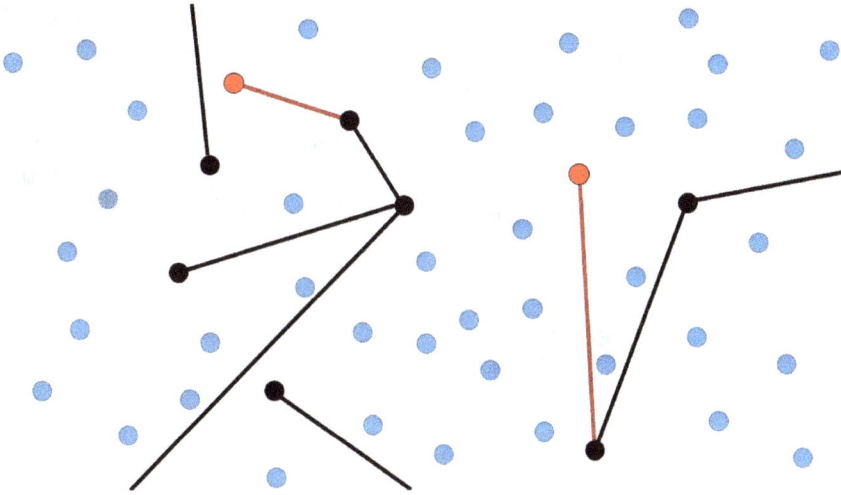

Fig. 10.6   New infections in the next step.

Now let's look at the new infections in the next step:

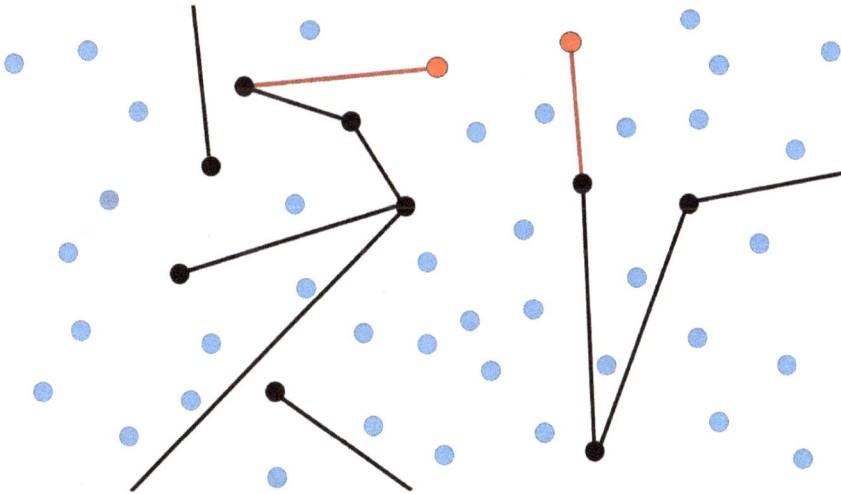

Fig. 10.7   Two more infections occurred.

The mean number of infections caused by each of the 2 infected persons of my previous picture (Fig. 10.6) is $\frac{1+1}{2} = 1$.

Farther away from $R = 0.75$ than before, but with fewer infected individuals, we should expect relatively larger random fluctuations.

Here we saw more infections than we might have expected; in other scenarios it might be fewer. It will occasionally happen that neither of two infected individuals transmits the virus to anybody else. After they recover, we would get the following picture:

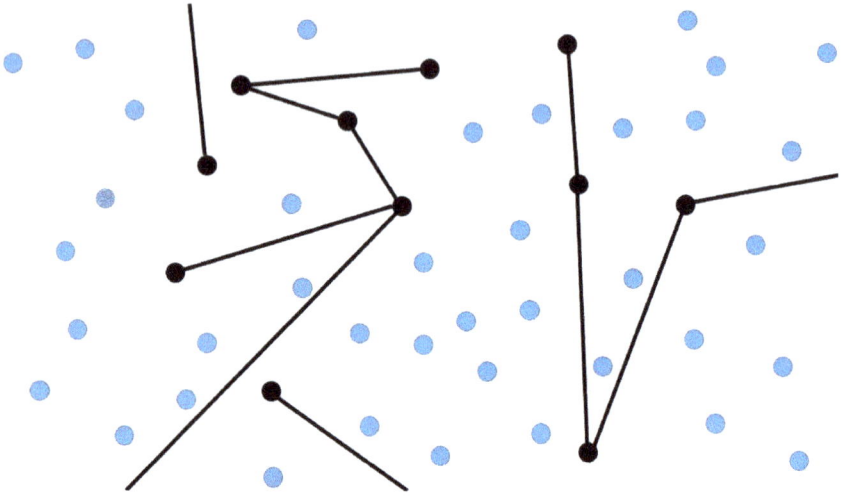

Fig. 10.8   No more transmissions occurred. The outbreak has run its course.

Bob: In this example, the outbreak fizzled out after a few steps. Even though several individuals brought the infection into the population.

Alice: Right. This is what our models predict for $R < 1$: Chains of transmissions will remain short, and an outbreak will fizzle out rather quickly.

Cindy: That's good. But in your example, the index case in the middle of your picture alone has caused a total of 4 other infections. I mean, directly or farther down a chain of transmissions. So this one infection from outside the population has made 5 people sick. Right?

Alice: In this example, yes.

Cindy: But 5 people out of 50, that is 10% of the population! And you said, Alice, that when $R_0 < 1$, then close to 0% of the population will experience infection. But here even with one index case we have 10%. This is not close at all to 0%.

Frank: Alice said, "large population". For once, I must defend those epidemiologists. They are thinking about populations of entire regions, states or countries, not of groups of only 50 people. Even in Athens county—the home of our university—with a population of about 65,000 people, 5 infections would be only 0.0077% of the population. Very close to 0%, if you ask me.

Alice: Thank you, Frank, for clarifying this for us!

Every new infection is regrettable. With 5 infections it is likely that at least one of them would involve great suffering. But 100% protection is not possible.

Epidemiologists need to study the spread of the pandemic on the scale of states, countries, or even the entire world. In our examples, I talk about a relatively small group of 50 people so that I can draw pictures. For such small populations, even one infection would be more than one percent of the population. But for very large populations, even all 11 infections in our last picture would be very close to 0%.

Let me summarize what we have learned today:

- The basic reproduction number R_0 can be interpreted as the average number of other people that an infected person has effective contacts with while being infectious.[62]
- When $R_0 > 1$, a single index case may start chains of transmission that will cause infections of a significant percentage of the population. This percentage, called the final size, will depend on R_0. For R_0 ranging from 2 to 3, it will be between 80% and 94% if no preventive measures are taken.
- More generally, we can think about the reproduction number R as the average number of susceptible people that a typical patient makes effective contact with while being infectious.

- As the proportion of susceptible people decreases over the course of an outbreak, R will typically also decrease, even if no control measures are adopted.
- When $R < 1$, chains of transmission will remain short, and a small outbreak that originates from outside the population will quickly fizzle out. For large populations, the introduction of an index case would then cause infections only in a very small percentage of its members.

Endnotes

[54] This is the definition of R_0 that can be found, with minor variations of the wording, in standard textbooks on mathematical epidemiology such as [2–4]. Of the ones mentioned here, Diekmann et al. [2] gives the most advanced and comprehensive treatment of the subject, while the book by Vinnycky and White [4] is the most accessible. A shorter introduction to the subject can be found in the book chapter [5].

[55] Relevant heterogeneities—that is, differences between people in the same population—are basically of two kinds. The first are physiological. Some people may shed more virus particles than others, or spread them farther [6]; some remain infectious for longer than others. The second kind are differences in how people make contacts. Some people are more gregarious than others and some professions require frequent contacts with many other people. These heterogeneities lead to overdispersion, where a small fraction of infectious people transmit the virus to many others, while most Covid-19 patients infect only one other person or nobody. See, for example [7]. Overdispersion complicates efforts to mitigate the spread of Covid-19 and needs to be incorporated in realistic predictive models. However, this requires a level of mathematical sophistication that goes beyond our exposition. For this reason, overdispersion will not be directly addressed in the dialogues.

[56] Introductions to epidemiological models based on contact networks can be found in the book chapter [8] and at the website [9].

For a comprehensive treatment of these models, see [10].

[57] These assumptions are technically called the assumption of homogeneity of hosts and of uniform mixing, respectively.

[58] Technically, Alice is assuming an SEIR-model for Covid-19 here. When re-infections can occur, an SEIRS model would be more appropriate. At the time of this conversation, in July 2020, no clear-cut cases of re-infection with Covid-19 had been documented. But later such cases were confirmed.[29]

[59] In the literature, the final size is usually represented as a proportion rather than a percentage. But here Alice talks about percentages to keep things more intuitive.

[60] These predictions would be obtained from SEIR-models with homogeneity of hosts and uniform mixing. See for example [9] for a technical description of how these numbers can be derived in a certain type of stochastic models.

[61] Technically, Alice is showing here the so-called generations of the infection for each index case.

[62] Covid-19 patients tend to be most contagious near the time of onset of symptoms and to a lesser degree later in the course of their illness. See, for example, Figure 1 of the survey [11]. Alice is implicitly assuming here that infectious individuals are uniformly contagious during the entire period of infectiousness. Such simplifying assumptions are often made in epidemiological modeling.

References

[1] Teixeira da Silva JA, Tsigaris P, Erfanmanesh M. Publishing volumes in major databases related to Covid-19. Scientometrics. Aug 28 [cited 2020 Nov 24]; 2020. https://link.springer.com/article/10.1007%2Fs11192-020-03675-3 DOI: 10.1007/s11192-020-03675-3

[2] Diekmann O, Heesterbeek H, Britton T. Mathematical tools for understanding infectious disease dynamics. Princeton: Princeton U Press; 2012. 520 p.

[3] Keeling MJ, Rohani P. Modeling infectious diseases in humans

and animals. Princeton and Oxford: Princeton U Press; 2008. 384 p.

[4] Vynnycky E, White R. An introduction to infectious disease modelling. Oxford: Oxford University Press; 2010. 400 p.

[5] Just W, Callender H, LaMar MD, and Toporikova N. Transmission of infectious diseases: Data, models, and simulations. In: Robeva R, editor. Algebraic and discrete mathematical methods for modern biology. London: Academic Press; 2015. p. 193–215.

[6] Camero K. What makes someone a COVID-19 superspreader? New study points to two features. Miami Herald 2020 Nov 20. [updated 2020 Nov 24; cited 2020 Dec 9]. https://www.miamiherald.com/news/coronavirus/article247328119.html

[7] Tufekci Z. This overlooked variable is the key to the pandemic. It's not R. The Atlantic 2020 Sep 30. [cited 2020 Nov 24]. https://www.theatlantic.com/health/archive/2020/09/k-overlooked-variable-driving-pandemic/616548/

[8] Just W, Callender H, LaMar MD. Disease transmission dynamics on networks: Network structure vs. disease dynamics. In: Robeva R, editor. Algebraic and discrete mathematical methods for modern biology. London: Academic Press; 2015. p. 217–235.

[9] Just W, Callender H, Drew LaMar MD. Exploring Erdős-Rényi random graphs with IONTW. QUBES. Community. Groups. Exploring Transmission of Infectious Diseases on Networks with NetLogo. 2015 May 9. [cited 2020 Dec 31]. https://qubeshub.org/community/groups/iontw/iontwmodules

[10] Kiss IZ, Miller JC, Simon PL. Mathematics of epidemics on networks: From exact to approximate models. Cham: Springer; 2017. 431 p.

[11] Eric A. Meyerowitz EA, Richterman A, Gandhi RT, and Sax PE. Transmission of SARS-CoV-2: A review of viral, host, and environmental factors. Ann Intern Med. 2020 Sep 17. [cited 2020 Dec 31]. https://www.acpjournals.org/doi/10.7326/M20-5008 DOI:10.7326/M20-5008

Chapter 11

What does "flattening the curve" do for us?

Alice, Bob, Cindy, and Frank meet on July 19, 2020. Economies around the world are slowly recovering from the sharp downturn during the lockdowns in March and April. The OECD area unemployment rate fell to 7.7% in July 2020, from 8.0% in June, but remained 2.5 percentage points above the rate in February.[63]

Cindy: When we read about "flattening the curve", is this referring to the trend curves we talked about?

Bob: I think so. I've read that this was the purpose of the lockdowns in our state and elsewhere. But I don't understand what this exactly means and what it would be good for in the long run.

Frank: You can say that! They couldn't keep people under lockdown forever. What was the point of imposing one?

Alice: Good questions! Let's look at the numbers of new infections in Ohio between March 13 and April 14 (Fig. 11.1).

The trend curve, also sometimes called epidemic curve, first steeply increases, then flattens out, and then slightly decreases near the end of this time frame.

Recall that the lockdown, or shelter-in-place order, in Ohio started on March 23 [2]. When we look more closely, we see that the trend curve bends upward until March 27.

Bob: This would be typical for exponential growth as I recall from our discussion a week ago. Or at least for nearly exponential growth.

Alice: Yes, this is what the data suggest. But on March 28 the trend curve became nearly a straight line. It peaked 2 weeks after the lockdown had been imposed and then started going down a bit. It was almost flat near the peak. That's where the expression "flattening the curve" comes from:

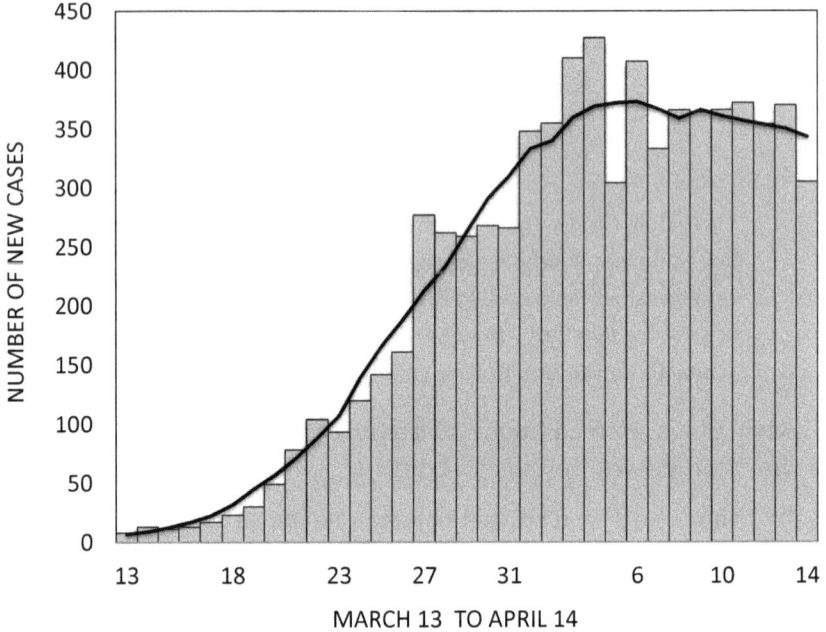

Fig. 11.1   Reported numbers of new infections in Ohio between March 13 and April 14. Based on data from the New York Times [1].

Bob: Well, the daily reported infections never reached 450 and it appears from the chart that weekly new infections peaked at around 2,500.

Cindy: This was well below the 45,000 threshold that we talked about last week. There were enough hospital beds available for all Covid-19 patients who needed one!

Alice: Right. The graph shows the immediate effect of the lockdown: It made sure that our healthcare system would not become overwhelmed.

Frank: Granted. But 2,500 is so much lower than our estimated threshold. This lockdown was overdone. During Spring Break, we got an email saying that the campus will be closed until the end of the semester and all classes will be online. And boom! I had lost my job in dining services. How am I supposed to pay tuition without a job?

Alice: I'm sorry to hear that, Frank! Yes, it was terrible news for all of us. Many people lost their jobs at the time, including many of us students.

Frank: Perhaps the state needed to do something, but definitely not locking up all people in their homes!

Alice: It is an interesting question whether our state could have done something less drastic. We may return to it some other time.

But first we need to understand precisely what the lockdown was supposed to accomplish and how this would fit into the strategy of limiting the spread of Covid-19 in the long run. We can best think about this in terms of the reproduction numbers R that we discussed last week.

Bob: But you had told us that the model based on $R_0 = 3$ would no longer be applicable when we are in a lockdown.

Alice: Correct! Recall that the reproduction number R is the average number of other people that an infected person will infect before recovering. We saw in our previous meeting how it depends on the average number of our effective contacts, which in turn depends on the total number and the intensity of our contacts. Near the start of an outbreak, without any control measures in place, it would be approximately equal to R_0.

Bob: But under lockdown, it would be a lot smaller, because people have a lot fewer contacts.

Alice: Exactly! The reproduction number R changes over time. In particular, it depends on the control measures that are in place.

Cindy: Could we treat this number R under lockdown as another constant? I mean, to keep the math simple?

Alice: Excellent suggestion, Cindy! To keep our discussion simple, we will assume that the reproduction number R under lockdown is a constant R_ℓ. It will be smaller than the basic reproduction number R_0, so that $R_\ell < R_0$.

Cindy: Can we make R_ℓ equal to 0? I think the math would then be really simple.

Alice: What would the equation $R_\ell = 0$ mean?

Bob: Then an average infected individual would infect 0 other people. It would mean that no more transmissions of the virus occur.

Cindy: And no more people will get sick! That's what I'd like to see!

Bob: Me too, Cindy. But this is unrealistic. We cannot cut all contacts. Even when we were under lockdown, some people still needed to go to work. And we still needed to do grocery shopping and keep essential appointments. So some new infections still occurred.

Alice: I agree. I would love to prevent absolutely all transmissions. But this is not possible. In practical terms we can only achieve a number R_ℓ that is smaller than R_0 but larger than 0.

Bob: Would it help to cut the reproduction number R to half of $R_0 = 3$ so that $R_\ell = 1.5$?

Alice: Unfortunately, this would not flatten the curve.

Frank: Why not?

Alice: If we change the reproduction number R from $R = R_0 = 3$ to $R = 1.5$, our model would still predict exponential increase.

If initially we had 10 infected people, then in the first week we would have about $1.5 \times 10 = 15$ new infections. And in Week 2 there would be about $1.5 \times 15 = 22.5$. That's a lot less than the 90 that we predicted for the model with $R = R_0 = 3$. But eventually, after about 21 weeks, the weekly numbers of new infections would cross the threshold 45,000 and overwhelm our healthcare system:

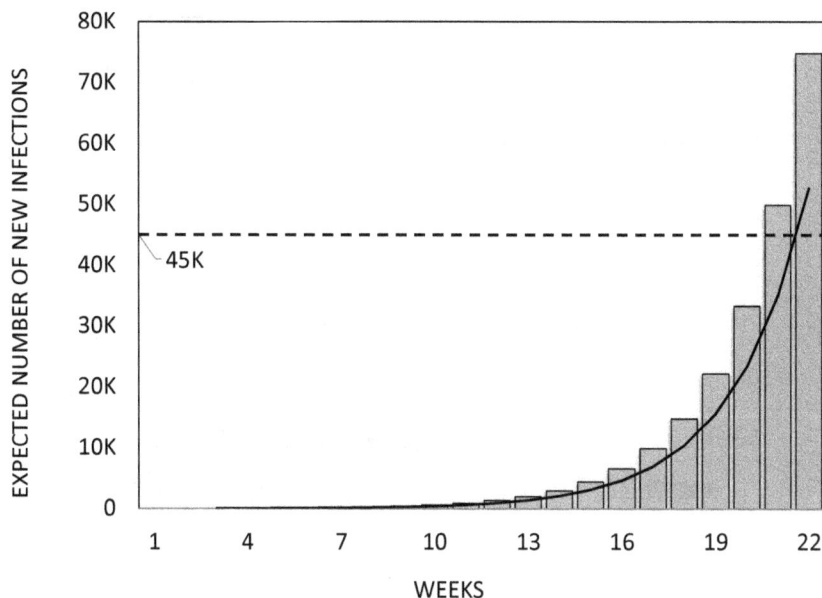

Fig. 11.2   Exponential increase of predicted weekly new infections with $R = 1.5$.

Cindy: Then we would still need to turn away sick people from hospitals. We cannot let this happen.

Alice: Right. We would have delayed the disaster by a few months, but not averted it.

Frank: But we wouldn't need to worry about anything yet for the first 10 weeks. In your graph, the numbers for these weeks are practically zero.

Alice: The slow growth in the first 10 weeks might have given us a false sense of security. But it would not have prevented the catastrophe.

Bob: Would the same pattern occur for any constant value $R > 1$?

Alice: That's exactly right! Let's look at a graph for $R = 1.1$:

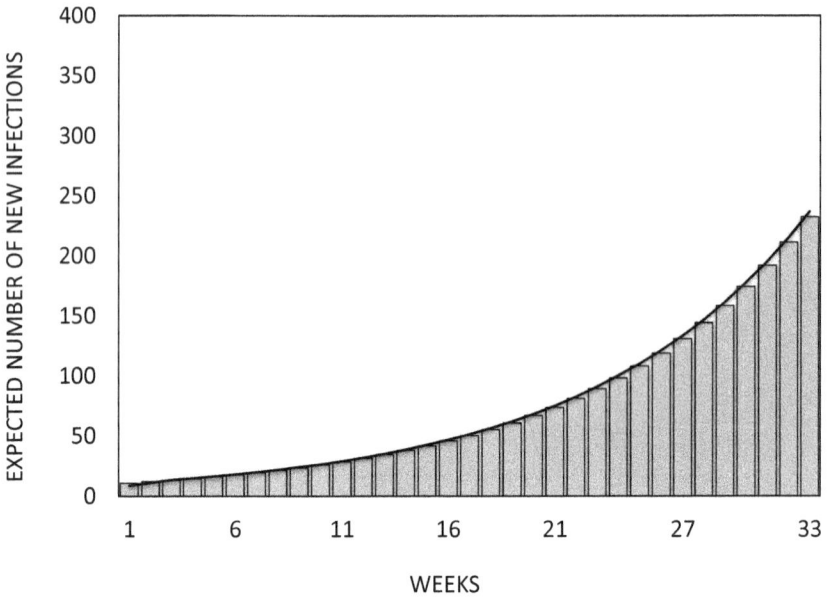

Fig. 11.3   Exponential increase of predicted weekly new infections with $R = 1.1$.

The scale on the vertical axis is different here than in my previous picture. We can see that for this value, the trend curve for new infections would grow very slowly for many weeks. But the trend curve bends upward, and if the pattern were to continue, the numbers would become intolerably large. When we see signs of nearly exponential increase, we need to act.

Cindy: So what if $R = 1$?

Bob: Would the model then predict the same number of infections week after week?

Cindy: And we would never need to turn away sick people from the hospital, right?

Bob: So, for controlling the spread of new infections, it might be enough to bring the reproduction number down to $R = 1$.

The trend curve will then be completely flat, like this:

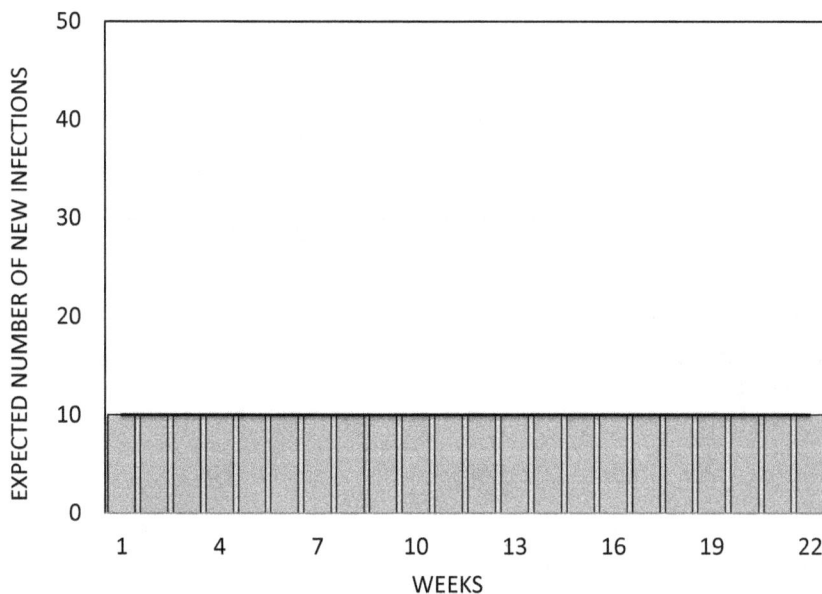

Fig. 11.4   Predictions of the model for $R = 1$.

Alice: In theory, yes. But we are talking only about a very simple model. Recall that the reproduction number R represents an average. In actual data, we would see some random fluctuations. And in practice it is very unlikely that R would be exactly equal to 1. It may easily creep up above 1 if it is equal or just a little below this number. So to be on the safe side, we would need $R_\ell < 1$ during the lockdown.

Then our models predict exponential decrease, also called called exponential decay, in the numbers of new infections per week.

Cindy: So with $R < 1$, the outbreak would then slowly fizzle out?

Alice: Right. This would happen for any fixed value $R < 1$.

Let's compare our predictions for $R \geq 1$ with the ones for $R < 1$. We will start with a hypothetical situation of 1,000 initially infected people instead of just 10. Let me show you two graphs. The first one for $R = 0.9$; the second for $R = 0.7$:

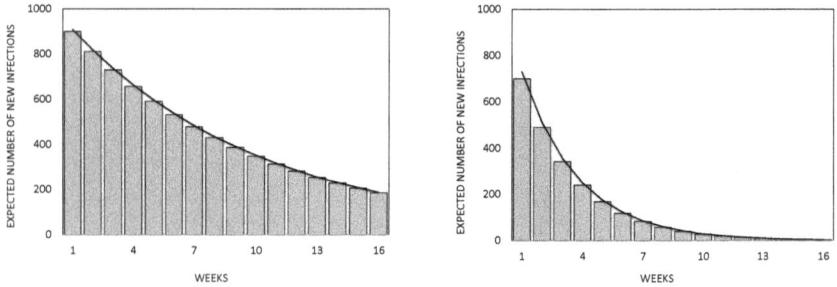

Fig. 11.5 Exponential decrease of weekly infections for $R = 0.9$ (left panel) and for $R = 0.7$ (right panel).

Cindy: And it would fizzle out faster if R is smaller?

Alice: Exactly! Let me summarize what all this means for the value of R_ℓ of the reproduction number for the time under lockdown.

By imposing a lockdown, we can avert the disaster of overwhelming the healthcare system, but only if we make sure that $R_\ell \leq 1$.

In practice, we need the number R_ℓ to be strictly smaller than 1; that is, $R_\ell < 1$. This is because we want to be safe from random effects and because we want the numbers of new infections to decrease rather than merely stay the same over time. When $R_\ell < 1$, our simple models predict that these numbers will decrease exponentially over time and will fizzle out.

Bob: But one cannot keep people under lockdown forever!

Alice: Of course not. At some time our state needed to re-open. This changes the reproduction number R again.

Cindy: So would the reproduction number after re-opening be still another constant? Like R_r?

Alice: Good notation, Cindy! To keep our discussion simple, we can think about it this way.

Bob: After lifting the stay-at-home order, people would have more contacts. And we saw last time that this would increase the reproduction number. So I think that we would then have $R_r > R_\ell$.

Cindy: But if we make $R_r > 1$, then we will get nearly exponential growth of new infections, as Alice called it. And our healthcare system will become overwhelmed some time later!

Alice: You have hit upon the key point, Cindy! We need to make sure that R_r, the average number of new infections caused by an infectious individual after re-opening, will not exceed 1. We can write this in symbols as $R_r \leq 1$.

Frank: Wait a minute! If $R_\ell = 1$ with a totally flat curve, and $R_\ell < R_r$, how could we possibly get $R_r \leq 1$?

Alice: Great observation, Frank! If $R_\ell = 1$, we could not get such an R_r. This is actually the most important reason why we need $R_\ell < 1$: We need to leave ourselves some wiggle room for re-opening in such a way that $R_\ell < R_r \leq 1$.

And when R_ℓ is a lot smaller than 1—for example, when $R_\ell = 0.7$ as opposed to $R_\ell = 0.9$—then there is more wiggle room for relaxing restrictions. In either case, a state or a country would need to be very, very careful about how to re-open so that R_r will not exceed 1.

Bob: I see. But let's take a step back and talk only about what happens during the lockdown. How would the weekly numbers of new infections change in our model when a lockdown with $R_\ell = 0.7$ is imposed?

Alice: I think you can explore this What-If scenario yourself, Bob. Give it a try!

Bob: So, let me assume again that initially there are 10 infected individuals and initially the outbreak grows exponentially with $R = R_0 = 3$ until Week 5, when the model predicts about 2,430 new infections.

Then a lockdown starts at the end of Week 5, so that R changes to $R_r = 0.7$. Now each infected individual will infect on average only 0.7 other persons, with some infecting nobody, and others infecting 1 or more others.

For Week 6, the model would only 1,701 new infections, for Week 7, only 1,191 new ones; and so on. Let me sketch a graph and share it on my screen:

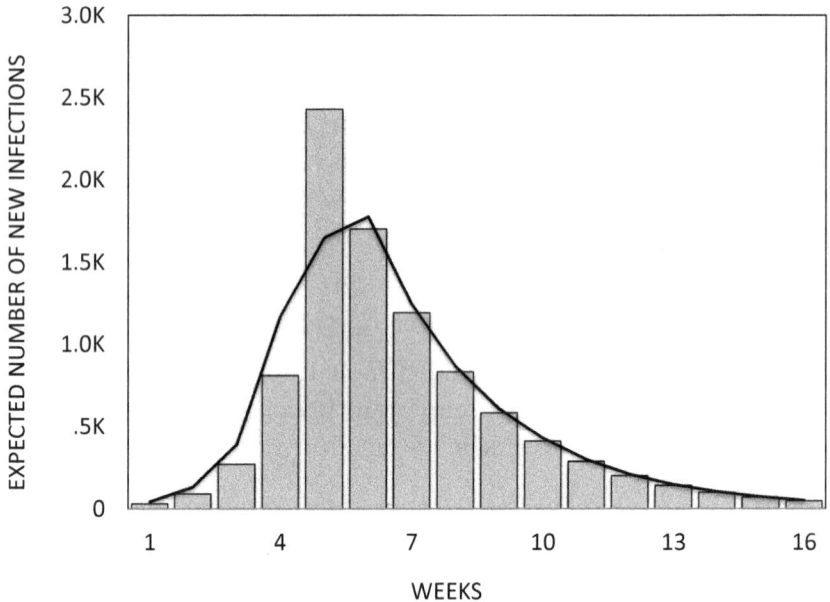

Fig. 11.6   Bob's model for the effects of a lockdown at the end of Week 5.

Cindy: Thank you, Bob, for explaining this so nicely! It looks like the trend curve would peak shortly after the time the lockdown is imposed and then decrease exponentially.

Frank: I don't quite buy this.

Bob: Why not?

Frank: I'm fine with the general pattern. But I think the peak would occur later than in Bob's graph.

Cindy: Why do you think so, Frank? I thought Bob's graph was right.

Frank: Bob had assumed that the lockdown would be imposed at the end of Week 5. So some people who got infected in this week would have already caused new infections before the lockdown. These would be detected only in Week 6, or perhaps even later. That's why. We probably would get something like this:

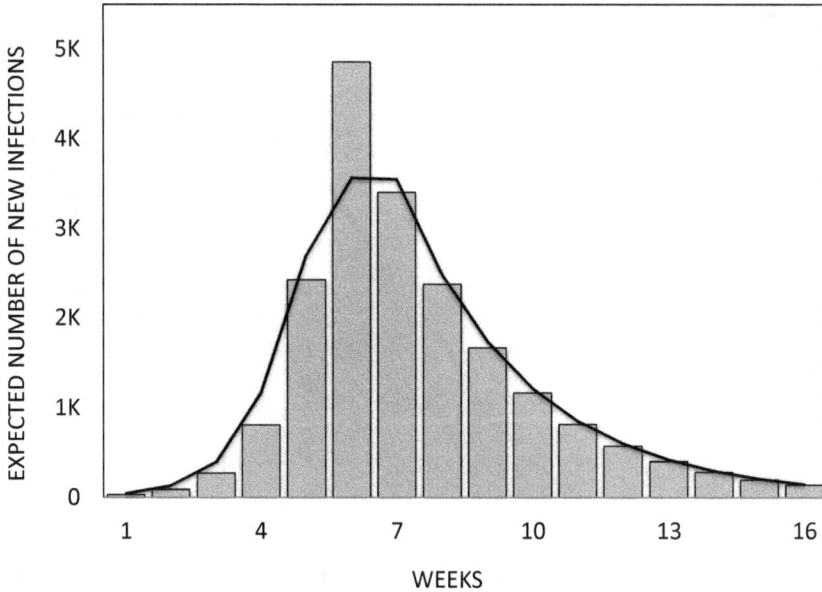

Fig. 11.7   Frank's model for the effects of a lockdown at the end of Week 5.

Alice: Very good point, Frank! For the reason you mentioned, we would predict some delay between the start of the lockdown and the actual peak. Let's look again at the data of daily new infections in Ohio until April 14 (Fig. 11.8).

They match our predictions fairly well: Nearly exponential increase before the lockdown on March 23, then flattening of the epidemic curve as in Frank's model, then a slight decrease of the curve.

Bob: But the peak in the number of new infections occurred only about 2 weeks after the lockdown started, even later than Frank had predicted.

Alice: Remember that the graph shows only the confirmed cases, the ones we know about because people got tested. This would typically occur only a week or more after exposure, and then a few more days would pass before the cases were recorded in the data base.

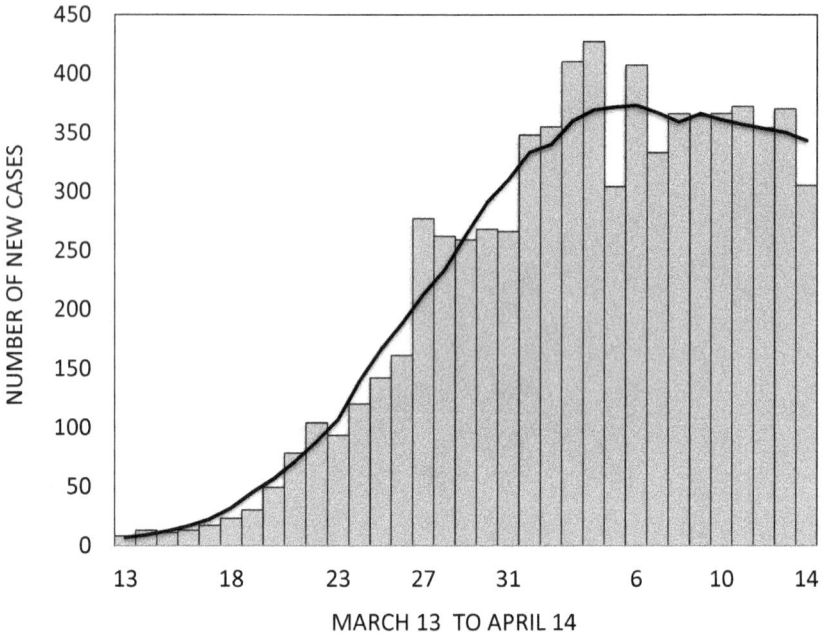

Fig. 11.8   Reported numbers of new infections in Ohio between March 13 and April 14.

Cindy: And the epidemic curve would then continue decreasing nearly exponentially after April 14. So the lockdown in Ohio was successful!

Alice: This is what our simple model predicts. But we need to be careful with jumping to conclusions based on a decrease for a few days after the peak. We should look at the data for Ohio after April 14 and see whether they confirmed this prediction.

Frank: Perhaps we can do this some other time.

What, exactly, do you mean by a "successful lockdown", Cindy?

Cindy: This was "flattening the curve", right? To make sure that the weekly numbers of new infections stay small enough so that the healthcare system can treat all people who might need hospitalization or even ventilators.

Alice: This is the immediate concern, yes. But we also need to bring the reproduction number R_ℓ down far enough below 1 so that the numbers of new infections substantially decrease and we can be sure that there is enough leeway for re-opening, with $R_\ell < R_r \leq 1$.

Bob: In other words, we want to make the epidemic curve look like the one on the left, not like the one on the right:

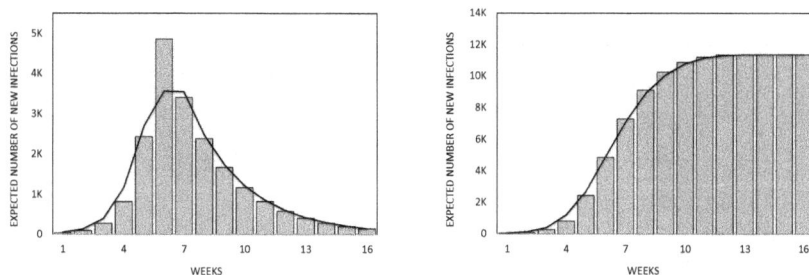

Fig. 11.9   General shape of the epidemic curve for $R_\ell < 1$ (left panel) and for $R_\ell = 1$ (right panel).

Alice: Very good illustration, Bob!

The phrase "flattening the curve" tells only part of the story. It should really be something like "flattening and pushing down the curve." But this would be too wordy.

The important thing is that now we all understand what is really meant by the shorter phrase: Making sure that the peak of the epidemic curve stays well below the capacity of our health care system, and that after reaching this peak it decreases. This will happen when the reproduction number R_ℓ during the lockdown satisfies the inequality $R_\ell < 1$.

Endnotes

[63] See [3]. The OECD (Organization for Economic Co-operation and Development) comprises 37 countries from North and South America to Europe and Asia-Pacific.

References

[1] Github Inc. nytimes/covid-19-data. [cited 2020 Sep 22].
https://github.com/nytimes/covid-19-data

[2] Johns Hopkins University of Medicine. Coronavirus Resource Center. Critical Trends. Impact of opening and closing decisions by state. [cited 2020 Sep 21].
https://coronavirus.jhu.edu/data/state-timeline

[3] Organisation for Economic Co-operation and Development. Unemployment rates, OECD—Updated: September 2020. [cited 2021 Jan 1].
https://www.oecd.org/newsroom/unemployment-rates-oecd-update-september-2020.htm

Chapter 12

How do social distancing and wearing masks help?

Alice, Bob, Cindy, and Frank meet on July 21, 2020. The worldwide total of confirmed Covid-19 infections has surpassed 15 million. But thanks to preventive measures like social distancing and wearing masks, the increase has slowed. In many countries, daily new infections remain low. Thailand, a country of nearly 70 million people, has reported only 81 new cases over the preceding 3 weeks [1]. Worldwide, there have been numerous protests against government regulations aimed at controlling the spread of Covid-19. Thailand saw large street demonstrations on July 18, 2020.[64]

Cindy: You already told us so many interesting things, Alice. But we have not talked about what we all need to do to fight the spread of Covid-19.

Bob: I think we have. We need to get the reproduction number R down to below 1. I recall that R was roughly the average number of people we make effective contacts with over a period of 10 days or so.

If we want to reduce the number of effective contacts, we need to reduce the total number of our contacts and change high-intensity contacts into low-intensity ones. That's what I understood from our discussions so far.

Cindy: I got that. But I mean: What does each of us need to do on a practical level? Can you tell us Alice?

Alice: Yes, let's start talking about practical steps today. These are called control measures or preventive measures.

Bob made a very important point: The control measures recommended by epidemiologists aim to reduce the number and intensity of contacts. Absolutely perfect protection is not possible. But if the basic reproduction number R_0 for Covid-19 is close to 3, we need to modify our contacts only in such a way that on average the number of people with whom we make effective contacts will be cut down to less than one third, perhaps to one fifth. Or to put it differently: We need to modify our contacts in such a way that about 80% of them that would normally be effective don't happen anymore or will no longer be effective.[65] Then the reproduction number R will be less than 1, and the spread of Covid-19 will be under control.

Bob: Lockdowns and closures of businesses or schools would be examples of control measures. Is that what we need?

Alice: These would be control measures with a heavy impact on the economy and our lives. I hope we don't need them if we adopt the ones that I want to talk about today: moving social life outdoors as much as possible, limiting the size of social gatherings, social distancing, and wearing masks.

Frank: In a free country, they shouldn't put such restrictions on people.

Bob: I don't like these restrictions either, Frank. But if this is what it takes to get people back into their jobs and us back into class, wouldn't you consider putting up with them? If the alternative is you know what?

Frank: Spit it out Bob: Another lockdown or hundreds of thousands of deaths from Covid-19.

I might put up with restrictions that make sense to me. If I clearly see what they are for. I will not follow a nonsensical rule just because some government official made it up.

Cindy: I think Alice is about to explain how these preventive measures work. Don't you want to listen to what she has to say, Frank?

Frank: Alright. Go ahead, Alice, with your lecturing.

Alice: I will tell you about these measures one-by-one so that we will more clearly see how they work. Let's start with moving social events outdoors as much as possible.

People are sociable. Social gatherings give us a sense of belonging to a group, to a larger community. Unfortunately, they often turn into superspreading events. This can happen when at least one infectious person interacts with a lot of susceptibles.

The most common transmission route of Covid-19 is through tiny droplets in the air that infectious people exhale. If a susceptible person gets directly hit by this air stream, there is a chance that he or she may become infected.

Recall that it takes a lot of virus particles to cause a new infection.[13] So the danger of exposure from a single such "hit" is very small. But when two people talk in close proximity for some time, there will be multiple such hits and a significant chance that the contact becomes effective.

Cindy: How can I picture these "hits" in my mind, Alice?

Alice: Let me draw a sketch and share it on my screen with you:

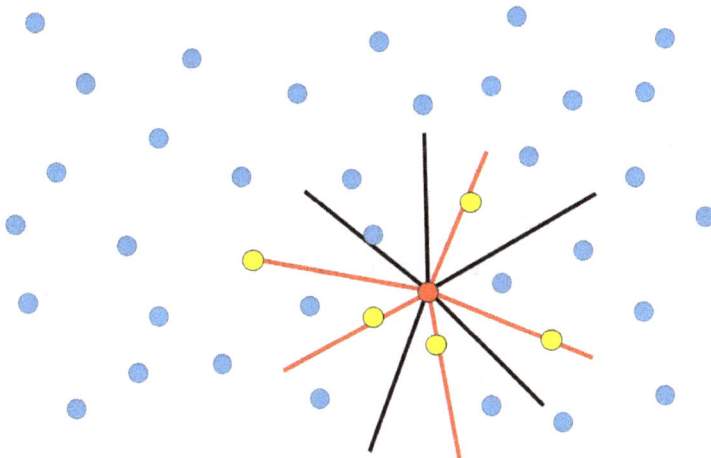

Fig. 12.1 A social gathering with one index case.

It shows a gathering of 40 people. Think of it as a large party. One of them is infectious. This will be the index case; let me call him Ingham again. The other 39 were susceptible at the beginning.

We can see here that Ingham will send exhaled air in all sorts of directions; perhaps by talking with different people at different times. Each of these airstreams has the potential of causing a new infection.

The picture shows five out of six people who were hit by one of these airstreams becoming exposed, while one lucked out and did not catch the disease. In reality, the proportion of those lucky ones may be higher. But also remember that my picture shows only a small fraction of the relevant airstreams.

Cindy: This would be terrible; five people infected at a single party!

Alice: There are many known cases where the number was even much higher, close to or even above 100. Such events are known as "superspreading events" or "superspreader events".[66] For reasons that scientists don't understand yet, some people seem to shed an unusually high number of virus particles.[67] In our example, Ingham would have been highly contagious, but not unusually contagious.

Bob: You said you would be talking about moving social gatherings outdoors. Is the one in your picture supposed to be outdoors or indoors?

Alice: My first picture (Fig. 12.1) is more characteristic for outdoor events, where droplets with virus particles quickly disperse. In indoor settings, these droplets hang around in the air for a lot longer and can cause an infection even without a direct hit, so to speak.

Moreover, in places like bars with music playing, people tend to talk more loudly, and the direct airstreams of their exhalations tend to travel farther.

Let me show in my next picture what might happen inside a bar.

In that picture (Fig. 12.2), the straight lines that represent direct airstreams are longer; this will happen when people talk more loudly. In my example, two additional transmissions were caused by this:

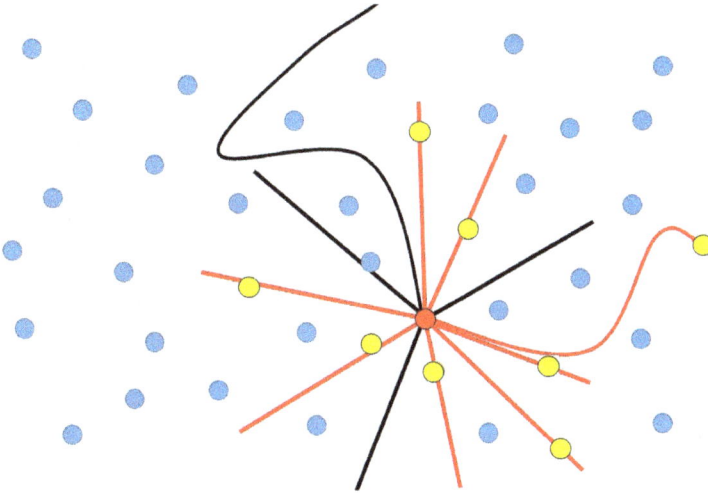

Fig. 12.2   A social gathering indoors with one index case.

The same effect may occur when people sing together, in a choir or a karaoke bar.

Cindy: Oh that's why you said choir practice is so dangerous! Now I see. But what are the squiggly lines in your picture?

Alice: They represent droplets that hang in the air for a long time and slowly travel in unpredictable directions. There will be some dispersal along the way even indoors, but much less than outdoors. I showed this graphically by making these lines a little thinner than the ones for the direct airstreams. Indoors these indirect hits may still lead to transmission of enough virus particles for causing a new infection. My picture illustrates this for one newly exposed person.

These are the two main reasons why bars and other indoor venues may become hotspots for the transmission of Covid-19.

Frank: Come on, Alice! After studying all day, five days a week, one needs to relax and talk with friends over a beer on the weekend.

If they close all the bars and fight tooth and nail against parties on our front porches, we students will have them in our basements. Enclosed spaces with poor ventilation. Same thing may happen as in your picture.

Alice: Yes, basements may be even worse hangouts than bars.

This is why I personally do not support closing all bars entirely. Consumption of alcohol is problematic though. Having too many drinks makes people careless. If you and your friends want to enjoy some beers together, choose an outdoor venue whenever possible. Outdoor seating in a bar. Somebody's front porch or backyard. If you want to really *talk* with your friends, choose a quiet place where nobody has to practically shout to be heard. A patio without music, for example. And make sure all of you limit the amount you drink to levels where you still make rational decisions.

When we compare my second picture with the first, we can see why epidemiologists recommend moving social life outdoors whenever possible. In this way, we will decrease the intensity of contacts without having to cut the ones that are most important to us. Remember that by decreasing intensity of a contact, we decrease the chances that it will become effective and lead to a transmission of Covid-19.

Cindy: So for an outdoor party, we would then have a situation like in the first picture you showed us. But there were already so many transmissions in this first picture!

Alice: Right.

Moving social gatherings outdoors will prevent some new infections, but not enough of them to decrease the reproduction number R below 1. And in a state like Ohio, it will work only for a few more months. When we go into November and December, with the weather becoming cold, gatherings outdoors will become much less of an option.

This is why we need additional preventive measures. One of them is limiting the size of social gatherings.

Let's look at my first picture again and then see what might have happened in the party of our first picture if only 20 people had attended instead of 40:

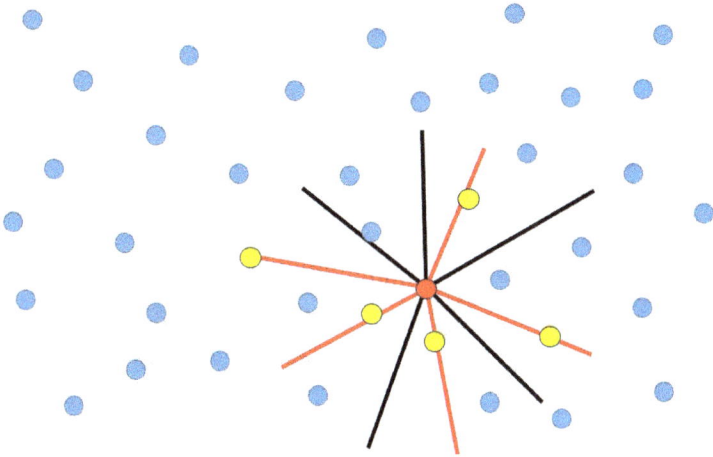

Fig. 12.3   An outdoor social gathering with one index case.

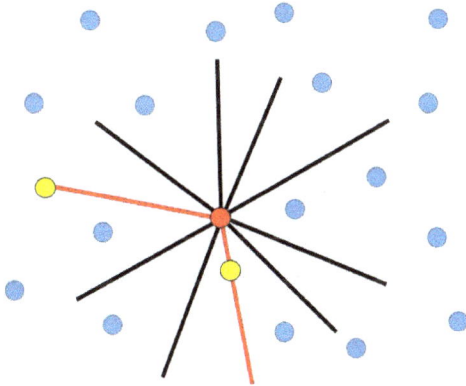

Fig. 12.4   A smaller social gathering outdoors.

Here I assumed that only two of the five people who became infected in the previous picture where present; the other three were among those who did not attend.

By limiting the size of the gathering we have not prevented all infections, but we could say that we have prevented this party from becoming a superspreading event.

Frank: But we shouldn't all be expected to cut our social life in half because of Covid-19!

Alice: We may need to dial down our socializing, but we don't need to give up on meeting other people. In my example, the other 20 people could have gone to a different party. None of them was infectious, so no transmissions would have occurred at the other party.

Frank: How would this work for bars? If they are all limited to half of their capacity, we would need to open an additional new bar for each existing one to make room for all customers!

Alice: Going to bars is not the only form of social life, Frank. Think for example of religious services. They also involve large gatherings of people. Many places of worship have increased the number of services they offer and simultaneously limited the size of the congregation permitted at any given service. This puts additional burdens on the clergy. But where it is possible, the spiritual needs of all members of the congregation can be met.

Cindy: Still, in the new picture with the smaller size of the gathering, two people got infected. That's two too many!

Alice: Yes, Cindy. Limiting the size of social gatherings alone will not prevent sufficiently many new infections, even when all gatherings were to take place outdoors.

Notice that in the above picture both people who caught the infection found themselves in airstreams full of virus particles because they happened to stand or sit too close to Ingham, our index case. Had they been farther away, they might have escaped infection.

Bob: So people should have kept farther away from Ingham.

Cindy: But how do we know who is infectious and who isn't?

Alice: In real life, we don't know. So we should stay sufficiently far away from everybody else. This is why epidemiologists recommend social distancing whenever possible; staying at least 6 feet away from all other people.[68]

Let's see what might have happened if all people in this gathering had followed this recommendation:

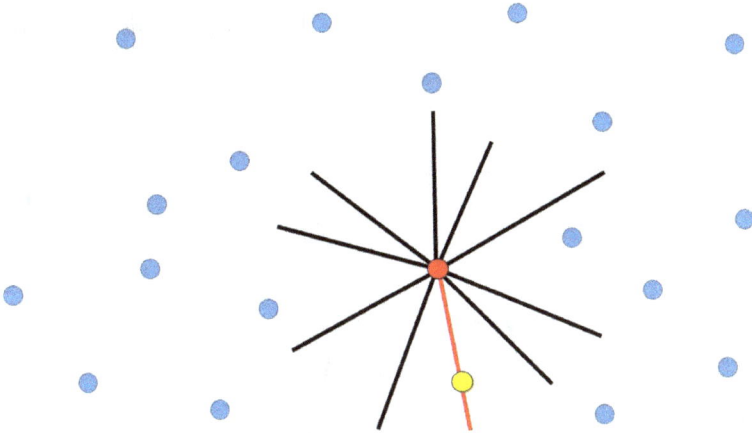

Fig. 12.5   A smaller social gathering outdoors with social distancing.

Here people have moved away more from each other; 6 feet or more in most cases. Some pairs seem still relatively close to each other; perhaps only 5 feet apart. This will occasionally happen. It is difficult to judge how far a distance of 6 feet actually is. And on occasion we will need to get closer than 6 feet; for example, when we pass somebody in a narrow spot. Also, even the distance of 6 feet is only a guideline; it is possible for droplets with virus particles to travel farther than that.

Social distancing will keep us fairly safe, but not 100% safe. In my picture, we still see one unlucky person, call her Sue again, who got too close to Ingham and became infected. Such transmissions will happen from time to time. Without additional precautions, they may happen too often for achieving our goal of keeping the reproduction number R below 1.

Cindy: If only these droplets with the virus would not travel quite that far! Then Sue would have avoided infection and would not have caught Covid-19 at this party!

Alice: There is a simple and very effective remedy: Wearing masks. They break and partially redirect the airflow during exhalation. They trap at least some of the virus particles in the breath.[69] They block most droplets and don't allow them to travel very far.

Let me show you in my next picture how this would look in our example:

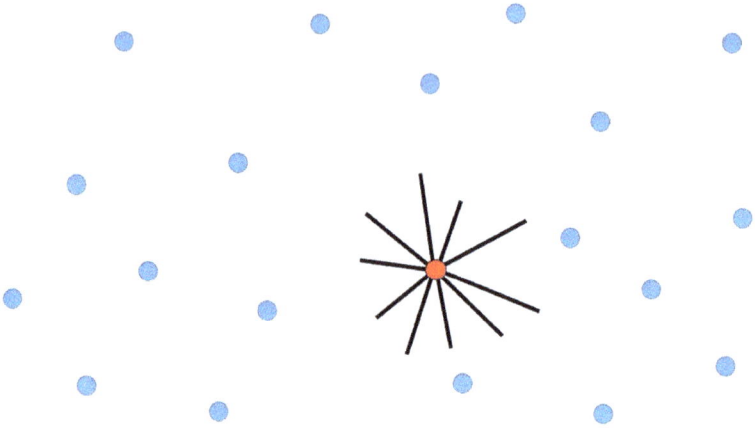

Fig. 12.6   A smaller social gathering outdoors with social distancing and wearing masks.

With masks, the air streams that people exhale do not travel very far. Had Ingham worn a mask, even somebody standing or sitting fairly close to him would have been reasonably well protected from droplets with virus particles.

Cindy: May we still become infected even with social distancing and wearing masks?

Alice: Yes. This is much less likely than without these precautions, but some transmissions will still occur. But usually the number of virus particles transmitted will be much smaller than without them. Studies have shown that when people got infected by smaller doses of virus during exposure, they were much less likely to develop severe symptoms and complications [2].

In this last picture, nobody got infected at the party, although there happened to be a person in the group who was unknowingly shedding virus particles. In combination, the preventive measures of limiting the size of the gatherings, moving it outdoors, social distancing, and wearing masks have prevented all Covid-19 transmissions in our example.

Bob: That's good. So how can we think about these control measures in terms of what we discussed earlier about contacts and reproduction numbers?

Alice: Limiting the size of the gathering reduced the number of contacts per person. The other three measures worked by reducing the intensity of contacts.

None of the four control measures we discussed here all by itself will be sufficient. But a combination of all four—together with readily available testing and sufficiently thorough contact tracing, isolation of confirmed cases, and quarantines of their close contacts—would bring the reproduction number R below 1 and keep it below 1.[70]

If R stays below 1, some new infections will still occur. But their numbers would decrease over time. At the price of relatively minor inconveniences, we will be able to lead reasonably normal lives. Most types of economic activity can resume. Kids will be able to go to school. And we will be able to study face-to-face on campus and meet with friends after class.

Cindy: If only all people would comply with these control measures!

Alice: Hoping for 100% compliance is as unrealistic as is expecting 100% protection from new infections. But near-universal compliance is needed to get the protection of the entire population that is achievable when the reproduction number R is below 1. Nobody can effectively protect him- or herself and their loved ones when the spread of the infection in the population is out of control.

Bob: I will admit that I was always thinking about preventive measures in terms of a tradeoff: Either we protect people's health, or we protect people's jobs. But the ones we talked about today protect people's health without direct adverse effects on the economy.

If they help in keeping businesses open, why would rational people not comply with them?

Alice: One important reason may be that many, perhaps most, people still think that we need to choose between either protecting peoples' health or peoples' jobs. The strategy proposed by epidemiologists aims at protecting both. But without enough compliance, we can protect neither.

Frank: Well, I can see your point. But I still have issues with these masks.

First of all, I don't see why it would be necessary to wear one outdoors while sufficiently far away from other people. Breathing fresh air may be more important than reducing a very tiny risk to a very, very tiny one.

Alice: I agree. Epidemiologists recommend that masks be worn in most indoor settings other than people's own homes and in outdoor settings when social distancing is not possible. Wearing one outside when you are all by yourself serves no purpose.

Frank: Second, I do think requiring people to wear masks crosses a line. At some point, we need to stand up for our personal freedom of choice.

Alice: I have a question: The U.S. gives us citizens the right to own guns. Would you agree that this right comes with the responsibility of owners to practice their use? So that when they might be needed for hunting or self-defense, they will hit their intended target and not an accidental bystander?

Frank: Very much so. That's what firing ranges are for.

Alice: So, when gun owners go to a firing range for target practice, do they randomly shoot in any direction that pleases them?

Frank: Don't be silly, Alice! People might get hurt or killed. There are important safety regulations that everybody needs to follow.
Rule 1: "Handle all firearms as if they were loaded." Rule 2: "Always keep the firearm pointed in a safe direction." The list goes on.[71]

Alice: Do these rules infringe upon our rights?

Frank: Don't play dumb Alice! You know as well as I do that they are just common sense.

Alice: Yes, I know.

With Covid-19 going around, infectious people are shooting tiny droplets full of virus particles into the air. These virus particles may kill somebody who accidentally gets into a stream of their exhaled air, or somebody farther down the resulting chain of transmissions.

As none of us can be absolutely sure that we are not infectious, we need to always handle our breath as if it were loaded, so to speak. We all need to breathe in order to live, and we have very limited control over where our exhaled air travels. So, unfortunately, much of the time we are shooting off these potentially loaded droplets into random directions.

Masks break the airflow, at least partially. It would not be too far off the mark to think about the mask as sending the airflow in a safe direction.

So, when we put on these masks, are we giving up an essential part of our freedoms, or are we exhibiting common sense?

Endnotes

[64] See [3] for a partial list of protests against preventive measures in various countries of the world. The street demonstrations in Thailand appear to have been triggered by the preventive measures against Covid-19, but the causes of dissatisfaction with the government were broader [4].

[65] With $R_0 = 3$, we would in theory need to reduce only the average number of people that we normally make effective contact with during a fixed time interval by 67%. But Alice is talking here about the number of contacts and takes into account the fact that multiple effective contacts with the same person can occur.

[66] The media and the scientific literature more frequently use the term "superspreader event", which has the same meaning as "superspreading event". Later in this text, only "superspreading event" will be used, as the term "superspreader" may also refer

a person who infects many others on multiple occasions. The survey [5] gives a list of well-documented superspreading events, including an overnight camp in Georgia, where 260 attendees subsequently tested positive [6].

[67] In November 2020 a paper [7] came out that examined possible reasons for these individual differences. See also [8] for a nontechnical description of this research.

[68] The term "social distancing" sometimes refers to the combination of all the control measures discussed in this chapter. Here the phrase is used in the narrower, more intuitive sense.

[69] The article [9] in the New York Times has nice visualizations that show in detail how masks filter virus particles.

[70] Empirical evidence for this claim will be discussed in Chapters 28 and 29.

[71] Actual firing ranges differ in how they phrase their rules and in which order they list them. But these lists usually include items similar to the ones Frank mentioned here.

References

[1] Worldometers.info. Dover, Delaware, U.S.A. COVID-19 Coronavirus Pandemic. [cited 2020 Nov 28].
https://www.worldometers.info/coronavirus/

[2] Mandavilli A. It's Not Whether You Were Exposed to the Virus. It's How Much. The New York Times 2020 May 29. [cited 2020 Dec 6]. https://www.nytimes.com/2020/05/29/health/coronavirus-transmission-dose.html

[3] Wikipedia: The free encyclopedia. Wikimedia Foundation, Inc. Protests over responses to the COVID-19 pandemic. [cited 2020 Nov 28]. https://en.wikipedia.org/wiki/Protests_over_responses_to_the_COVID-19_pandemic

[4] Wikipedia: The free encyclopedia. Wikimedia Foundation, Inc. 2020 Thai protests. [cited 2020 Nov 28].
https://en.wikipedia.org/wiki/2020_Thai_protests

[5] Eric A. Meyerowitz EA, Richterman A, Gandhi RT, and Sax PE.; Transmission of SARS-CoV-2: A review of viral, host,

and environmental factors. Ann Intern Med. 2020 Sep 17. [cited 2020 Dec 31]. `https://www.acpjournals.org/doi/10.7326/M20-5008` DOI:10.7326/M20-5008

[6] Szablewski CM, Chang KT, Brown MM, Chu VT, Yousaf AR, Anyalechi N, et al. SARS-CoV-2 transmission and infection among attendees of an overnight camp—Georgia, June 2020. MMWR Morb Mortal Wkly Rep. 2020 Aug 7. [cited 2020 Dec 9]; 69:1023–1025. `https://www.cdc.gov/mmwr/volumes/69/wr/mm6931e1.htm` DOI:10.15585/mmwr.mm6931e1

[7] Fontes D, Reyes J, Ahmed K, Kinzel M. A study of fluid dynamics and human physiology factors driving droplet dispersion from a human sneeze. Phys Fluids 2020 Nov 12. [cited 2020 Dec 9]; 32:111904(2020) `https://aip.scitation.org/doi/10.1063/5.0032006` DOI: 10.1063/5.0032006

[8] Camero K. What makes someone a COVID-19 superspreader? New study points to two features. Miami Herald 2020 Nov 20. [updated 2020 Nov 24; cited 2020 Dec 9]. `https://www.miamiherald.com/news/coronavirus/article247328119.html`

[9] Fleisher O, Gianordoli G, Parshina-Kottas Y, Patanjali K, Peyton M, Saget B. Masks work. Really. We'll show you how. The New York Times 2020 Oct 30. [cited 2020 Dec 9]. `https://www.nytimes.com/interactive/2020/10/30/science/wear-mask-covid-particles-ul.html`

Chapter 13

How can we make re-opening safe?

Alice, Bob, Cindy, and Frank meet on July 24, 2020. Reported new infections in the U.S. have been increasing over the previous month, but have started to decrease in several states, including Arizona and Texas. Massachusetts, where new infections have remained low, issues an order that requires travelers coming into the state to produce a negative test result or quarantine for 14 days [1].

Bob: I am reading a lot about a second peak of Covid-19 infections in the U.S. What can you tell us about it, Alice?

Alice: The trend curve for new infections in the U.S. increased rapidly between mid-June and mid-July. It is still increasing, but has been pretty flat for the last week. So we may be nearing a second peak. And that second peak will be more than twice as large as our first peak in early April.[72]

Bob: Last time, we discussed how preventive measures like social distancing, wearing masks, and limiting the size of social gatherings can reduce the number of effective contacts. This would then lead to a reduction of the reproduction number R. And we had seen earlier that when we keep this number R below 1, the number of new infections would decrease, and we could lead reasonably normal lives.

Seems with this second peak it didn't work out that way. Why not?

Alice: Let's talk about this today. First, let's remind ourselves how the proposed strategy was supposed to work in terms of numbers of new infections over a long time frame.

Recall that the reproduction number R is the average number of other people that an infectious individual will infect before recovering. It depends on many factors and may change over time.

In our earlier discussions, we had assumed for simplicity that early in the outbreak this number R was constant with $R = R_0 = 3$. This model then predicted exponential increase of the numbers of weekly new infections.

When a lockdown is imposed, the value of R changes to $R = R_\ell < 1$, with the epidemic curve first flattening, then reaching a peak some time after the lockdown starts, and then exponentially decreasing.

Cindy: This was all before re-opening, right?

Alice: Right. After re-opening, the reproduction number R changes again, to some value R_r with $R_\ell < R_r < R_0$. The key to successful re-opening is making sure that $R_r < 1$. Then our model predicts numbers of weekly new infections that look like this:

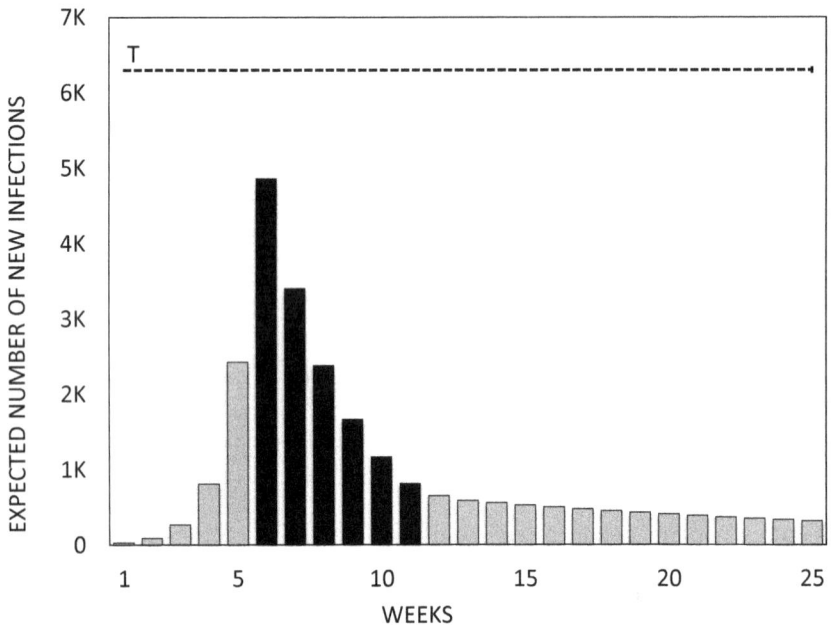

Fig. 13.1 Predicted numbers of weekly new infections when $R_\ell < R_r < 1 < R_0$. The weeks of the lockdown are shown in black.

As we discussed previously, there would be some delay between the starting time of the lockdown and its effect, so that the numbers are still higher in Week 6 and Week 7 than they were in Week 5. For similar reasons, there will be a delay between the time when the lockdown ends and the time when the full effect of relaxing the restrictions shows up in the data.

Frank: Wasn't the curve supposed to flatten early in the lockdown?

Alice: This flattening would show up in graphs of daily rather than weekly data. Also, the very simple model that I used for making this graph assumes that all restrictions of the lockdown are put in place simultaneously. In many states and countries, these restrictions were imposed more gradually [2]. This would lead to a flatter curve around the peak.

But most importantly, we can see that, after re-opening, the numbers of new infections would still decrease, but more slowly than during the lockdown. My simple model predicts exponential decrease; in actual data, it would only be nearly exponential.

Cindy: What is this number T with the dashed horizontal line in your graph, Alice?

Alice: This represents a threshold for the number of new infections that we don't want to cross. In our earlier discussions, we calculated such a threshold from the number of available hospital beds in Ohio. But it could also be imposed by some other limiting resource, like the number of ICU beds. So I simply call it T and don't put a particular number on it.

Cindy: Like, when we look at the infections in another state or country, with a different number of hospital beds? The value of T would then not be the same as in Ohio, but we get the same general picture, right?

Alice: Right. The number would be different, but we could still call it T. By using letters for unknown numbers, scientists make their models more flexible. The same model can then be used in a variety of slightly different situations.

Bob: So what if the reproduction number after re-opening were $R_r = 1$ instead of $R_r < 0$? I think the predicted numbers of new infections would then level off instead of exponentially decreasing further. Like in this graph:

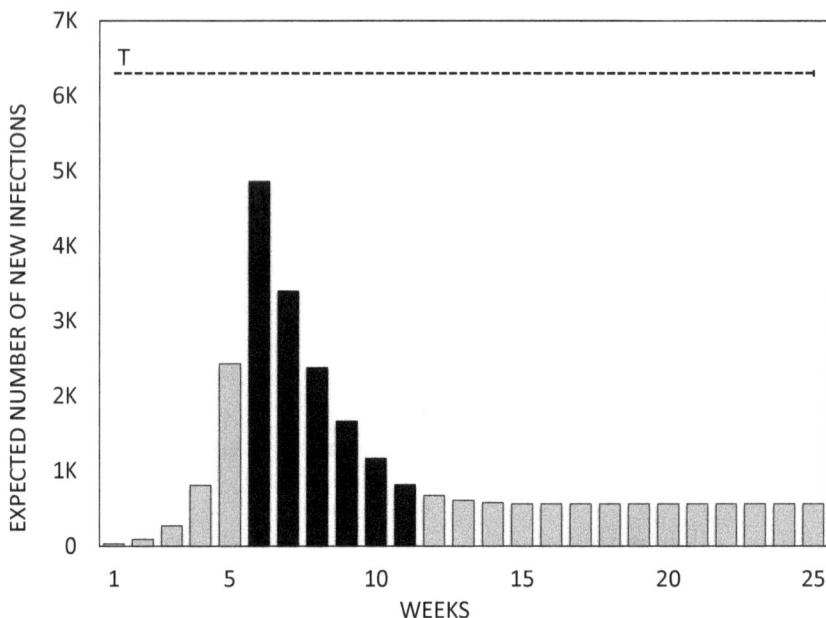

Fig. 13.2   Predicted numbers of weekly new infections when $R_\ell < R_r = 1 < R_0$. The weeks of the lockdown are shown in black.

Alice: Yes, this is what our model would predict for $R_r = 1$.

Let's assume we had a choice between these two scenarios. Which one would we prefer? The one that I showed you, for $R_r < 1$, or the one that Bob showed us, for $R_r = 1$?

Bob: Both would keep the numbers of new infections below the threshold T.

Cindy: But with $R_r < 1$, there would be fewer new infections, with fewer people having to go to the hospital and fewer people dying!

Alice: Good observation, Cindy! In general, the smaller the value R_r of the reproduction number after re-opening, the fewer infections we will see in the long run.

Bob: On the other hand, doesn't making R_r smaller require more restrictions? Including ones that may hurt the economic recovery?

Alice: Generally speaking, yes.

Frank: So they should re-open with $R_r = 1$, or even slightly bigger than 1. More than enough jobs have already been lost.

Cindy: But Frank, when $R_r > 1$, even just a little bigger, then we would see exponential increase of the numbers of new infections. Or maybe I should say nearly exponential increase.

And after some time, the numbers of new infections will cross this threshold T that we wanted to avoid in the first place! Let me try to draw a graph for this and share it on my screen:

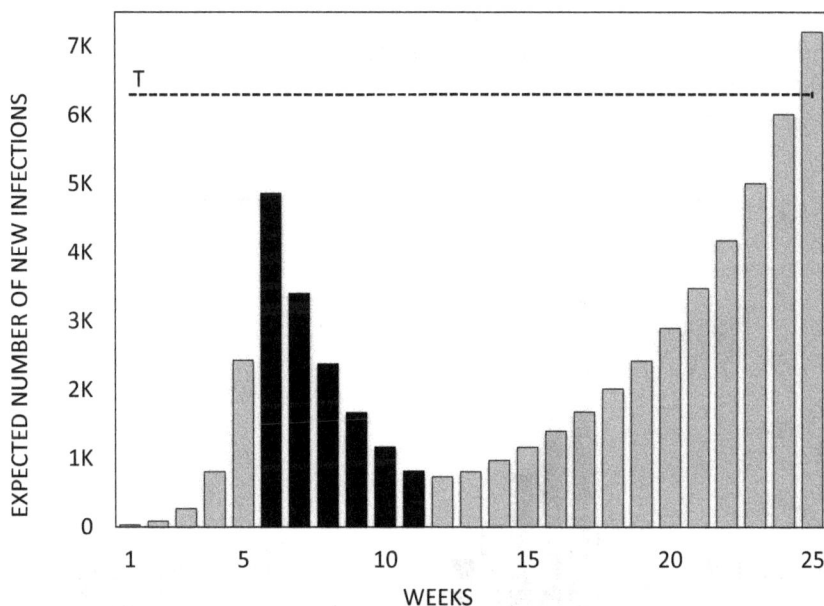

Fig. 13.3 Predicted numbers of weekly new infections when $R_\ell < 1 < R_r < R_0$. The weeks of the lockdown are shown in black.

Alice: This is correct, Cindy. The right half of your picture looks similar to what we saw in many states and in the U.S. as a whole between mid-June and mid-July. Many states re-opened too quickly by relaxing too many restrictions at once. This pushed their reproduction numbers back above 1 and we saw nearly exponential increase in the numbers of new infections.

Bob: Is this what they mean by second peak? That after re-opening the reproduction number R_r is again bigger than 1?

Frank: But Cindy's graph doesn't show any second peak.

Alice: It doesn't. Our modeling so far only shows the cause of the increase after the lockdown. It is the inequality $R_r > 1$.

Cindy's graph shows what would happen if the reproduction number after re-opening remained a constant larger than 1. If we observe such a nearly exponential increase, some corrective action will be necessary. This will change $R_r > 1$ again, to some value $R_r^- < 1$, and we will see a second peak, as in this picture:

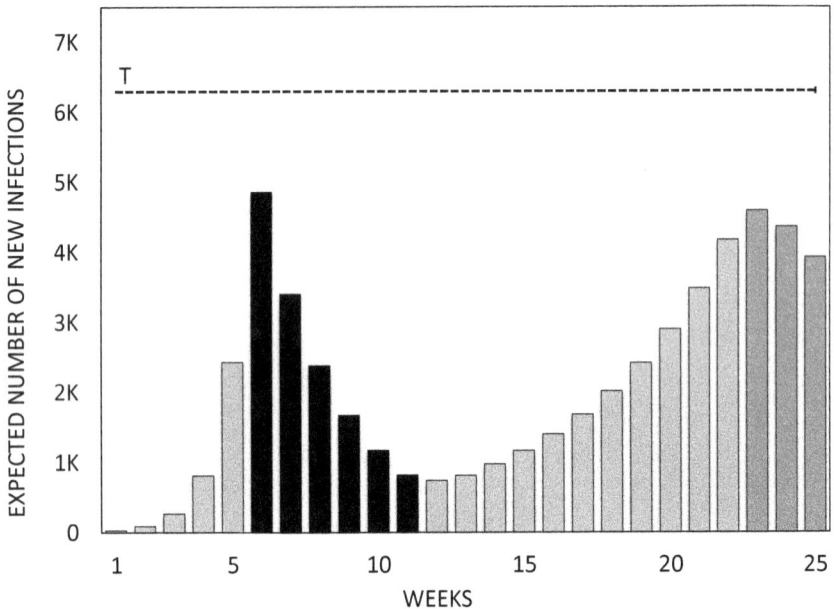

Fig. 13.4   Predicted numbers of weekly new infections when $R_\ell < R^- < 1 < R_r < R_0$. The weeks of the lockdown are shown in black; the weeks after corrective action in darker shade.

Frank: "Corrective action" as in "The state imposes tighter restrictions again?" Give me a break!

Alice: It was necessary in a number of states. For example, on June 26, Florida closed the bars. On the same day, Texas also closed bars and a number of other businesses. On June 29, Arizona prohibited large gatherings and paused the operations of bars, gyms, movie theaters, water parks and tubing rentals [2].

This seems to have worked. The spread slowed down, and the numbers of new infections seem to be near a second peak.

Bob: But businesses need a stable environment to prosper! When it goes like a seesaw—suddenly close one day, then re-open a few weeks later, then close again after a couple of months—who could do any planning of expenses and revenue?

Alice: I agree. It is very unfortunate when businesses or schools need to close again after re-opening. We don't want this to happen.

Re-opening has to be done very carefully so that the new value R_r does not go above 1. This will also be true for re-opening our university, not only for re-opening of states. In practice, it is impossible to keep R_r exactly at 1; this is an important reason why we want it to be strictly below 1.

Frank: But for states it didn't go well, as you just told us.

Alice: In some states, it didn't. Other states, like Massachusetts or New Hampshire, so far did not need to impose new restrictions inside their states.

Bob: But I've read that Massachusetts announced some restrictions today.

Alice: Yes, they did. But this one requires travelers coming into the state to produce a negative test result or quarantine for 14 days [1]. There have been no new restrictions inside the state since they re-opened.

Bob: You are saying that some states did well; other states didn't. What made the difference?

Alice: There certainly were a number of factors. A very important one was whether or not a state followed the guidelines of the federal government and the CDC for reopening.[73]

Let me discuss here two important components of these guidelines. One recommendation was that states should re-open in phases; that is, not relax too many restrictions at once. We can see now why: This gradual approach gave states some time to observe what happened after the first phases of re-opening and then either relax more restrictions if things went well or delay the next phases if they didn't. In this way they could better avoid this see-saw effect of lifting restrictions and then re-imposing them again.

Frank: But states did re-open in phases! So why are the media now writing that some states re-opened too soon?

Alice: There were other parts of the federal recommendations that some states did not follow.

The one I want to talk about today is that states should see a decrease over at least 14 days in the numbers of reported new infections before starting to re-open. For example, the governor of Kansas announced on April 30 that the state will start re-opening on May 4, while the numbers of reported new cases had increased from 63 on April 15 to 187 on April 29 [2].

Bob: That sounds bad for Kansas. How about Ohio? We looked at the data when we talked about flattening the curve. There was already a decrease between April 6 and April 14. So why did Ohio wait until May 1 with phasing in re-opening and not start on April 20? And why does it need to be a decrease over 14 days? Wouldn't one week be enough?

Alice: Very good question! We had looked at the data only until April 14 and seen a decrease of new infections over a one week, between April 6 and April 14. In general, we cannot reliably infer what is going on by looking at the data for just a few days. When we study them over a longer time frame, we can.

Let's look at the data on infections in Ohio for a longer period, until June 5. In this chart for Ohio, we see some ups and downs, with an overall downward trend since April 20. This gives us much more confidence in the success of the lockdown in terms of R_ℓ having been less than 1:

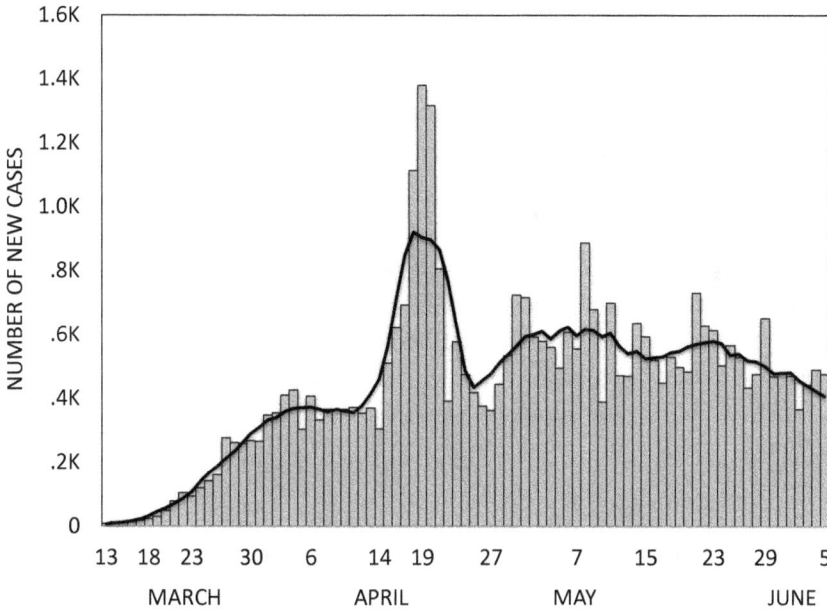

Fig. 13.5 Reported daily new infections in Ohio between March 13 and June 5. Based on data from the New York Times [3].

Frank: Wow! There was a huge peak around April 19, shortly after the initial peak that we had looked at when you showed us the data until April 14. Your model did not predict this. What do you say now, Ms. Epidemiologist?

Alice: Remember that we can discuss here only the very simplest models. The models that are used in real decision-making incorporate factors that can lead to such effects. Ohio's Department of Health actually predicted on April 14 that the peak would occur on April 19.

Cindy: But what caused this terrible spike?

Alice: Covid-19 can spread like wildfire in certain hotspots where many people live or work in close proximity. Examples of such places are cruise ships, meat-processing plants, and prisons. The rapid spread in such hotspots may show up as spikes in the data. The peak you see here mostly counts confirmed cases in two Ohio prisons when the inmates were tested [4].

The spread inside a hotspot can then spill over into the general population and cause a larger outbreak. It is possible that the large outbreak in northern Italy in March started among Chinese migrant workers in Italy's fashion industry [5]. Their cramped living quarters and workspaces could easily have been a hotspot for coronavirus transmission. Another example is the rapid increase in new cases that Singapore experienced in early April. The country had been extremely successful in containing the spread of Covid-19 throughout March. The second wave in April was triggered by local outbreaks in dormitories where migrant workers live in crowded conditions [6].

Bob: How should we think about spread inside a hotspot in terms of reproduction numbers?

Alice: Very simple models like the ones we've discussed so far assume that the virus spreads evenly among the entire population. This shows us the big picture, but the real world is more complicated. For example, the virus spreads faster in cities where there is a large population density than in more sparsely populated rural areas.

It might help if we think about the reproduction number R inside a given hotspot as a separate constant R^h that is specific to that place. So R^h is then the average number of infections caused by an infected person inside that hotspot. Similarly, we can use the symbols R_ℓ^h and R_r^h for the reproduction numbers in that hotspot during the lockdown and after re-opening.

Bob: Are you saying that we might have had $R_\ell < 1$ statewide during the lockdown, but inside those prisons it could still have been $R_\ell^h > 1$?

Alice: Yes. This helps us understanding why there could still be large local outbreaks even though R_ℓ was below 1 statewide.[74]

Frank: Well, a shelter-in-place order wouldn't have made any difference inside a prison. I can see that.

Cindy: So what can be done to help these people who work in prisons or meat-processing plants? And those prisoners? They were convicted to serve some time, but not convicted to contract a deadly disease!

Alice: This is a difficult question. Some states have released non-violent prisoners, at least temporarily, to reduce density inside these facilities, but the overall reduction in the prison population appears to be small.[75] Nobody seems to have a good answer right now what to do about meat-processing plants or whether it can be safe to go on a cruise in the near future.

The most important example of potential hotspots where many people live close together and where many local Covid-19 outbreaks have occurred are nursing homes.[76] This is very troubling. The elderly people who live in nursing homes are especially vulnerable to developing severe symptoms and dying from Covid-19. On the one hand, one wants to do everything to protect them from becoming infected and restrict visits of their families. But this will make them feel even more isolated than they already are. For most of them, their greatest joy in life is seeing their grandchildren and great-grandchildren. Do we want to take this away from them?

Frank: I have another question. Wouldn't a university campus also fit your description of a hotspot? It is a place where there are many people in close proximity.

Cindy: But Frank, you cannot compare our beloved university to a prison!

Alice: Not to a prison. We are all here because we want to be here. But somebody has compared university campuses to landlocked cruise ships. Making sure that our campus does not become a hotspot for Covid-19 transmission is a very important concern.

Bob: But our campus is not like a cruise ship either! Once a cruise ship leaves port, there is not much one can do to get away from other passengers. But we have a large campus with beautiful wide open spaces, and we can keep our distance while hanging out with other students.

So we might be able to keep R_r^h below 1. I am talking about the reproduction number inside our university when we came back in fall. Then we can study and socialize in a reasonably normal way. And they won't close down our school again.

Alice: Very well put, Bob! I was not saying that our university will be a hotspot of Covid-19 transmission, I was only saying that there is a real danger that it may become one. And to prevent that danger, to keep Ohio University safe and open, we all need to do our part.

In terms of the models we discussed today, this means keeping R_r^h below 1. This will make sure that the numbers of new infections don't grow and stay within acceptable bounds.

In more practical terms, it means social distancing, wearing masks, and socializing outdoors as much as possible. It also means frequent hand-washing and following guidelines for quarantining and getting tested.

Cindy: Please tell us about frequent hand-washing, Alice! I think this is very important.

And when should I quarantine myself? How often should I get tested?

Alice: Let's discuss in our next meetings how these control measures contribute to keeping all of us safe.

Endnotes

[72] The 7-day moving average for daily new infections in the U.S. was in fact almost flat between July 19 and July 25. It reached its peak at 66,781 cases on July 25 and then started decreasing. In comparison, the first major peak of this trend curve was reached on April 10 at 31,709 cases [7].

[73] The guidelines that Alice is referring to here where announced by the U.S. federal government on April 16, 2020. The official document bears the logos of both the White House and the CDC [8].

[74] For a detailed mathematical explanation why smaller local outbreaks can still occur even when $R < 1$, see [9].

[75] For more details about Covid-19 infections in correctional facilities, see [10]. The article mentions that prisons and jails in the U.S. experienced declines in total population (approximately 11% of the incarcerated population) in the first half of 2020, but that these reductions appear to be mainly the result of declines in arrests, jail bookings and prison admissions related to lockdowns and the closure of state and local courts. The numbers of people being held in jails began climbing again over the summer [11].

[76] According to [7], as of December 11, 2020, more than 35% of deaths from the virus in the United States have been tied to nursing homes and other long-term care facilities. The same website also tracks cases in other potential hot spots in the U.S., including prisons and college campuses.

References

[1] Department of Public Health, Massachusetts. COVID-19 Travel Order. 2020 Jul 24. [cited 2021 Jan 2]. https://www.mass.gov/info-details/covid-19-travel-order

[2] Johns Hopkins University of Medicine. Coronavirus Resource Center. Critical Trends. Impact of opening and closing decisions by state. [cited 2020 Sep 21]. https://coronavirus.jhu.edu/data/state-timeline

[3] Github Inc. nytimes/covid-19-data. [cited 2020 Jun 6]. https://github.com/nytimes/covid-19-data

[4] Zuckerman J. Nearly 80% of inmates have COVID-19 at two Ohio prisons. Ohio Capital Journal 2020 Apr 23. [cited 2020 Dec 11]. Regionally available from: https://ohiocapitaljournal.com/2020/04/23/nearly-80-of-inmates-have-covid-19-at-two-ohio-prisons/

[5] Rudan I. A cascade of causes that led to the COVID-19 tragedy in Italy and in other European Union countries. J Glob Health. 2020 Apr 3 [cited 2021 Jan 2]; 10(1):010335. http://www.jogh.org/documents/issue202001/jogh-10-010335.htm

[6] Chang N, Tjendro J. Singapore sees record daily spike of 120 COVID-19 cases, 'significant number' linked to

worker dormitories. Channel News Asia 2020 Apr 5. [cited
2020 Dec 11]. https://www.channelnewsasia.com/news/
singapore/covid19-singapore-record-daily-spike-120-
new-cases-workers-dorms-
12611132?cid=h3_referral_inarticlelinks_24082018_cna

[7] The New York Times. Covid in the U.S.: Latest map and
case count. [cited 2020 Dec 11]. https://www.nytimes.com/
interactive/2020/us/coronavirus-us-cases.html

[8] U.S. Federal Government and Centers for Disease Control and
Prevention. Opening Up America Again 2020 Apr 16.
https://www.whitehouse.gov/openingamerica/

[9] Moore C. R-naught is just an average: The transmission rate
varies widely, and outbreaks can be surprisingly large even when
the epidemic is subcritical. Santa Fe Institute 2020 Apr 27. [cited
2020 Oct 18]. https://www.santafe.edu/news-center/news/
transmission-t-024-cristopher-moore-on-the-heavy-
tail-of-outbreaks

[10] Editorial Board. America is letting the coronavirus rage through
prisons. The New York Times 2020 Nov 21. [cited 2020
Dec 11]. https://www.nytimes.com/2020/11/21/opinion/
sunday/coronavirus-prisons-jails.html

[11] Widra E. Visualizing changes in the incarcerated population
during COVID-19. Prison Policy Initiative 2020 Sep 10. [cited
2020 Dec 11]. https://www.prisonpolicy.org/blog/2020/
09/10/pandemic_population_changes/

Chapter 14

How dangerous is it to touch surfaces?

Alice, Bob, Cindy, and Frank meet on July 27, 2020. All over the world, huge efforts are being put into frequent cleaning of high-touch areas to prevent the transmission of coronavirus. The Atlantic magazine publishes an article titled *Hygiene Theater Is a Huge Waste of Time. People are power scrubbing their way to a false sense of security [1].*

Cindy: It's really scary to press an elevator button or turn a doorknob these days! So many people touch them all the time. Just thinking of all the coronavirus particles that might sit there makes my stomach turn. I can wear my mask, and I can keep a distance from others. But how can I possibly avoid touching anything?

Bob: I worry about that too, Cindy. But perhaps it's not so bad. In public buildings, high-touch areas are now being cleaned a lot. Sometimes you can clean a surface yourself by wiping it down with sanitizing tissue before you touch it.

Frank: Nobody can constantly clean all surfaces. Sometimes we need to touch a doorknob right after another person did. But I wonder how dangerous touching contaminated surfaces really is. I think people make too much fuss about cleaning them.

Alice: Good questions! Let me illustrate how transmission of the coronavirus through touching surfaces actually works. It involves several steps.

Think about an infectious person; let's call him Tom. He would have lots of virus in his lungs and saliva, but not normally on his hands. But if Tom coughs or sneezes into his hands, many virus particles will spray there. This would be Step 1 of the transmission.

Tom may then push down a bar that opens a door while the virus particles are still on his hands. Some of the virus particles on his hands will get on the bar, where they will persist for a while. This would be Step 2.

Virus particles can survive outside the body only between a few hours and a few days, depending on the surface they land on.[77] But this will be long enough before the next person, call her Mandy, opens the same door by pushing the same bar down with one of her hands. Then some of the virus particles left by Tom on that bar will get on Mandy's hand. This would be Step 3.

But the virus particles that cause Covid-19 cannot enter Mandy's the human body through the skin. They can enter our bodies only through mucous membranes. If Mandy touches her face in an area near her mouth, nose, or eyes, some virus particles from her hand will get on her face or directly on these mucous membranes. Then they could enter her body and infect her with Covid-19. This would be Step 4.

Cindy: I don't even want to think about the virus particles traveling from Tom's nose or mouth all the way into Mandy's mouth. This is so gross. Yuck!

Alice: Yes, it really is yucky. Fortunately, we have this instinctive aversion to touching dirty surfaces; this sense of "Yuck".

We are trained from kindergarten to avoid touching dirty surfaces and wash our hands if we do. Most people will readily comply with recommendations to wash our hands more frequently and thoroughly, to clean surfaces, and to avoid touching them. This helps in the fight against Covid-19.

But if you really think about it: Wouldn't it be every bit as yucky if the virus particles got into Mandy's mouth directly through droplets in the air that Tom exhales?

Cindy: That's also gross. But ... but somehow Mandy picking it up from a dirty surface *feels* more yucky. Am I being irrational?

Bob: I don't know whether this is rational. Would it be more likely to get Covid-19 by directly inhaling droplets or through touching surfaces? Can you tell us, Alice?

Alice: Many people feel the same way as you do, Cindy. But catching the virus through directly inhaling droplets is *a lot* more likely than through touching surfaces.

Epidemiologists have a lot of evidence for this. For example, there is a famous study[78] of an outbreak in a skyscraper in Seoul, South Korea that happened in March. On one side of the 11th floor of the building, about half the members of a call center got sick. In a call center, people sit close together and talk a lot. So we can be pretty sure that the transmissions in this call center occurred directly through the air. But less than 1% of the other people in the building contracted Covid-19, even though more than a thousand workers and residents shared elevators and were surely touching the same buttons within minutes of one another.

Frank: Sounds plausible. But the story you told us about Tom and Mandy also sounded plausible. So why would transmission through contaminated surfaces be a lot less likely?

Alice: Recall that the transmission from Tom to Mandy involved four steps. At each step, only a small fraction of the virus particles were transferred from one surface to the next. It takes a fairly large number of virus particles to actually cause an infection, most likely at least hundreds of them.[13] We can be pretty sure that it often happens that *some* virus particles are transmitted from one person to another through touching the same surface. But when their numbers diminish at each step, it is very, very unlikely that enough of them will make it through all the steps to cause a new infection.

Bob: But if Tom and Mandy were to shake hands, there would only be three steps. Would transmission then be more likely?

Alice: Much more likely than by touching the same surface. That's why people should avoid shaking hands.

Cindy: I'm confused. Are you saying that we should not worry at all about catching the coronavirus through touching contaminated surfaces? Only avoid shaking hands?

Alice: That's not what I meant. I only wanted to say that we should worry a lot more about transmission of Covid-19 through droplets that travel in the air.

So we should not be paranoid about catching the disease from touching a contaminated surface. But we should exercise common sense and take reasonable precautions to avoid this route of transmissions.

Frank: Why? You just said it is very, very unlikely that a story like the one about Tom and Mandy will actually lead to an infection. So, really, why worry about it at all?

Alice: The problem is that that during each day, we make many, many contacts. Let me show you a picture that illustrates different types of contacts:

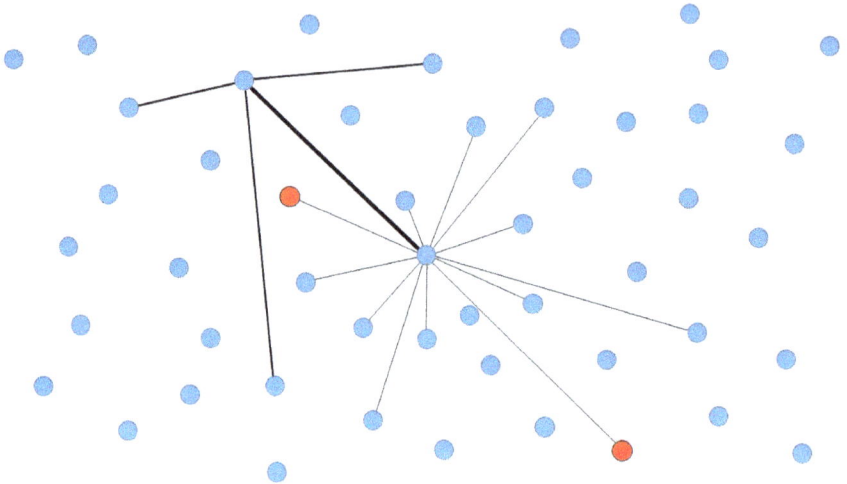

Fig. 14.1   Direct and indirect contacts.

A few are high-intensity with a large chance of being effective and potentially leading to a new infection. Like working all day in the same office. Let's call the person in the middle Mandy again. The picture shows one high-intensity contact for her, perhaps with her office mate.

Many more contacts are low-intensity and have a much smaller chance of being effective. Like riding in the same elevator for half a minute. My picture also shows a few low-intensity contacts for Mandy's office mate.

And then there are these indirect contacts with a very, very low intensity. Like touching the same elevator button. In my picture, we see a number of contacts that Mandy made when she touched the elevator on her way to the office. These contacts are very low-intensity, but they are with a lot of other people.

When we touch a surface, we indirectly make contact simultaneously with many people; with all those who have touched it not so long ago. Some of them are likely to be infectious. Every single such indirect contact with an infectious person is very, very unlikely to lead to transmission of enough virus particles. So we should not become paranoid whenever we touch a surface.

But we typically touch many surfaces during a day and make many, many such indirect contacts. One of them may eventually cause an infection. This is still a lot less likely overall than becoming infected by inhaling droplets full of virus particles, but not impossible. So it makes sense to cut the chances of getting infected through indirect contacts even further.

Cindy: How can we best do this, Alice? I mean, if we really do need to touch something?

Alice: There are several methods. To see how they work, let's look at the steps of the transmission in my story about Tom and Mandy one by one.

Step 1: Tom coughs or sneezes into his hands.

Tom could have prevented virus particles from getting on his fingers by covering his nose and mouth with his elbow instead of his hands. The elbow would also have blocked more droplets full of virus particles from escaping into the surrounding air than Tom's hands, where they may slip through his fingers. Covering up with the elbow is very effective, because it also cuts the potential for airborne transmission.

Similarly, had Tom worn a mask, it would have further blocked the virus from traveling to his hands, to his elbow, or into the surrounding air.

Step 2: Tom touches the bar that opens a door while the virus particles are still on his hands.

Tom could have avoided transmission at this step by washing his hands between sneezing into them and touching the bar. Washing hands with soap and water for 20 seconds is very effective. It gets rid of all virus particles.

If soap and water were not immediately available, Tom could have used hand sanitizer instead. This is not quite as effective as thoroughly washing one's hands, but nearly so and works well enough in most situations.

Step 3: Mandy, opens the same door pushing the same bar down with one of her hands.

She might have opened the same door by pushing the bar with another part of her body instead of her hands. Some virus particles might have gotten on her clothes in the process, but this would have added at least one more step to an already very, very unlikely route of transmission.

Mandy could also have avoided the transmission if she wiped down the bar before touching it.

Bob: In a public building, the institution might already clean such high-touch areas more frequently than they used to. This might also have prevented the transmission.

Frank: But only if they cleaned after Tom had opened the door and before Mandy did. Come on! How likely would that be?

Alice: Very unlikely if hundreds of people go through the same door each day. Epidemiologists would be the last people to discourage frequent cleaning of high-touch areas in public buildings. It will make us feel more comfortable and will prevent the spread of a variety of other diseases. But in reality, it doesn't do much in terms of preventing Covid-19 transmissions. If an institution has a choice between putting resources into more cleaning or into improving ventilation, they should improve ventilation.

Step 4: Mandy touches her face after touching the bar.

Again, the transmission in this step would have been entirely avoided had Many thoroughly washed her hands before touching her face.

And Mandy would have been entirely safe if she had not touched her face. We all touch our faces many, many times during the day. We usually don't realize how often we do this, and it is very difficult to kick the habit. But we can train ourselves to do it less often if we pay attention to it. Wearing a mask will greatly help, as it discourages us from touching the face near our mouth and nose. And wearing glasses discourages us from touching near the eyes.

Cindy: So nothing bad will happen if I do get some Covid-19 virus particles only on my fingers?

Alice: Most likely not. Don't panic if you suspect that it might have happened. If you wash your hands or use hand-sanitizer before touching your face, you will be safe.

Don't touch a surface if you don't have to. As much as possible, avoid touching your face. Don't shake hands. Wash your hands thoroughly and frequently, for at least 20 seconds, with soap and water.

These precautions will keep you and others safe from contracting Covid-19 through contaminated surfaces.

Endnotes

[77] Viable SARS-CoV-2 virus was isolated for up to 72 hours from various surfaces; the longest reported viability was on plastics and stainless steel, with half-lives around 6 hours [2].

[78] The outbreak in the call center in South Korea was studied in [3]. Our description of it is adapted from the one given in the article [1] of the Atlantic, which argues that heightened cleaning efforts have little effect on the spread of Covid-19 and are largely a waste of resources. The New York Times article [4] makes a similar point. The survey [5] describes several case studies of presumed transmission through contaminated surfaces (called fomites in the medical literature), but found no conclusive evidence for it. The authors conclude: "Direct contact and fomite transmission are presumed but are likely only an unusual mode of transmission."

References

[1] Thompson D. Hygiene theater is a huge waste of time. People are power scrubbing their way to a false sense of security. The Atlantic 2020 Jul 27. [cited 2020 Dec 11]. https://www.theatlantic.com/ideas/archive/2020/07/scourge-hygiene-theater/614599/

[2] van Doremalen N, Bushmaker T, Morris DH, Holbrook MG, Gamble A, Williamson BN, et al. Aerosol and surface stability of SARS-CoV-2 as compared with SARS-CoV-1 [Letter]. N Engl J Med. 2020 Apr 16 [cited 2020 Dec 11]; 382:1564–1567. https://www.nejm.org/doi/10.1056/NEJMc2004973 DOI:10.1056/NEJMc2004973

[3] Park S, Kim Y, Yi S, Lee S, Na B, Kim C, et al. Coronavirus Disease Outbreak in Call Center, South Korea. Emerg Infect Dis. 2020 Aug [cited 2020 Dec 11]; 26(8):1666–1670. https://wwwnc.cdc.gov/eid/article/26/8/20-1274_article?fbclid=IwAR3FIvI5POY_84oCFUqlI9UYOOEN3X39tZ_EC37mv3MOXpnG2mxWeJOWLwI DOI:10.3201/eid2608.201274

[4] Ives M, Mandavilli, A. The coronavirus is airborne indoors. Why are we still scrubbing surfaces? The New York Times 2020 Nov 18. [cited 2020 Dec 11]. https://www.nytimes.com/2020/11/18/world/asia/covid-cleaning.html

[5] Eric A. Meyerowitz EA, Richterman A, Gandhi RT, and Sax PE. Transmission of SARS-CoV-2: A review of viral, host, and environmental factors. Ann Intern Med. 2020 Sep 17. [cited 2020 Dec 31]. https://www.acpjournals.org/doi/10.7326/M20-5008 DOI:10.7326/M20-5008

Chapter 15

How do isolation and quarantine help?

Alice, Bob, Cindy, and Frank meet on July 29, 2020. Daily reported infections have been increasing since the start of the pandemic, but now seem to be stabilizing around 260 thousand [1]. Control measures that include isolating of confirmed cases and quarantining their close contacts appear to have prevented further increase of new infections.

Cindy: When we talked about safe re-opening, we discussed what we need to do to remain safe after our return to campus: We need to wear our masks, practice social distancing, and frequently wash our hands. And you also mentioned quarantine, Alice. Can you tell us more about that today? How does it work?

Alice: Isolation and quarantine are also very important for limiting the spread of infections. Both work by making sure that an infected person has as few contacts as possible while being infectious. In most cases, the person should stay in a separate room and not interact with other people during the period of isolation or quarantine unless it is absolutely necessary.

Cindy: Then what is the difference between an isolation and a quarantine?

Alice: The difference is that people with symptoms or confirmed Covid-19 infections should go into isolation, and their close contacts should go into quarantine. Here the phrase "close contact" does not refer to an interaction between two people, but to a person who is known to have had a highly intense contact with an infected individual during a time when that individual very likely was infectious. Epidemiologists make this distinction because there are slight differences in the rules for quarantine and isolation. For example, two people in quarantine should never share the same room, because we don't know for sure whether one of them or both are actually infected. But two people with confirmed infections can isolate themselves together, because they can no longer infect each other. They need to stay away from everybody else though.

Most importantly perhaps, the CDC recommends[79] that quarantine last 14 days from the time of the last contact with the infected person. In contrast, isolation can end already after 10 days if the person has been symptom-free for at least 24 hours.

Frank: Why is that? Why are there stricter rules for people in quarantine even though they may not even be infected?

Alice: Both rules aim at cutting chains of transmissions, at making sure that the person does not transmit the infection during the period when he or she might be infectious. Recall that most Covid-19 patients remain infectious for up to 10 days. It usually takes 4 days or more after exposure before an infection leads to symptoms or can be confirmed by a test. That's when isolation starts and why it usually needs to last only 10 days.[80] But quarantine may need to include the additional 4 days before infections could normally be confirmed.

Bob: So, when an infected person goes into isolation, would this be in your models like putting that person into the removed state earlier, before the actual recovery? And when a person goes into quarantine, would this be like putting that person into the removed state right away?

Alice: Yes, Bob! At least temporarily, especially for quarantine. The quarantined person may not actually be infected and will then not be immune after leaving the quarantine. Isolation and quarantine quite literally remove a person from all potential chains of transmissions while they last.

To illustrate how isolation and quarantine work in terms of contacts, let me show you some pictures of a small group of people who interact on a regular basis. In the first one, we see the contacts that they might normally have each day:

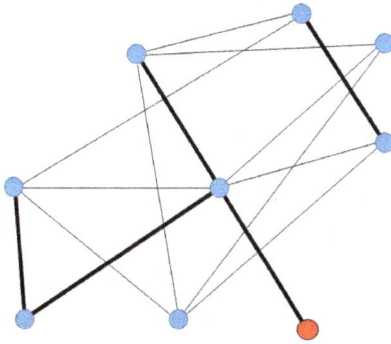

Fig. 15.1   Regular contacts among a small group of people.

The person in the lower right corner, call him Ingham again, is infected. The one in the middle, call her Emily, has high-intensity contacts with Ingham. This is like in our first conversation about contacts where we had assumed that Emily is Ingham's girlfriend.

Now assume that both Ingham and Emily discover that Ingham is infected; either because Ingham developed symptoms or because he took a test. Ingham would then need to isolate himself, and Emily would go into quarantine:

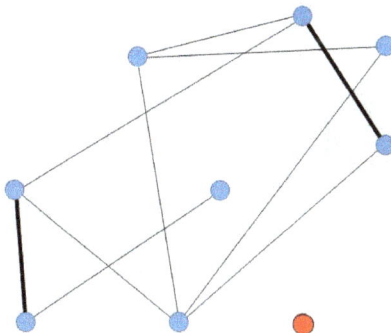

Fig. 15.2   The contacts in this group while Ingham is in isolation and Emily is in quarantine.

Emily would have been at high risk of having been infected by Ingham. But my picture (Fig. 15.2), she did not actually contract Covid-19 and is still susceptible.

Ingham and Emily would also have cut contacts with people outside of this group, but my pictures don't show these.

Cindy: Why is there still one line from Emily to another person in your picture? Wouldn't she need to cut all contacts when in quarantine?

Alice: In theory yes, but in practice this is not possible. A quarantined person cannot go shopping or do things around the apartment outside of her room. Someone needs to look after Emily. For example, her mother would. Contacts between family members are normally high-intensity, as I had shown by the thick line between Emily and her mother in my first picture. But now Emily's mother needs to take proper precautions, like wearing a mask and staying six feet away from Emily when she brings her food and other essentials. This will make the contacts low-intensity, as shown by a thin line here.

After 14 days, Emily would end her quarantine. Ingham would also have recovered by then and ended his isolation:

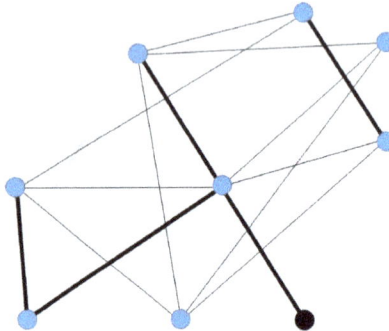

Fig. 15.3   After Ingham's isolation and Emily's quarantine end, regular contacts resume.

The people in our picture could then resume their usual contact pattern, and no further infections would have occurred.

Cindy: That's good! But I feel so sorry for Emily. It must have been so hard for her to sit all alone in that room for two weeks and worry whether she would get sick!

Frank: Yeah! And it wasn't even necessary. The isolation of Ingham would have been sufficient to prevent all further infections in this group.

Alice: This is true in my first example. But in real life Emily would not have known this.

Let me now show you pictures for a scenario when Emily had been exposed to the infection before Ingham isolated himself:

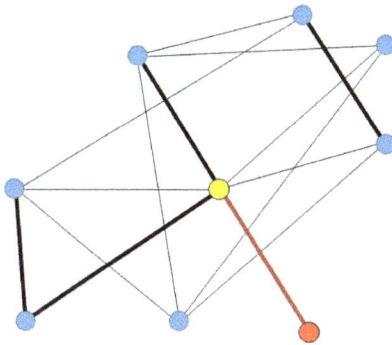

Fig. 15.4   Emily has been exposed through contact with Ingham.

In contrast to the first example, let's now assume that Emily does not quarantine herself when Ingham goes into isolation.

Bob: So, she would then maintain all her contacts?

Alice: Except for the one with Ingham, who did go into isolation.

Cindy: And she would put other people at risk!

Alice: Yes, she would.

Let's fast-forward 4 days. Emily has no symptoms, which is shown with pink salmon color, but has infected her mother:

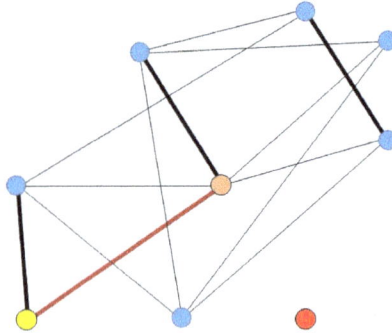

Fig. 15.5　Emily did not quarantine herself and has infected her mother by Day 4.

Let's fast-forward another week:

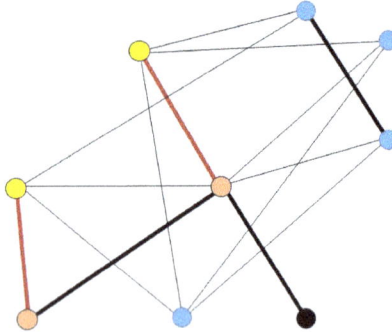

Fig. 15.6　By Day 11, Emily and her mother have caused further infections. Ingham has reached the end of his isolation period.

Now Ingham has recovered. He has reached the end of his isolation period and can make contacts. In the meantime though, both Emily and her mother have transmitted the infection to other people.

Bob: That's bad.

Alice: After the last day that was recommend for a quarantine, the picture will look like this:

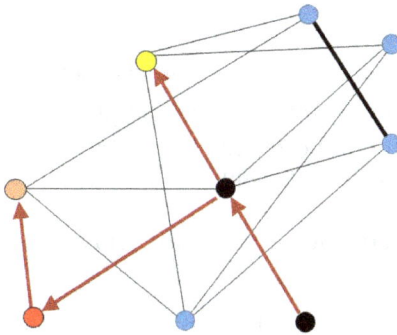

Fig. 15.7 Transmissions without quarantine up to Day 15.

We see that without quarantine, Emily has become part of two chains of transmissions. In my example, she remained asymptomatic and her mother developed symptoms only after infecting another person. Emily's mother and the people further down these chains of transmission may suffer severe symptoms or even die.

Had Emily gone into quarantine, on that same day the picture would have looked like this:

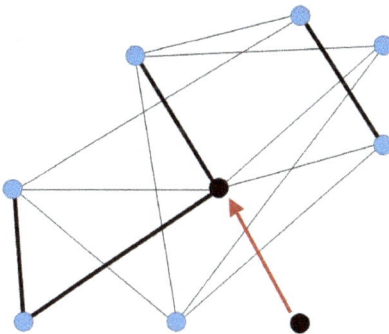

Fig. 15.8 Transmissions up to Day 15 when Emily quarantines herself.

The quarantine would have cut short the two chains of transmissions that we saw in the previous picture (Fig. 15.7). This is what quarantine can do for us.

Bob: But Emily did not actually know whether or not she had been exposed. When in quarantine, Emily cannot go to work and may lose income. Wouldn't it be better to quarantine Emily only if she knew that she really was infected?

Alice: This would boil down to Emily only isolating herself, not going into quarantine.

Emily can find out about her infection only if she develops symptoms or takes a test. We will talk more about tests next time. But let me mention that it is unlikely that she could find it out from a test earlier than 5 days after exposure. Also, symptoms also start on average not earlier than 5 days after exposure.

So let me modify my example and assume that Emily developed symptoms 5 days after her last contact with Ingham and then isolated herself. As in the previous example, she might already have infected her mother by then. For Covid-19, infectiousness typically starts 2 days before the onset of symptoms and such transmissions happen a lot.

In this scenario, right after Emily notices symptoms, she would cut her contacts and the picture would look like this:

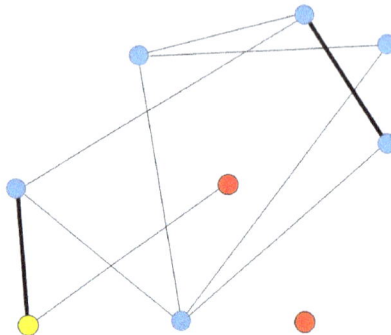

Fig. 15.9   Emily goes into isolation after developing symptoms on Day 5.

When Emily leaves isolation, the picture would then look like this:

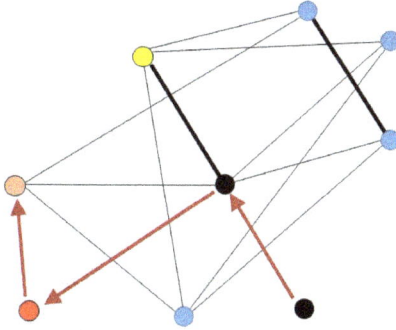

Fig. 15.10   Transmissions without quarantine up to Day 15. Here Emily and her mother isolated themselves only after developing symptoms.

Only one of Emily's two chains of transmission has been cut.

Bob: Well, this is less effective; I can see this now. And it would not have worked at all if Emily had remained asymptomatic throughout, as in your second scenario.

Frank: But when close contacts of infectious people go into quarantine, they cannot go to work and cannot lead a normal life. Even though they may not even be infected. What a waste!

Cindy: Quarantine may prevent many infections and even deaths though! As we don't know for sure who really has been infected and who hasn't, we should be cautious and quarantine ourselves when we had a close contact with an infected person.

Frank: How about if that person only showed symptoms and wasn't really infected?

Alice: That's why epidemiologists recommend that people who show symptoms take a test. In our example, when Ingham notices symptoms, he should take a test and isolate himself, while Emily quarantines herself. If the test shows an infection, then Ingham should stay in isolation and Emily in quarantine as in our first example. If the test shows no infection, Ingham can end his isolation and Emily can leave her quarantine.

Bob: Yes, this would be most effective in terms of preventing new infections. And it may make it a lot easier for both Ingham and Emily in case the symptoms were not really caused by the coronavirus.

But for that the test results need to come back very quickly. When people have to wait two weeks for the test result, the test will be completely useless!

Alice: Exactly! A quick return time for the test results is crucial. Let's talk more about tests next time.

Frank: It's still not clear to me who actually should go into quarantine. To Emily and Ingham in your examples, it may have been obvious that they had a close contact. And Ingham would of course have told her about his symptoms or test result. But in many situations we don't even know who the person we had close contact with even was, or whether that person was infected.

Alice: Very good question, Frank! We often can find out through contact tracing. We should talk some other time about how this works.

Endnotes

[79] The CDC website gives more details at [2] and [3]. These recommendations are subject to change. They also may differ slightly from country to country and even between localities within a country.

[80] Infectiousness may last longer than 10 days after onset of symptoms, especially in severe cases that require hospitalization [4]. The healthcare provider may then recommend isolating for longer than 10 days [2].

References

[1] Worldometers.info. Dover, Delaware, U.S.A. COVID-19 coronavirus pandemic. [cited 2020 Nov 27].
https://www.worldometers.info/coronavirus/.

[2] Centers for Disease Control and Prevention. COVID-19. Isolate if you are sick. [cited 2021 Jan 2]. https://www.cdc.gov/coronavirus/2019-ncov/if-you-are-sick/isolation.html

[3] Centers for Disease Control and Prevention. COVID-19. When to quarantine. [cited 2021 Jan 2].
https://www.cdc.gov/coronavirus/2019-ncov/if-you-are-sick/quarantine.html

[4] Eric A. Meyerowitz EA, Richterman A, Gandhi RT, and Sax PE. Transmission of SARS-CoV-2: A review of viral, host, and environmental factors. Ann Intern Med. 2020 Sep 17. [cited 2020 Dec 31]. https://www.acpjournals.org/doi/10.7326/M20-5008 DOI:10.7326/M20-5008

Chapter 16

How do COVID-19 tests work?

Alice, Bob, Cindy, and Frank meet on August 1, 2020. After the recent second peak of Covid-19 infections in the U.S., universities around the country are re-evaluating their plans for re-opening in Fall Semester. There is much debate about effective policies for testing students returning to campus. Ohio University has just announced that it will re-open in two phases.[81]

Bob: Did you see the messages from the OU President and Provost? Sounds like only a few classes will meet face-to-face until the end of September in Phase 1 and nobody knows yet how many students will be allowed back into the dorms in Phase 2 and which classes will remain online throughout the semester.

Frank: I sure did. What are they thinking? In engineering, we have lab courses, and they can't be taught online.

Alice: I also have lab courses. I heard they want to re-schedule them so that all the work in the labs can be done during Phase 2.

Bob: What's the point of re-opening in two phases and then perhaps squeezing some courses into half the time?

Alice: I'd love to return to campus and to my lab as soon as possible. On the other hand, I'm glad the university will re-open in phases. It's like re-opening of states: Start by relaxing some restrictions; let some students back on campus. Collect some data on Covid-19 infections; see how it goes. Then decide what will be possible in Phase 2. It's much better to take a gradual approach than risking a situation where we would run out of rooms set aside for quarantining students and then be forced to close campus again and move all instruction online.

Frank: Not that again! We need to complete these courses in real labs. I'm with you on that one, Alice.

Cindy: The message from the Provost also mentioned availability and turnaround time of tests. I think this is very important. Can you tell us today more about tests, Alice?

Alice: Yes. We can find out who is infected by testing people for Covid-19. Isolation and quarantine will work well only if the tests are reliable and if people get their test results back as quickly as possible.

Frank: Yeah. But often test results come back only after two weeks when the quarantine would be over anyway. This makes them totally useless. Worse than useless if the result is wrong. And that also happens a lot!

Bob: I'm with you, Frank! Nobody should be forced to pay for a test when they have to wait longer than a couple of days for the result.

Why does it take days rather than minutes for test results to come back? And why can it take even a week or longer?

Cindy: But some test results come back very quickly. I've heard that they produce them even in Athens, our university town.[82]

I think I should take such a test every week or so, just to be on the safe side. But if the test comes back with the wrong result, this would be so scary! So I don't know. Alice, can you tell me how often I should get tested?

Alice: Important questions, all! Let's talk about them today.

First we need to understand some terminology. When a test shows a Covid-19 infection, then we say that the test was positive. If the result does not show a Covid-19 infection, then we say that the test was negative.

Cindy: But if a test comes back and says "You are infected", this would be horrible and not positive at all!

Alice: I agree. This medical jargon of calling a test result "positive" if it detected an infection is unfortunate and emotionally disturbing.

But the terminology is what it is. If we want to make sense of the information, we need to look past the emotions.

As Frank had mentioned, a test may give the wrong result. There are two possible types of errors: A false positive test shows an infection for a person who in reality has not been infected with Covid-19, and a false negative test fails to detect an infection that in fact has occurred.

Bob: Why do some tests give such false positive or false negative results?

Alice: A test may come out false positive if it does not accurately distinguish between Covid-19 infections and infections by similar viruses. Therefore, we say that a test that gives a lot of false positive results has low specificity.

A test may overlook some infections if there are relatively few molecules that the test is supposed to detect. Too few for the test to spring into action, so to speak. So we say that a test that gives a lot of false negative results has low sensitivity.

Frank: Let me try to understand this from the opposite angle: High specificity would then mean that the test only rarely gives false positives and high sensitivity that it only rarely gives false negatives.

Alice: Correct. Specificity and sensitivity are usually expressed in terms of the percentages of false positive and false negative results of the test. Lower percentages are better.

There are many different tests on the market, and manufacturers constantly improve their quality. I will not talk about actual percentages for particular tests here; by the time you may need to take a test, these numbers might have changed. But when you have a choice between different tests, look up how their rates of false positives and false negatives compare.

Cindy: So when I have a choice between several different tests, I always should take the one with the lowest percentage of false negatives and false positives, right?

Alice: Usually, this will be the better one. But it may also depend on why you would want to take the test.

First, let's suppose that you wake up one morning with a fever and a cough. It may be a common cold, or it may be Covid-19.

Cindy: Then I should take a test and stay home until the result comes back!

Alice: Yes, you should, Cindy. Let's assume you have a choice between two tests; let me call them Test A and Test B. To keep matters simple, let's also assume that both have the same specificity and will give false positive results for 2% of the people who have not been exposed to Covid-19.

But let's assume that Test A has a false negative rate of 5% and Test B has a false negative rate of 25%. This means that Test A fails to detect Covid-19 for 5% of people who are in fact infected, while Test B has lower sensitivity and fails to detect the infection for one quarter of infected people.

Cindy: Then I would take Test A of course! Why would anybody want to take Test B given such a choice?

Alice: Suppose the result of Test A will come back only after two days, while the result of Test B will come back in less than an hour?

Cindy: I see. That may be a problem. While I wait for the result of Test A, I could not go to class and might need to reschedule important appointments. And I would be so scared all the time while I wait for the result.

Test B comes back right away. But if it is negative, then I still might have Covid-19. If my symptoms are mild or quickly disappear, I would then believe I don't have Covid-19, go to class, meet friends, or visit my grandma. But I would pose a danger to all of them. Especially to my grandma. She is already 70 years old and has diabetes.

So I would rather take Test A, wait a few days for the results, and make sure I don't have Covid-19.

Alice: This would be the right decision, Cindy. Even with Test A coming back negative, you would not have 100% certainty that you don't have Covid-19. This test also gives some false negative results. But much less often; only 5% of the time.

So you want to maintain some caution even when Test A comes back negative. Stay home as much as possible until 24 hours after all symptoms disappear, and be super cautious about visiting your grandma over the next couple of weeks. She really wants to see you, so please don't stop visiting her altogether. But perhaps you can reschedule your next visit or at least limit close physical contact. The most important thing for grandma is to know how much you care about her.

Cindy: I can explain to her that with Covid-19 going around this means keeping a little distance. She will understand.

Alice: Now let's suppose you find out that another student tested positive for Covid-19. A couple of days ago you had talked with this student who was not wearing a mask. For less than 15 minutes, maybe five. And you don't remember how close you were standing; perhaps four or five feet. A situation that does not quite meet the definition of the CDC of somebody having been in "close contact" who should go into quarantine.[83] But similar enough so that there was a substantial chance of transmission. What would you do then, Cindy?

Cindy: You mean, it would be, like, a toss-up whether or not I should go into quarantine? I would be so scared and would be super cautious over the next couple of weeks.

But maybe not go into a real quarantine, because I guess this kind of thing will happen a lot when we get back to campus. And I cannot sit all the time in my room. I need to go to class, go shopping, and meet friends sometimes. So I would take a test and find out, or at least ease my worries. Then I can decide what to do about the quarantine.

Alice: This would be a wise decision. Given a choice between the two tests that I described, which one would you take? Test A or Test B?

Cindy: I would take Test B, because it gives me the result faster, and I could resume my normal life right away if the test comes back negative. Especially if I have some important appointments coming up during those two days. With Test B, I would not be quite sure that I really did not catch Covid-19 from that other student, but as you described the situation, the chances of catching it would have been low in the first place. And Test A would not give me perfect certainty either. So I think Test B may be good enough in such a situation.

Alice: This sounds reasonable, Cindy. So when would you take the test?

Cindy: I would take it right away, of course! I really would like to know as soon as possible.

Alice: This would seem to be the natural thing to do. But it may not be the best timing.

Even the most sensitive tests can detect infections only a few days after exposure. Think about it this way: A new infection typically occurs when a person inhales a few droplets full of virus particles. Each droplet contains many, many of them. But these droplets are also very, very tiny compared with the size of an entire human body. So the number of virus particles transmitted from another person is imperceptible to any test.

After transmission, the virus particles multiply inside the body until there are enough of them to make a person sick. This usually takes a few days and is the reason why we don't have any symptoms and don't spread the virus around to other people right after exposure. When people become infectious, after the end of the latency period, there will be many, many more virus particles inside their bodies. And this is when tests will be able to detect them.

Even the best tests can have a high false-negative rate when taken too soon after exposure. A study[84] has found that sensitivity of tests tends to be low during the first 4 days after exposure and is highest on Day 8. So if you decide to take a test because you are worried about having been exposed during a specific encounter or social event, don't get tested earlier than 5 days after the potential exposure. In the meantime, isolate yourself as much as possible. Start being super-careful on Day 3 after the potential exposure; this is when most people become infectious.

Cindy: I see. But most of the time we don't know that a person who we talked with had Covid-19. And we need to talk with other people once in a while.

So I think we all should take tests regularly. Perhaps once every week. This will keep us safest.

Alice: Testing everybody once a week would certainly help in detecting most infections early and preventing many transmissions.

Bob: But that would require more than 330 million tests each week in the entire U.S. Are that many tests even available?

Alice: Far from it. Currently between 5 and 6 million people are tested in the U.S. each week.[85] We would need to scale up our testing capacity by a factor of at least 50 if we wanted to test everybody once a week. This may not be feasible in the near future.

There is also a less obvious problem with testing everybody. The likelihood of becoming infected is actually very small for most people. With all our preventive measures currently in place, in Ohio it may be something like 1 in 500 per week. At least for people who are behaving very cautiously and are not very often in close contact with infectious people. Does this description sound like you, Cindy?

Cindy: I hope so! I try to be as careful as possible!

Alice: Now suppose you take a test and it comes back positive. What would you think, Cindy?

Cindy: This would be so awful! It would mean that I am infected with Covid-19, that I may get terribly sick, and may infect others. Or I may even already have infected others before I got the test result. I would be devastated!

Alice: Couldn't it also be the case that your test was false positive? In the example that I gave you, the false positive rate was 2%. So it would happen to some people, right? Couldn't this have been the case with your test, Cindy?

Cindy: It could, but how likely would that be?

Alice: Very good question, Cindy! Let's look at it first in this way: A false positive rate of 2% means that one in every 50 tests that are given to people without Covid-19 comes back positive. If you never get infected but take a test with false positivity rate 2% each week for a whole year, over 52 weeks, then on average how many of these tests will come back false positive, Cindy?

Cindy: Do you mean I should expect a positive result for about 1 of them?

Alice: Right. For every single test, the chances of coming back false positive are small. But with so many tests over the entire year, they add up.

Cindy: But if I do get a positive result? Wouldn't it then be more likely that is is a true positive than a false positive?

Alice: Now let's look at a single test that did come back positive.

It might mean that you did in fact catch Covid-19, despite exercising caution all the time. In Ohio, we currently have on the order of 10,000 new weekly reported cases in a population of roughly 11 million. The actual weekly rate of new infections may be several times higher, but for exceptionally careful people it should be no more than twice the reported average. This puts your chances of this happening to you in a given week at less than 2 in 1,000, Cindy.[86] We can express them as a probability of at most 0.002.

Or it might mean that the test was false positive. This would happen if you did not catch the infection during the week—which by our assumptions has a probability of at least 0.998—and the test result showed infection.

Cindy: With a 2% false positivity rate, this would happen with probability of $1/50 = 0.02$, right?

Alice: Yes. So your probability of getting a false positive test result in any given week are about 0.998×0.02, very close to 0.02.

Cindy: It would then be nearly 10 times more likely than that the test result is a true positive and shows that I'm really infected!

Alice: Yes, this follows from our assumptions. The actual probabilities may be a little different, depending on how specific the test is, how much of Covid-19 is going around at the time, and how careful you really are.

But under most such assumptions, if you take a test despite having very small chances of being infected, a positive test result will be more likely a false positive than a true positive. If you test positive, you should then take another test to confirm the possible infection or override the first test, as the case may be. While waiting for that second result, you should go into quarantine, and you should try not to worry too much.

Cindy: So I will miss class for a couple of days, most likely unnecessarily. And that last part, the one about not worrying too much, will be the hardest of all.

Alice: Yes. False positive results can be nerve-racking. This is the second reason why testing everybody on a weekly basis would be problematic.

Bob: But shouldn't healthcare workers be tested regularly?

Alice: The calculation changes for healthcare workers and others who are regularly in close contact with potentially infected people. They have a much higher chance of becoming infected during a given week. People in these professions should get tested on a regular basis.

Cindy: But wouldn't this also be true for all students when face-to-face classes resume? You told us that universities may become hotspots for Covid-19 transmission. Then we students will also be at a very high risk!

Alice: There are a lot of discussion about this right now. Universities have very carefully re-designed classroom space and put policies in place to ensure safety on campus. The biggest potential danger that may turn them into hotspots for Covid-19 would be careless behavior of some students after class. Especially during large parties without social distancing. Regular testing of students should help limit the spread of Covid-19.

Frank: So let them test us regularly instead of requiring these masks and all that social distancing.

Alice: You touched on another potential problem with regular testing of students, Frank. When students get tested regularly, as long as the tests come back negative, they may no longer believe that there is a need to take other precautions. But even with weekly testing, some transmissions will still happen between the end of the latency period of about 3 days and the next test. There will also be many false negative results.

In other words, regular testing may give a false sense of security. Then it would turn into a double-edged sword. Many new infections will be avoided as more cases will be detected. But other infections will happen precisely because some students might feel safer than they really are and might become careless.

Bob: Interesting. I never thought about it in this way.

But you have not told us yet why it takes so long for some test results to come back.

Alice: I will, but first we need to talk about three different types of tests.

The first are PCR tests. They are the most reliable ones. A PCR test will detect whether there are traces of the genetic material of Covid-19 viruses in a swab taken form a person's nose or throat. If there is, we can conclude that the person is currently infected.

Bob: By "genetic material", do you mean the RNA?

Alice: Yes. Some viruses use DNA as their genetic material, but coronaviruses use RNA.

There is one problem with trying to detect traces of the viral RNA: There are only very small amounts of it, even in the swabs taken from infectious people. So before we can actually detect these small amounts, we need to make a lot of copies of this particular RNA. This is possible by a neat biochemical trick called the polymerase chain reaction, or PCR. That's where these tests get their name from.

However, the trick is not easy to pull off; only well-equipped labs with specially trained personnel can properly perform it. And it takes a few hours before a PCR produces enough copies of the viral genetic material for the actual test to detect.

In theory, the results of a PCR test can be obtained within a few hours in the lab. But most PCR tests are taken at locations at some distance from the nearest qualified lab. It will take some time to ship the sample taken from the patient to the lab before the technicians can perform the PCR. When things go smoothly, the results of a PCR test should come back within two days. But there are shortages of some chemicals needed for the procedure, of lab equipment, and of technicians trained to perform the PCR. Some labs have backlogs, which cause delays. This is why in some regions of the U.S. people have to wait a week or even longer for the result of a PCR test.

The second kind are the so-called antigen tests. Similarly to PCR tests, they also detect whether a person is currently infected. But instead of viral RNA, they detect certain proteins of the virus. This difference matters, because viral proteins are easier to detect and do not require amplification by a PCR.

Thus for antigen tests, the samples do not need to be shipped to a lab, and we usually can get results very fast, within less than an hour. That's why antigen tests are also called rapid tests.

But since there is no amplification involved in the process, antigen tests need to look for very, very tiny amounts of protein. So their sensitivity is lower than for PCR tests; they give more false negative results.

Bob: Can we then think of Test A in your example as a PCR test and of Test B as an antigen test?

Alice: You got the picture, Bob! But I made up the percentages of false negatives and false positives in my example just to give you numbers that are easy to understand. For actual tests, they could be very different. I only wanted to illustrate the principle.[87]

Finally, there are serological tests or antibody tests. Their name almost sounds like "antigen tests", but they are very different. They do not detect molecules of the virus, but so-called antibodies that the immune system has produced as a defense against the virus during an actual infection. Antibodies would be found in the bloodstream, and the sample is obtained by drawing some blood from the patient.

That's why these tests are called serological tests.

The antibodies make a person immune to re-infection, and we hope that they will hang around in the bloodstream for a long time. We don't know yet how long that would be, but we do know it would be at least for several months.[29]

Frank: But couldn't these antibodies have been produced at any time before the test was taken? If they hang around even after the patient has recovered, how would we know from an antibody test whether a person is currently infected?

Alice: We don't. Only diagnostic tests, that is, PCR tests or antigen tests, will tell us whether an individual is currently infected. If an antibody test comes back positive, we know that the person has been infected at some previous time, but we have no idea when. In particular, we don't know whether the person is still infectious.

Bob: What's the point then of giving an antibody test if it cannot tell whether the person is currently infected?

Alice: Antibody tests have other uses. We may talk about one of them next time.

Endnotes

[81] The last two sentences and other information about re-opening of Ohio University and other colleges in the U.S. are based on first-hand knowledge of the author.

[82] The first FDA emergency approval for the antigen, or rapid, test in the U.S. was granted on May 9, 2020 [1]. The test had been developed by the Quidel corporation, and was in fact being produced at the time of this conversation at a facility of this company located in Athens, Ohio.

[83] Alice is referring here to the CDC's definition of a close contact that requires quarantine. This concept will be further discussed in Chapter 19 on contact tracing.

[84] A study [2] found that over the 4 days of infection before the typical time of symptom onset (Day 5), the probability of a false-

negative result in an infected person decreases from nearly 100% on Day 1 to about 67% on Day 4. On the day of symptom onset, the median false-negative rate was 38%. It decreased to about 20% on Day 8 (3 days after symptom onset), then began to increase again, from around 21% on Day 9 to around 66% on Day 21.

[85] This estimate is based on data from [3] for late July and early August.

[86] During late July, on the order of 10,000 new weekly cases in a population of roughly 11 million were reported for Ohio [4]. While actual weekly incidence may have been up to 7 times higher than reported incidence,[91] it is not unreasonable to assume that for exceptionally careful individuals it would be at most twice the reported average incidence for the state.

[87] It should be strongly emphasized that actual false positive and false negative rates differ between tests offered by a variety of manufacturers. They also depend on the time after exposure when the test is administered [2] and other factors and are likely to improve as better tests become available. Therefore, Alice very carefully labels the numbers she used for illustrative purposes as "made up", although her false negative rates are actually consistent with the numbers quoted in the Fox News article [5].

References

[1] U.S. Food and Drug Administration. Coronavirus (COVID-19) update: FDA authorizes first antigen test to help in the rapid detection of the virus that causes COVID-19 in patients. May 9, 2020. [cited 2020 Dec 12]. https://www.fda.gov/news-events/press-announcements/coronavirus-covid-19-update-fda-authorizes-first-antigen-test-help-rapid-detection-virus-causes

[2] Kucirka LM, Lauer SA, Laeyendecker O, Boon D, Lessler J. Variation in false-negative rate of reverse transcriptase polymerase chain reaction–based SARS-CoV-2 tests by time since exposure. Ann Intern Med. 2020 Aug 18 [cited 2021

Jan 3]; 173(4):262–267. `https://www.ncbi.nlm.nih.gov/pmc/articles/PMC7240870/` DOI: 10.7326/M20-1495

[3] Johns Hopkins University of Medicine. Daily state-by-state testing trends. [cited 2020 Sep 28]. `https://coronavirus.jhu.edu/testing/individual-states/usa`

[4] Worldometers.info. Dover, Delaware, U.S.A. COVID-19 coronavirus pandemic. [cited 2020 Sep 28]. `https://www.worldometers.info/coronavirus/`

[5] McGorry A. Are coronavirus rapid tests accurate? Fox News 2020 Aug 18. [updated 2020 Oct 2; cited 2021 Jan 2]. `https://www.foxnews.com/health/coronavirus-rapid-tests-accuracy`

Chapter 17

How to estimate the ratio of actual to reported numbers of infections?

Alice and Bob meet on August 4, 2020. The worldwide total of reported Covid-19 cases surpasses 19 million [1], a number equal to the entire population of the country of Romania. It is generally believed that the actual numbers of Covid-19 infections are several times higher. On the previous day, a study came out that showed a ratio of 6:1 between reported cases and actual cases in Italy [2].

Bob: Alice, you told us that the actual numbers of Covid-19 infections may be 10 times higher than the reported numbers. I can see why the actual numbers would be higher than the reported ones. But if infections are not reported, there are no data on them. Without data, how could one possibly estimate this ratio of 10:1 of actual to reported cases?

Alice: Good question, Bob! There actually are data that we can use for estimating this ratio.

Last time we talked about serological or antibody tests. A positive result of such a test does not show whether the person is currently infected, but it shows whether the person has been infected at any time in the past.[88]

Now let us do one of our What-If thought experiments and assume that we would ask everybody in a given country to take a serological test today. What would the results of these tests tell us?

Bob: They would give us the total number of Covid-19 infections in that country until today.

Alice: Not the exact number, because there would be some false positives and some false negatives. And not until today. Remember that it takes the immune system a few days after exposure to the virus to build up enough antibodies for the test to detect. If all these tests were given today, they would give us a fairly accurate picture of the total number of Covid-19 infections until the end of July.

Bob: But no country can give millions and millions of tests to all of its people on one day!

Alice: Right. Epidemiologists would not ask everybody to take the test, but only a representative sample that includes people from large cities, from rural areas, young people, older people, people like health care workers who are at high risk for contracting the disease, people at medium risk, and people at low risk who don't have many contacts with others. All these groups should be included in the sample in the same proportion as in the overall population. So the sample needs to be fairly large; perhaps on the order of 50,000 to 100,000 people.

Bob: Can even that many people get tested on a single day?

Alice: It's not absolutely necessary to conduct all these tests on one day. Since we are trying to estimate the total number of infections that occurred over several months, the estimates will still be fairly accurate if people in the sample take these tests over a period of a couple of weeks.

Bob: But if researchers ask people in their sample to participate, would they actually volunteer to take these blood tests? I doubt that many would.

Alice: This is a potential problem in all studies based on a sample of volunteers. We cannot expect everybody to join the study. But if the proportion of those who do participate is sufficiently large, we still get a representative sample.

Such large-scale studies were successfully conducted in Italy and in Spain. In Spain, more than 80% of those that could be contacted by the researchers agreed to participate. The study enrolled over 60,000 volunteers.[89]

Bob: An amazing participation rate! These tests would not benefit the volunteers personally, but only indirectly all people in their country. Seems the people in Spain are very public-spirited.

What did these studies find?

Alice: Let me talk about the one in Italy first. It was done at the end of July, and the results just came out [2].

The researchers were able to recruit 64,660 volunteers from all over the country. Based on the proportion of serological tests that detected antibodies against Covid-19, the study concluded that around 1.5 million people in Italy would have been infected with Covid-19 at some time before the end of July. This corresponds to about 2.5% of the population of Italy, which is close to 60.5 million.

In late July, the total number of confirmed Covid-19 cases in Italy was around 245,000 [1]. Thus, the actual number of total Covid-19 infections was about 6 times higher than the total number of reported cases.

Bob: Let me see whether I got this right: Would it mean that in Italy, for every new infection that got reported in late July, there were 5 other new infections at roughly the same time that were not reported?

Alice: Not necessarily. The study only shows that on average there were about 5 unreported infections for every infection that got reported until late July. The ratio of 6:1 is an average over the entire period since the start of the pandemic in Italy. For new infections that occurred in late July, the ratio would likely have been smaller.

Bob: Why would that be?

Alice: In March and early April, the Italian health care system was overwhelmed [4]. There were shortages of everything, including tests for Covid-19. That's also the time when the bulk of infections were reported in Italy. It would certainly also have been the time when most actual infections occurred.

Let's look at the daily reported infections in Italy until the end of July:

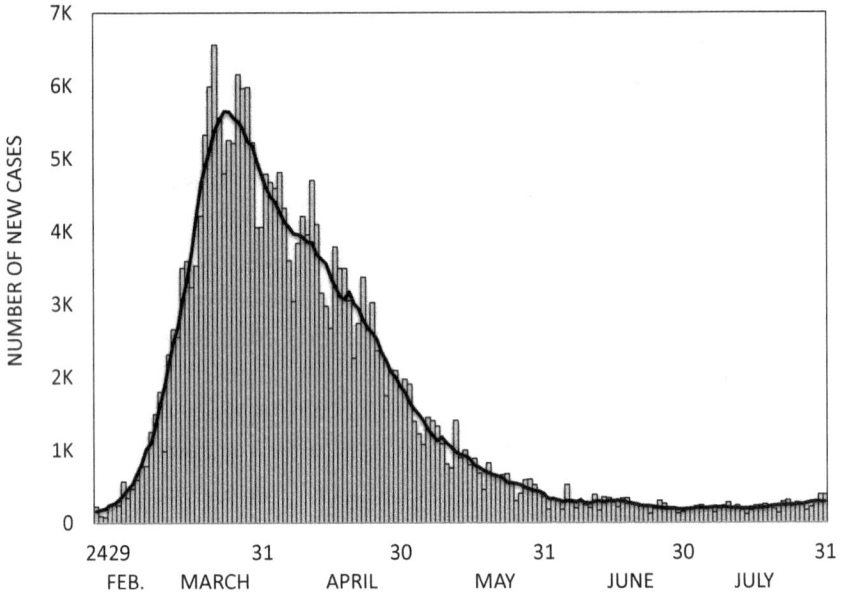

Fig. 17.1   Daily reported infections in Italy until July 31. Based on data published by the Italian Ministry of Health [3].

Bob: Do you mean that at the time when most of the infections were reported in Italy, the ratio of unreported to reported infections would have been larger than in July?

Alice: Yes, this seems very plausible. Italy's numbers of new infections had come down a lot by the end of May. Many more tests per confirmed case are being done recently, which would most likely result in a smaller ratio of unreported to reported infections. The average ratio of 6:1 reflects more closely the situation in March and April.

Therefore, I suspect that for infections that occurred in July, this ratio would be smaller. But we cannot tell from this study whether it was much smaller or just a little smaller. Remember that a positive antibody test only confirms an infection that occurred some time in the past, but does not tell us whether this happened very recently.

Bob: Could one estimate the current ratio between actual new infections and reported new infections by conducting similar large-scale studies? Perhaps by using diagnostic tests that detect current infections?

Alice: In principle, yes, but in practice it would be very difficult. The proportion of currently infected people is much smaller than the proportion of people who have been infected since the start of the pandemic. To obtain accurate estimates, one would then need even larger sample sizes than in studies based on antibody tests.[90]

Bob: I've read that the CDC estimates that the ratio between actual and reported total infections in the U.S. has been about 10:1 so far [5]. If this is true, can we then assume that for current new infections the ratio would also be smaller? By the same argument as you gave for Italy?

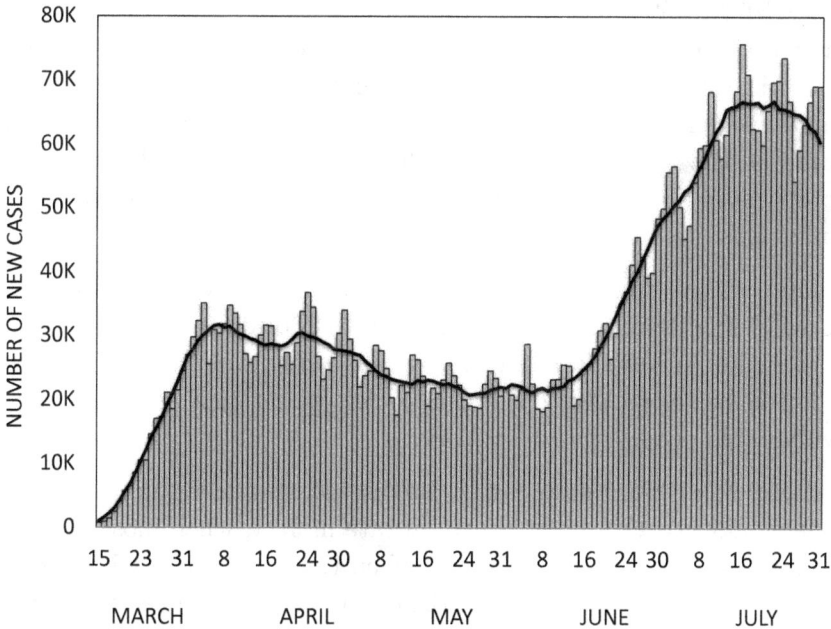

Fig. 17.2   Daily reported infections in the U.S. until July 31. Based on data from the New York Times [6].

Alice: Well, let's look at the chart of daily reported infections for the entire U.S. (Fig. 17.2) that I just showed you. We also had large numbers of infections in April, when tests were very scarce. So the ratio of actual to reported infections would likely have been highest at that time. Now we test many more people, and I would expect a smaller ratio.

In May, infections came down a bit in the U.S., but not nearly as much as in Italy. Eventually they went up again, and we saw a second peak in late July, a much larger one than the first.

Bob: So, if a large-scale study as in Italy were conducted in the U.S. right now, it might mostly detect infections that occurred during the second peak.

Alice: Probably. Therefore, the calculated overall ratio to the ratio of infections during the month of July might be closer in the U.S. than these two ratios would be in Italy.

The ratio may be different in different states though. In the Northeast, in states like New York, the numbers of new infections look more like the ones for Italy that I showed you earlier. In states like Florida, the second peak was much, much larger than the first. I'm pretty sure that in New York, the overall ratio of actual to reported infections was much higher than in Florida.[91]

Bob: Interesting. I just read an article on the mortality from Covid-19 in Florida and New York.[92] In Florida it has been much lower than in New York, and the author wrote that this was because Florida has been doing a much better job at protecting its most vulnerable people than New York.

Alice: As we learn more about the disease, treatment improves, and one would expect a higher survival rate in July, when most cases in Florida occurred, than in March, when the pandemic hit New York very hard. But I think most of the difference between the two states is simply due to the fact that the reported numbers of mortality are a percentage of the reported cases, which is technically known as the case-fatality rate. But we normally think of mortality as a proportion of infected people who die from the disease. This is technically known as the infection-fatality rate.

If the ratio between actual and reported cases has in fact been much higher in New York than in Florida, it is not clear whether the infection-fatality rate in Florida really has been lower than in New York. We will need to wait for more data to come out before we can really know how mortality differed in these two states.[93]

Bob: Has the U.S. conducted similar nationwide serological studies as Italy and Spain?

Alice: Not until now, and I am not aware that one is being planned.

Bob: So how did the CDC come up with its estimate if there were no such studies?

Alice: By using other sources of data. For example, there is a study[94] of blood samples that were collected during routine medical exams from March 23 through May 12, 2020. Such samples are somewhat representative of the entire population, but not quite. In this study, the samples came mostly from several large cities; so rural areas were under-represented. Also, young and healthy people take routine medical exams less often than older people; so this group might also be under-represented in the study. But as long as we are trying to obtain very rough estimates, studies like this one can give us sufficiently good information.

Bob: I have another question: Can we use studies like the ones you described for estimating the percentage of people who remain asymptomatic during a Covid-19 infection?

Alice: Yes. Spain conducted such a study [7–9].

In contrast to the Italian study, it was done in two rounds: First, the participants were tested for antibodies between April 27 and May 11. Then most of the same participants were tested again in a second round three weeks later, between May 18 and June 1.

Based on the first round, it was estimated that 5% of the people in Spain had been infected with Covid-19 at some time prior to the study; for the second round, the study gave an estimate of 5.2%. These estimates were about 10 times higher than the total percentages of people in Spain who had reported a Covid-19 infection up to that time. This is quite similar to what the CDC estimated for the U.S.

The participants in the Spanish study were also asked to carefully monitor any possible symptoms over the weeks between the two rounds. Persons who tested negative in the first round and positive in the second would then report whether or not they had experienced symptoms. Based on these reports, it was estimated that about 33% of all Covid-19 cases remain asymptomatic.

Endnotes

[88] Estimates of cumulative incidence based on antibody tests as described in this chapter are based on the assumption that antibodies remain in the bloodstream at sufficiently high levels when the test is taken. As immunity wanes over time, this assumption may not be satisfied in the long run. But it appears to be true for at least 5 months [10], which is a sufficient time span for the studies described in this chapter.

[89] More precisely, 66,805 of 81,294 successfully contacted individuals who were asked to participate in the first round of the study [7], and 68,480 of 83,524 successfully contacted individuals who were asked to participate in the second round volunteered [8].

[90] Another important issue is that one needs reliable estimates of the false negative and false positive rates for the tests being used. This is true regardless of whether they are antibody tests or diagnostic tests. But as was discussed in Chapter 16, with low prevalence, diagnostic tests may come out more often false positive than true positive. So these estimates would need to be very precise for diagnostic tests if they were to give an accurate picture of actual prevalence in a random sample.

[91] Alice's hunches were confirmed by the subsequent study [11]. Its authors concluded from their statistical analysis that until July 25, less than 10% of the U.S. population had experienced Covid-19 infections. During the same time frame, Covid-19 infections had been confirmed for roughly 1.3% of the U.S. population.

This translates into a ratio of around 7:1 between actual and re-ported infections; lower than the 10:1 estimate that was derived from the earlier study [12].

[92] Bob may be referring to an article like [13] by the Heritage Foun-dation, a conservative think-tank. The author of this article en-tirely ignores the distinction between the reported case-fatality rate and the actual infection-fatality rate.

[93] Figure 2 in the survey [11] suggests that, by July 25, more than 1 in 3 residents of New York state but fewer than 1 in 20 residents of Florida may have experienced infection; a ratio of roughly 7:1. If these data based on their samples translate into reasonably accurate statewide estimates, the infection-fatality rate until the end of July may have been 40% higher in Florida than in New York.

[94] Harvers et al. [12] estimated that, for 7 of the 10 sites for which they analyzed data, over 10 times more SARS-CoV-2 infections occurred than the number of reported cases.

References

[1] Worldometers.info. Dover, Delaware, U.S.A. COVID-19 corona-virus pandemic. [cited 2020 Aug 21].
https://www.worldometers.info/coronavirus/

[2] Bartoloni M. Gli italiani colpiti dal Covid sono 1,5 milioni, metà in Lombardia: letalità scende al 2,5%. A Bergamo uno su 4 ha gli anticorpi. Il Sole 24 Ore 2020 Aug 3. [cited 2020 Aug 21]. https://www.ilsole24ore.com/art/gli-italiani-colpiti-covid-sono-15-milioni-meta-lombardia-letalita-scende-25percento-ADftekh?refresh_ce=1

[3] Github Inc. Dati COVID-19 Italia. [cited 2020 Sep 26].
https://raw.githubusercontent.com/pcm-dpc/COVID-19/master/dati-andamento-nazionale/dpc-covid19-ita-andamento-nazionale.csv

[4] Horowitz J, Buciarelli F. The lost days that made Bergamo a tragedy. The New York Times. 2020 Nov 29. [Updated 2020 Dec

6; cited 2020 Dec 6]. `https://www.nytimes.com/2020/11/29/world/europe/coronavirus-bergamo-italy.html`

[5] Centers for Disease Control and Prevention. CDC Newsroom. Transcript for the CDC telebriefing update on COVID-19 2020 Jun 25. [cited 2020 Oct 22]. `https://www.cdc.gov/media/releases/2020/t0625-COVID-19-update.html`

[6] Github Inc. nytimes/covid-19-data. [cited 2020 Sep 25]. `https://github.com/nytimes/covid-19-data`

[7] Pollán M, Pérez-Gómez B, Pastor-Barriuso R, Oteo J, Hernán MA, Pérez-Olmeda M, et al. Prevalence of SARS-CoV-2 in Spain (ENE-COVID): a nationwide, population-based seroepidemiological study. Lancet 2020 Aug 22. [published online 2020 Jul 6; cited 2021 Jan 3]; 396(10250):535–544. `https://www.thelancet.com/journals/lancet/article/PIIS0140-6736(20)31483-5/fulltext` DOI: 10.1016/S0140-6736(20)31483-5

[8] Spanish Ministry of Health. Estudio ENE-COVID19: Segunda ronda estudio nacional de sero-epidemiología de la infección por SARS-COV-2 en España. Preliminary report 2020 Jun 3. [cited 2020 Dec 29]. `https://www.mscbs.gob.es/gabinetePrensa/notaPrensa/pdf/04.06040620180155399.pdf`

[9] Pérez P. España sigue sin inmunidad frente al coronavirus. El Mundo. Salud. 2020 Jun 4. [cited 2020 Dec 29]. `https://www.elmundo.es/ciencia-y-salud/salud/2020/06/04/5ed8e530fdddffda998b4675.html`

[10] Wajnberg A, Amanat F, Firpo A, Altman DR, Bailey MJ, Mansour M. Robust neutralizing antibodies to SARS-CoV-2 infection persist for months. Science 2020 Dec 4 [cited 2020 Jan 3]; 370(6521):1227–1230. `https://science.sciencemag.org/content/370/6521/1227.full` DOI: 10.1126/science.abd7728

[11] Anand S, Montez-Rath M, Han J, Bozeman J, Russell Kerschmann R, Beyer P, et al. Prevalence of SARS-CoV-2 antibodies in a large nationwide sample of patients on dialysis in the USA: a cross-sectional study. Lancet 2020 Sep 25. [cited 2020 Sep 25]; 396(10259):1335–1344. `https://www.thelancet.com/journals/lancet/article/PIIS0140-6736(20)32009-2/fulltext` DOI: 10.1016/S0140-6736(20)32009-2

[12] Harvers FP, Reed C, Lim T, Montgomery JM, Klena JD, Hall AJ, et al. Seroprevalence of antibodies to SARS-CoV-2 in 10 sites in the United States, March 23–May 12, 2020. JAMA Intern Med. 2020 Jul 21, 2020. [cited 2021 Jan 3]; 180(12):1576–1586. https://jamanetwork.com/journals/jamainternalmedicine/fullarticle/2768834 DOI:10.1001/jamainternmed.2020.4130

[13] Badger D. When it comes to COVID-19 deaths, Florida is no "New York". The Heritage Foundation 2020 Jul 29. [cited 2020 Dec 11]. https://www.heritage.org/public-health/commentary/when-it-comes-covid-19-deaths-florida-no-new-york

Chapter 18

Was the recent increase in reported COVID-19 infections caused by more testing?

Cindy and Frank join Alice and Bob in their meeting on August 4, 2020. In the U.S., the daily numbers of reported Covid-19 infections have declined somewhat from their peak in late July, but are still almost three times as high as they were two months earlier.[95] Simultaneously, the number of tests performed in the U.S. increased from 477,333 on June 3 to 800,718 on August 3 [1].

Bob: Welcome to our meeting, Cindy and Frank!

Thank goodness daily new infections in the U.S. are now coming down from that peak at the end of July.[72] Alice just told me this second peak may have been so much higher than the first because we now do much more testing than in April. So the actual numbers of daily infections may have been even higher around that first peak than they are now.

Frank: That's what I thought. I think this increase in June and the so-called second peak of infections in July may all have been because we now do much more testing. I already asked about this in our first meeting back in June.

Alice: And I got some data and graphs from the internet right after that meeting to answer this question. But we first talked about other things. Let me show them to you now.

Here is a graph of the daily new infections in Ohio until the time when we had our first meeting:

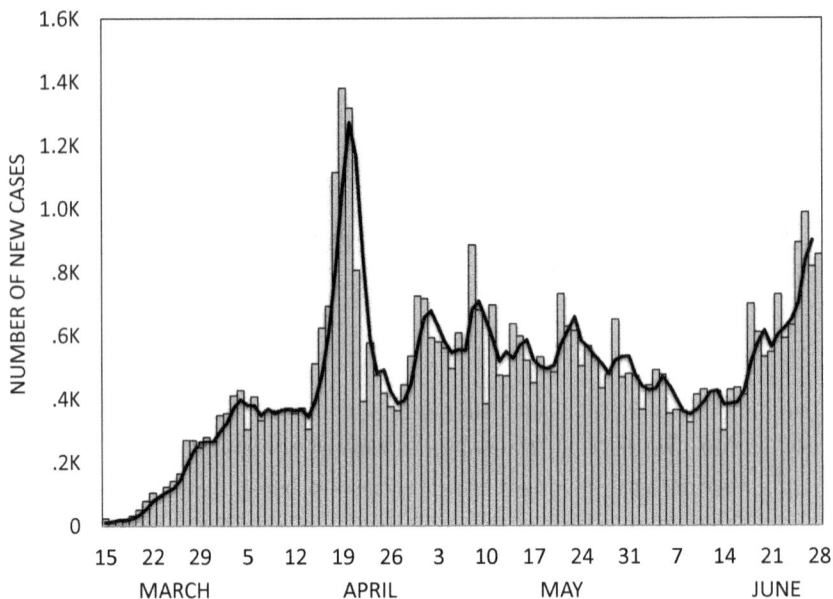

Fig. 18.1   Reported daily new infections in Ohio until June 28, 2020. The graphs on reported daily new infections in this chapter are based on data from the COVID Tracking Project at The Atlantic [2].

Cindy: The increase at the end of June looks so scary!

Frank: Back when we first met, I thought this was just because of more testing. And from what Bob just told us, it sounds I was right.

Cindy: But Frank, more testing doesn't lead to more infections! We test more because we want to prevent transmissions. More testing will decrease the number of new infections.

Alice: Let's not get into a heated argument. Let's sort things out slowly. Cindy, can you remind us how tests can prevent new infections?

Cindy: We talked about this. When people get tested, we will know who needs to go into isolation and who should go into quarantine so that they will not spread the coronavirus further. The more people get tested, the more new infections will be prevented.

Frank: I got that. But you are talking about avoiding exposure of someone who might have contact with a person who should be in isolation, or of someone further down the chain of transmissions. This would only prevent transmissions that might have happened after the person took the test.

If more tests are given, say, on June 26, these tests will not decrease the number of infections reported on June 26.

Bob: But they will help reduce the number of new infections in the next days and weeks; I would agree with Cindy here. And they also will show whether a person with symptoms really has Covid-19. If not, the person can end the isolation and go to work.

Frank: Sure. But as Alice has told us, the numbers of new infections that get reported are only a fraction of the actual numbers. If a larger number of test results are reported for a given day, all else being equal, a larger number of new infections will also be reported for that day.

Alice: You all explained it very well. The reported numbers of daily new infections are influenced by a number of factors, and we need to tease them apart if we really want to understand what is going on. Frank, can you explain to us what you mean by "all else being equal"?

Frank: Let's suppose we have a stable situation in some state, with 10,000 new infections every day. But since we cannot test everybody each day, we will detect only a fraction of these new infection; let's say 10% of them, or 1,000 new infections per day. This would be the case if we also give the same number of tests every day over a couple of weeks.

Now let me give you one of those What-If scenarios and assume that the actual number of new infections remains the same, but testing is increased. Let's say 20% more tests are given in the second week than in the first. Or that the number of tests has increased by a factor of 1.2 if you want to look at it in this way. Then the number of new infections that get detected and reported will also increase by the same factor 1.2.

And this would show up in the graph as a 20% increase in the number of new infections for Week 2 over Week 1. Some people may panic, although the spread of new infections would not have changed at all.

Bob: And some may even want to impose new restrictions. This would be totally unnecessary.

Cindy: But what if all else is not equal?

Frank: This wouldn't change my point. New infections could even decrease by 5%, or by a factor of 0.95, from Week 1 to Week 2. If testing were to increase by a factor of 1.2, we would still see an increase in the numbers of reported new infections, although the number of actual new infections has gone down.

More precisely, reported infections would increase by a factor of $1.2 \times 0.95 = 1.14$, or 14%.

Bob: Interesting. But reported infections would increase less than the number of tests. I think this would show that the actual numbers of new infections went down.

Cindy: But what if the number of actual infections really has gone up, for example, by 10%?

Frank: This would be by a factor of 1.1. If testing had increased by a factor of 1.2, we would then see an increase by a factor of $1.2 \times 1.1 = 1.32$, or 32% in the number of reported new infections.

Cindy: But Frank, in your example, the increase of 32% in the number of new infections is much larger than the increase of 20% in the number of tests. So we can see right from this comparison that the actual number of new infections in the population would have also increased.

Alice: Very good observation, Cindy! When the number of reported new infections increased *faster* than the numbers of reported test results, we can infer that the actual number of new infections also increased.

Conversely, as Bob had noticed earlier, when the numbers of reported new infections increased *slower* than the numbers of reported test results, we can infer that the actual numbers of new infections decreased.

Cindy: This sounds really quite simple!

Frank: Still, in the last example, there was only a 10% increase in the number of actual new infections, while reported new infections increased by 32%, which is totally overblown. So if we look at the reported numbers of new infections while testing has increased, we may get a misleading picture.

Alice: I almost agree with you, Frank. But I would add one little word to what you just said: If we *only* look at the reported numbers of new infections, we may get a misleading picture.

Cindy: What else do we need to look at, Alice? If only there was a way to calculate whether the actual infections are really going up or down and by how much. I am sick and tired of all this uncertainty.

Alice: There is actually a very simple and fairly reliable method for estimating by how much the actual number of new infections is going up or down. And Frank has basically already told us how it works.

Frank: Who, me? I said you can't tell if the number of tests changes.

Alice: You said that when the actual daily numbers of infections don't change, but the number of tests is increased by 20%, the number of positive tests—that is, the number of tests that detect an infection—will also increase by 20%. Why would this be?

Frank: Because the percentage of these positive tests would be proportional to the number of actual infections in the population. By "proportional" I mean that if the number of actual infections was twice as high, the percentage of positive tests also would be twice as high. But if the actual number of new infections stays roughly the same, this percentage would also stay roughly the same.

Alice: Exactly. So wouldn't you agree then that the change in the percentage of positive tests might give us a fairly reliable picture of the change of actual new infections in the population?

Frank: I guess this does follow from my argument.

Alice: This percentage of tests that come back positive is sometimes called the positivity.

Let's calculate it for your last example, where the number of tests increase by 20%, or a factor of 1.2, from Week 1 to Week 2, while the number of new reported infections increased by 32%, or a factor of 1.32.

When we divide 1.32 by 1.2, we get an increase of $1.32/1.2 = 1.1$, or 10%, in the percentage of positive tests from Week 1 to Week 2.

Cindy: This is exactly what we had assumed about the increase in the actual numbers of new infections!

Alice: That's what I meant. The change in the percentage of positive tests gives us a fairly reliable estimate of the change of actual daily new infection. And it is easy to calculate.[96]

Cindy: Let me try this for Frank's second example where the number of tests increased by 20%, the number of actual new infections decreased by 5%, and the number of reported new infections increased by 14%.

So we need to divide a factor of 1.14 for the 14% increase in reported infections by a factor of 1.2 for the increase in the number of tests. Then we get $1.14/1.2 = 0.95$. Is that right?

Alice: Very well done, Cindy! In this example, the percentage of positive tests in Week 2 is only 95% of what it was in Week 1. This shows a 5% decrease in the percentage of positive tests from Week 1 to Week 2; exactly the same as Frank had assumed for the decrease in the actual numbers of new infections.

Bob: Neat! Now I'm wondering whether this actually happened anywhere. I mean, tests and reported new infections increased, while actual numbers of infections decreased.

Frank: For that we would need numbers of tests performed, but it seems nobody is making these numbers public. Those politicians and health experts are hiding something from us.

Alice: Most news outlets focus on the reported numbers of infections. This is unfortunate, because they don't give us the full picture.

But the data on testing are readily available online. I'll show you some graphs that I adapted from such sources right after our first conversation on June 29.

Let's start with data on reported numbers of new infections in the state of Connecticut:

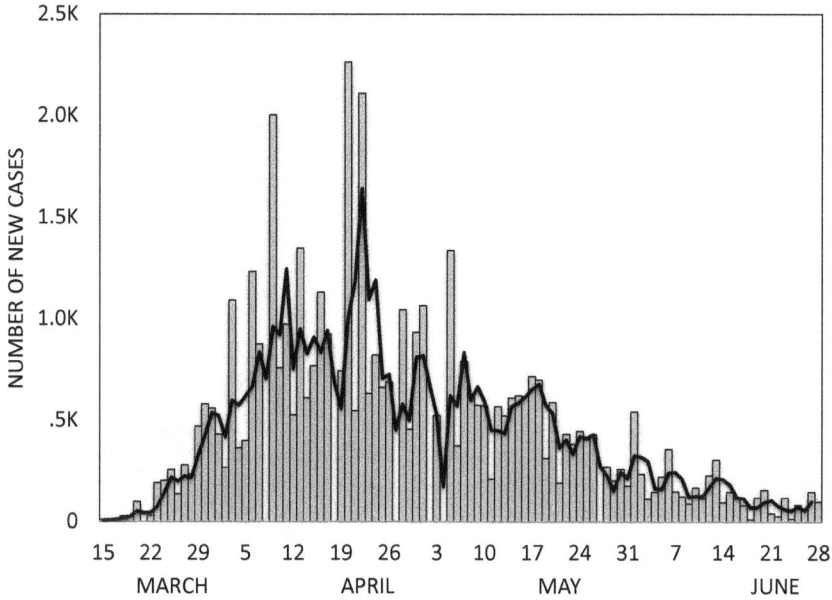

Fig. 18.2   Reported daily new infections in Connecticut until June 28, 2020.

Cindy: Wow! They have brought down their numbers a lot more than our state of Ohio.

Alice: Yes. The strategy for limiting the spread of Covid-19 has been working very well in Connecticut, at least so far. They went into lockdown on March 23, the same day as Ohio, but started re-opening only after May 20, nearly three weeks later than Ohio did [5].

Cindy: But there is an uptick over the last 4 days on this graph.

Bob: It could be due to more actual infections or to more testing. We would not know from this graph alone.

Alice: Now let's look at a graph that shows the numbers of tests, the numbers of positive tests, and the 7-day moving average for the percentage of positive tests until June 28 in the state of Connecticut:

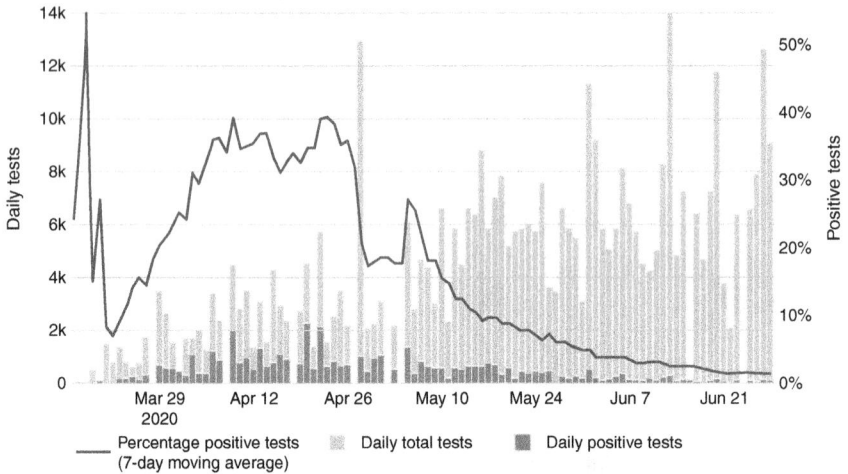

Fig. 18.3   Testing volume and percentage of positive tests in Connecticut until June 28, 2020. The graphs on testing volume and percentages of positive tests in this chapter were adapted from the Coronavirus Resource Center at Johns Hopkins University [4].

Bob: The trend curve for the percentage of positive tests keeps going down, at least so far. So this would show that the actual numbers of new infections also keep going down.

Frank: See what I meant? The numbers of tests over those last three days were very high, and this explains the uptick. There is nothing to worry about in the state of Connecticut.

Alice: I would agree that so far this state has been very successful in dealing with the epidemic. But this doesn't mean that the people in this state can let down their guard. Things may still change for the worse later if they become careless.[97]

Bob: I can see that they had a huge spike in early March and then a very high percentage of positive tests in April.

Alice: Yes. The reason for the early spike is that at the time the first tests became available, they were given only to very sick people.

The high percentages in April tell me that the reported numbers for this month probably underestimated the actual numbers much more than they do now. Bob and I talked about this earlier today.

Next let's look at the reported numbers of new infections until June 28 in the state of Florida:

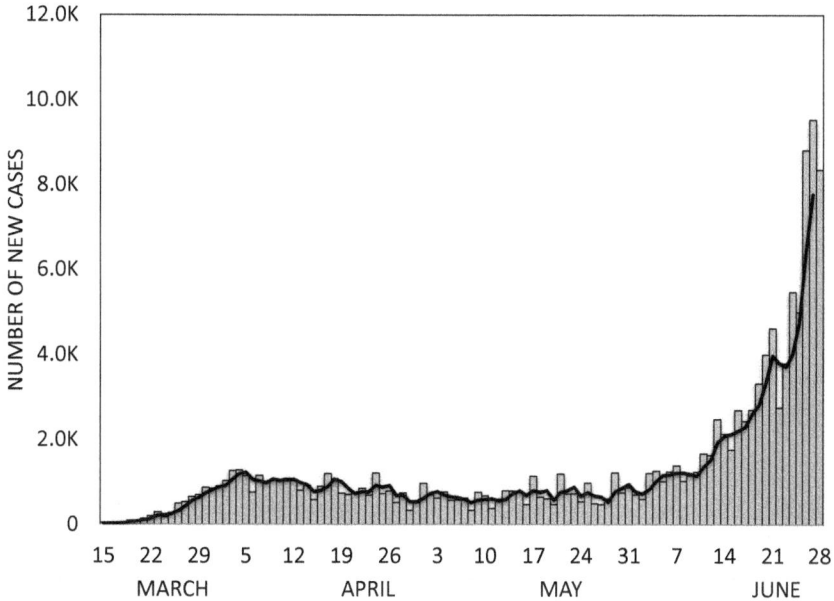

Fig. 18.4   Reported daily new infections in Florida until June 28, 2020.

Cindy: This looks so horrible! Terrifying! One cannot explain away this increase over the last few weeks because there was more testing!

Bob: If in fact there was. But Cindy, we cannot draw any conclusion based on this graph alone, even if it does look horrible. Alice needs to show us the graph that has the data on testing before we can see what really had been going on.

Alice: Yes, Bob. Let me show the graph for numbers of tests and percentage of positive tests in Florida:

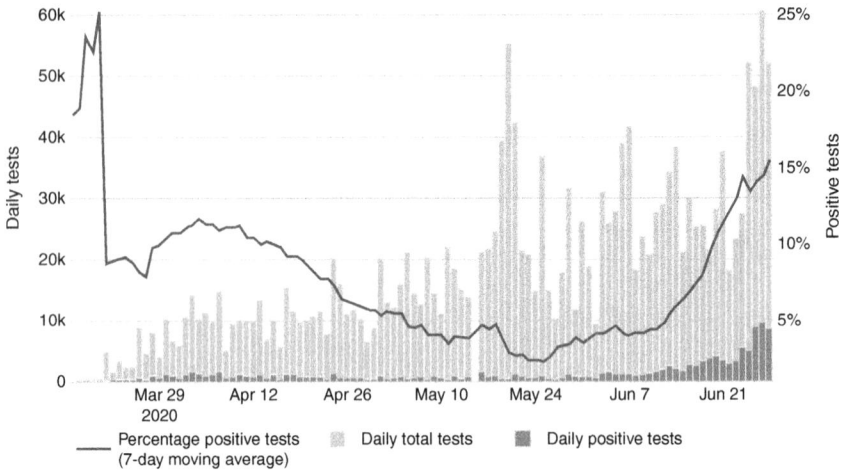

Fig. 18.5   Testing volume and percentage of positive tests in Florida until June 28, 2020.

Frank: Well, testing did go up in Florida at the end of June. But I can see it didn't go up nearly as much as the reported number of new infections.

Bob: And during the second half of June, the percentage of tests that came back positive was increasing a lot. This would mean a large increase in the actual number of new infections. Seems it was high time for the state to do something about it.

Alice: In fact, on June 26 the governor ordered the shutdown of bars [5]. This seems to have helped to some extent. The positivity rate in this state may have peaked by now.[98]

Cindy: I feel so sorry for the people of Florida.

And what was going on in June in our own state? Can we talk about Ohio now?

Alice: Yes, Cindy! In my first picture (Fig. 18.1), we saw that reported new infections in our state rapidly increased in our state during the second half of June.

And now let's look at the testing data for Ohio until June 28:

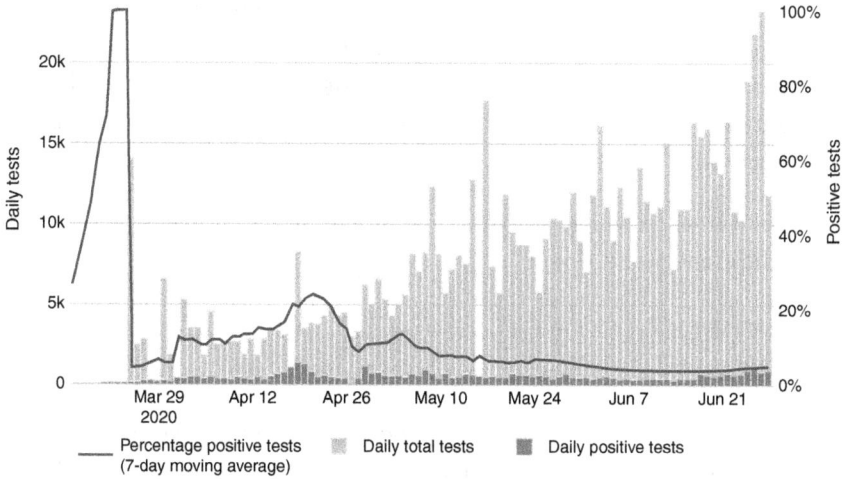

Fig. 18.6   Testing volume and percentage of positive tests in Ohio until June 28, 2020.

Frank: Testing went up a lot, and this largely explains the increase in new infections.

Bob: But not entirely. There was a definite upward trend in the percentage of positive tests over the last 2 weeks of June. Not nearly as steep as in Florida, but an increase nevertheless.

Alice: Right. Our percentages of positive tests slowly decreased until mid-June or so, and then started increasing slightly. This shows that actual numbers of new infections were also increasing at the time. Not nearly as much as reported new infections, but the trend was still concerning. On July 8, the Governor signed a health order requiring face coverings in public in the most affected counties [5]. This successfully reversed the trend. Reported new infections increased until July 17 and then started decreasing [6].

Cindy: That's good. And it may have helped that we did a lot more tests so that people who really got infected we would isolate themselves and their close contacts would go into quarantine.

Bob: Glad we are past that peak. And we can all see now that there was a real increase in the number of actual new infections in Ohio and in Florida.

It's really quite simple: When reported numbers of new infections increase faster than the number of tests, then there is also an increase in the the actual number of new infections. And the change in the percentage of positive tests shows us how fast actual new infections are increasing.

Frank: Or decreasing, for that matter, if the percentage of positive tests happens to go down.

Endnotes

95 According to Worldometer [3], the 7-day moving average of daily reported Covid-19 infection was 22,275 on June 3 and 62,521 on August 3, 2020.

96 This will be true only as long as there are no significant changes in the policies governing testing or in the kinds of tests being used. On the other hand, it is worth pointing out that these estimates do not require knowledge of the ratio between actual and reported infections. Neither can the method described here be used for determining this ratio. It only can estimate the change in actual infections, not their absolute magnitude.

97 By the time of this conversation, August 4, the percentage of positive tests in Connecticut had in fact gone up, but only very slightly. It remained well below 2% throughout the summer.

98 See Chapter 22 for a more detailed discussion.

References

[1] University of Oxford. Oxford Martin School. Our World in Data. Total COVID-19 tests. [cited 2020 Dec 12].
https://ourworldindata.org/grapher/full-list-total-tests-for-covid-19?time=2020-02-20..latest

[2] The Atlantic Monthly Group LLC. The COVID Tracking Project. The data. [cited 2020 Dec 30].
https://covidtracking.com/data

[3] Worldometers.info. Dover, Delaware, U.S.A. COVID-19 coronavirus pandemic. [cited 2020 Dec 12].
https://www.worldometers.info/coronavirus/

[4] Johns Hopkins University of Medicine. Coronavirus Resouce Center. Daily state-by-state testing trends. [cited 2020 Jun 29].
https://coronavirus.jhu.edu/testing/individual-states/usa

[5] Johns Hopkins University of Medicine. Coronavirus Resource Center. Critical Trends. Impact of opening and closing decisions by state. [cited 2020 Oct 25].
https://coronavirus.jhu.edu/data/state-timeline

[6] The New York Times. Ohio Covid Map and Case Count. [cited 2020 Oct 25]. https://www.nytimes.com/interactive/2020/us/ohio-coronavirus-cases.html

Chapter 19

What is contact tracing and how does it help?

Alice, Bob, Cindy, and Frank meet on August 11, 2020. Contact tracing is of crucial importance for limiting the spread of Covid-19, but requires an enormous workforce. It has been estimated that the U.S. alone needs as many as 100,000 contact tracers, but only about 37,000 were available in mid-June, and the number has barely grown since then.[99]

Frank: They tell us to go into quarantine when we had close contact with an infected person. But how would we know whether that person was infected?

Bob: Good friends would tell you if they test positive.

Frank: Sure. But if the person wasn't a good friend?

Alice: This is where contact tracing comes in. The goal is to first identify all recent contacts of the patient who tested positive and then notify them about the possible exposure to the virus.

Bob: But each of us makes so many contacts every day! How could one possibly remember all of them? Often we don't even know the name of the guy who was standing close to us.

Cindy: Right! I worked at a supermarket checkout last summer and served hundreds of customers per shift. I didn't know any of them.

Alice: Yes, each of us makes many, many contacts during a day, and we often don't know whom we got close to.

Any of these contacts could in principle lead to a transmission. But this is unlikely, except for the most intense ones. The goal of contact tracing can only be to identify these most intense contacts. For this reason, the CDC and similar agencies in other countries have singled out contacts that would be most high-intensity. These are called close contacts.

I don't want to go into too many details here how a close contact is defined; it slightly differs from country to country and may change over time as we learn more about how Covid-19 is spreading. Let me only mention the most important category from the CDC website: "A close contact is anyone who was within 6 feet of an infected person for at least 15 minutes."[100]

Cindy: I'm confused. This sounds like a "close contact" is a person. I thought a close contact was something that happened between two people.

Alice: The word "contact" can refer to an interaction between two people or to a person. This may be a little confusing. In our discussion, we will try to keep the two meanings straight.

Contact tracing has two steps; let's discuss them separately.

The first step is called case investigation. If somebody tests positive, he or she has an interview with a contact tracer. The contact tracer interviews the patient and tries to obtain the information about all close contacts of the patient prior to taking the test or developing symptoms, whichever came first. The interview is conducted in such a way as to reveal relevant information while protecting the privacy of all involved to the extent possible. To make this work, contact tracers need to undergo training and strictly follow an established protocol.

Cindy: But what if the infected patient had close contacts after developing symptoms or while waiting for the test results? Wouldn't those also put other people a risk?

Alice: Yes, this is an important concern. For this reason, people should isolate themselves as soon as they develop symptoms or between taking the test and finding out about the result.

Bob: This may be very difficult if it takes a long time for the test results to come back.

Alice: Yes. Let's assume here that people do isolate themselves when they show symptoms and that test results come back without a time lag. The real world is more complicated, but this will make it easier for us to understand how contact tracing is supposed to work.

Cindy: I still think that more people should count as close contacts. What if two people work in the same office all day? Wouldn't there be a great risk of transmission, even when they never get within 6 feet of each other for long?

Alice: Yes, there would. Contact tracing can never identify all close contacts that posed a risk of transmission. But one can try to find more of them by expanding the definition. This is sometimes called wide-net contact tracing. As we talk, many universities are considering such procedures.[101] For example, when a student who lives in a dorm becomes infected, all students who live on the same floor might be at an elevated risk. The university may establish a policy that requires testing and quarantining all of them.

Bob: But this may send a lot of students unnecessarily into quarantine. We are coming to campus for going to class and meeting interesting people, not for sitting all by ourselves in a room for two weeks! And who is going to pay for training all the contact tracers and for the tests? If the university does, then they will raise tuition, and higher education will become more expensive than it already is. One has to draw the line somewhere.

Alice: I agree with you, Bob. One has to find a reasonable tradeoff between what would prevent as many infections as possible and what is economically feasible. Universities around the world are struggling with finding the best balance. And so are entire countries. The CDC's definition of a close contact draws such a line; other countries or particular institutions may draw their lines differently.

Frank: But what if we come back to campus and there are a lot of cases? With this wide-net contact tracing, they will try to keep all students of entire dorms locked up inside their rooms for weeks. Good luck with that! And the university will still make them pay rent and tuition. That's unfair.

Cindy: But Alice told us that if we all wear our masks and practice social distancing, there won't be many cases. If a student doesn't do this and puts other students at risk, those may end up in isolation and quarantine. So I think it is very unfair to other students if any of us doesn't wear a mask or parties a lot.

Alice: Very well put, Cindy! Bob and Frank also made important points. Casting a wide net for identifying contacts will be feasible only if the number of infections is low enough. Then the burden of going into quarantine and the costs of testing and contact tracing will be limited to the contacts of only a few sporadic cases. Contact tracing will then be very effective. Together with isolation and quarantine, it will cut enough chains of transmissions to keep the number of new infections low and manageable.

This applies to entire countries as much as to universities. When the daily numbers of new infections are as high as they currently are in the U.S., casting a wide net in testing and contact tracing would be prohibitively expensive. It can't be done, and too many new infections will remain undetected.

Bob: Which means the number of new infections will remain high and restrictions will remain in place for a long time. A few days ago, I heard on NPR that we currently have only about 40% of the workforce needed to do enough contact tracing [1]. It really ticks me off when I think about what we have to put up with. In other countries, they can already do business almost as usual, because their numbers are low. But here we cannot, and they may slap new restrictions on us at any time when our numbers go up even more.

Frank: Be that as it may. I have two more questions. First of all, what if the patient who tested positive does not know who they had contact with?

Alice: This is another complication. When we meet a person in a bar, for example, most of the time, we don't exchange phone numbers afterwards. And when we sit next to somebody on a long bus trip, we may not even talk to this person.

To make identifying contacts in such situations possible, restaurants ask their customers to leave a phone number on record. Also, digital technology can be used to identify contacts by checking which cell phones were in close proximity at the time of the reported contact. This is called digital contact tracing.[102]

Frank: That goes too far. Why should the healthcare system be allowed to snoop on our whereabouts? We have a right to privacy, and they are trying to take it away from us.

Alice: I also worry about the loss of our privacy, Frank. Whenever we visit a website, whenever we carry a cell phone, our moves online and offline are being recorded by internet service providers or phone companies. Legal protections of what companies can do with these data are very weak. We know they are stored, analyzed, and sold to advertisers. We have very little control over what else is being done with these data.

Frank: The government will use them to snoop on us and control us, obviously.

Alice: I'm afraid of that, too. In the case of contact tracing, it is possible to restrict the use of cellphone data to the ones that are generated by special apps that users voluntarily install on their phones. This would be in their best interest, as they would more likely be alerted about having been in a high-risk situation.

Frank: I wouldn't install the app on mine. I won't give voluntary consent to anybody snooping on my whereabouts.

Alice: I feel the same way. But the only way to not give such consent is to not carry a cellphone at all and not go online. Would you go that far, Frank?

Frank: Come on, Alice! That's impossible.

Alice: I agree. There are no good solutions to this problem right now. But we need to be aware of it and try to figure out what we can do to protect our privacy.

Let me only say this about contact-tracing apps: I find it inconsistent to be against the use of cellphone data for the particular purpose of restricting the spread of a potentially lethal disease while not being concerned about collection and storage of such data by companies who can do who knows what with them.

Frank: I didn't say I am not concerned about the bigger problem; in fact, I am. I just don't see what anybody can do about it.

But let me come to my second question: You said that during the interview the contact tracer would try to find out the contacts that happened "prior" to taking the test or when symptoms started. What do you mean by this? How far back into the past would they dig?

Alice: Important question! We are obviously most concerned about people whom the patient might have infected before showing symptoms. Symptoms often start a day or two after the end of the latency period, after the patient becomes infectious. For this reason, in most protocols for forward contact tracing, a period of 48 hours prior to onset of symptoms or taking the test is being investigated.

Bob: Why do you call this "forward" contact tracing, Alice?

Alice: Because this procedure can identify only those people whom the patient might have infected. As symptoms typically start around 5 days after transmission, if we want to find the person from whom the patient caught the infection, we need to identify all contacts over the last week or so. This attempt to find the source of the infection is called backward contact tracing.

Bob: But this would require investigating a lot more contacts and would be three times more expensive than forward contact tracing alone. Would it actually help to do both forward and backward contact tracing?

Alice: We will talk about the effects of both methods on the spread of the disease.

So far, I have only told you about the first step, the case investigation. In the second step—which is actually the step that is technically called contact tracing—the contact tracer attempts to reach all contacts that were identified during the case investigation. These people are then alerted about having had a close contact with an infected individual, but without being told who that infected person was.

They are being advised about going into quarantine and, depending on the policies of the particular health care system or institution, about taking a test.

Bob: Will these close contacts actually take the call? If it comes from a number they don't recognize, they may think it's a junk call.

Alice: Not all attempts to reach these contacts are successful; some will not answer the calls, and some will not comply with the recommendation. This decreases the effectiveness of contact tracing and can be a big problem.

Let's look at a small population of people who are all susceptible, except for one index case. The following picture shows some of their contacts. I have drawn only close contacts that could be identified during contact tracing:

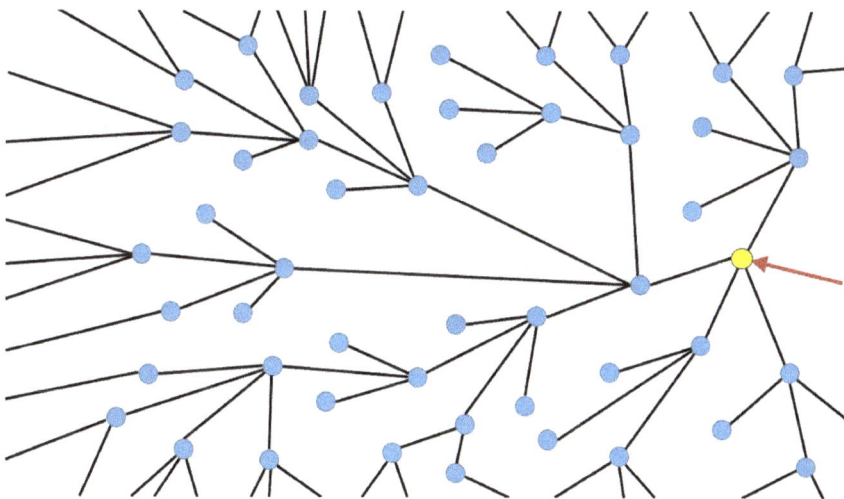

Fig. 19.1 A small population with one index case. Only relevant close contacts are shown.

I'll try to keep matters as simple as possible for our discussion. Most of the time, I will assume that all relevant close contacts can be identified, can be reached, and will comply with recommendations about quarantine and testing.

Cindy: Yes, Alice, please keep it simple! It already sounds so complicated with all this tracing forward and backward and testing or not.

Alice: To keep matters as simple as possible, much simpler than they would be in reality, I will assume in my pictures that each of these close contacts will lead to a transmission if there is no quarantining of contacts or isolation of infected patients. Without these control measures, after some time, each of these people would have experienced infection, and many of them would have infected others outside of this population. As in the following picture:

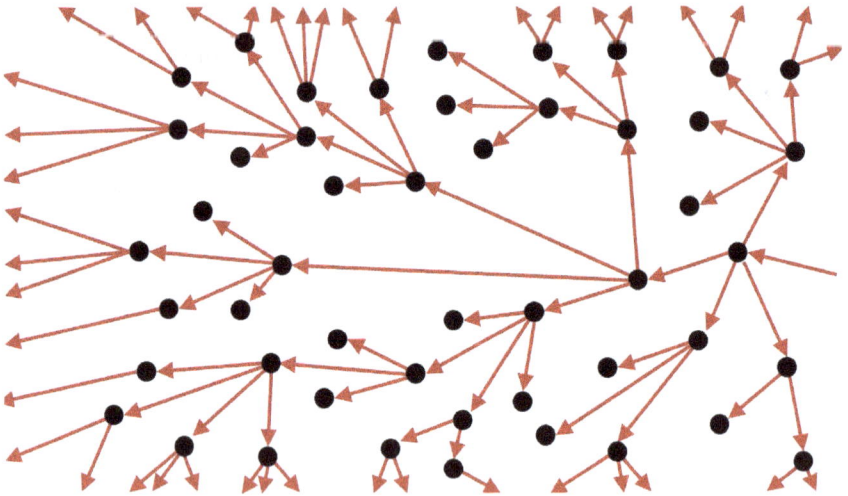

Fig. 19.2   Spread of infections without contact tracing, isolation, or quarantine.

Cindy: This looks so scary!

Alice: Yes, it does. The black color indicates that the person has reached the "removed" state where they no longer can infect others. But each black dot represents a different personal story. Many patients may have experienced only mild symptoms or none at all, others will have suffered through a lot, some may still battle with long-term effects such as brain fog. Some of them may have been hospitalized, and some may have even died.

Bob: So what would happen with quarantining close contacts that are identified in contact tracing?

Alice: Let's look at a time when some chains of transmission had already been started. The index case, let me call him Ingham again, is still asymptomatic, but has already infected three other people. One of them, let's call him Symon, has developed symptoms after infecting two other people:

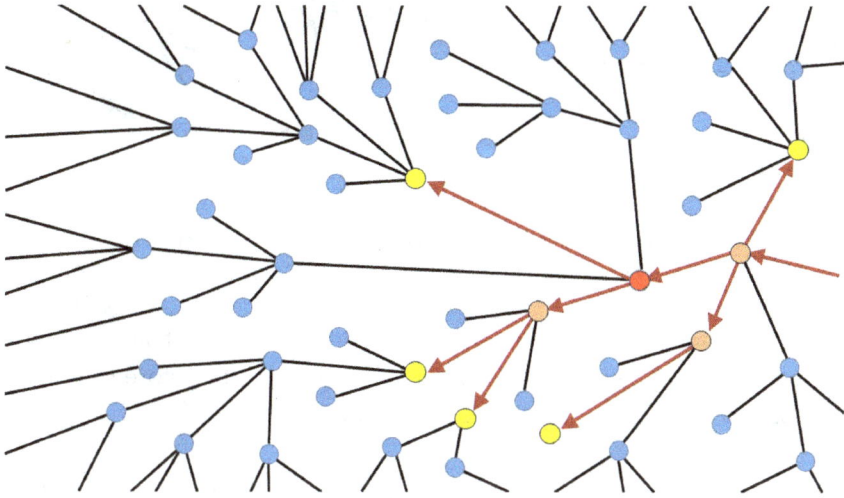

Fig. 19.3 Several chains of transmissions have been started. Ingham remains asymptomatic, but Symon has developed symptoms.

Then Symon gets tested and goes into isolation. This cuts Symon's contacts with others who are still susceptible.

Cindy: These would be he two people connected to Symon with black lines in Fig. 19.3, right?

Alice: Right! Let me call them Layla and Lane. They would be the ones with whom Symon would have had close contact after becoming symptomatic had he not gone into isolation. Symon's isolation protects them. I'll show this by removing two black lines from Fig. 19.3:

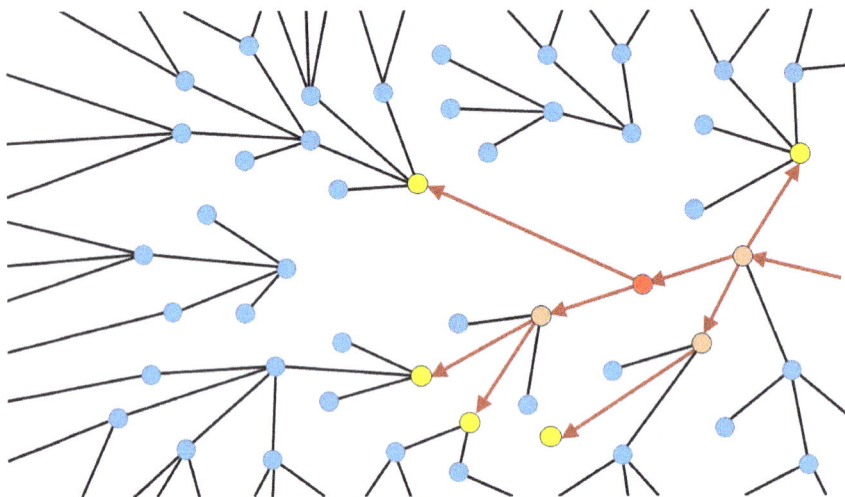

Fig. 19.4   Symon went into isolation and cut all close contacts.

After Symon received his positive test result, contact tracing might have identified all close contacts during the 48 hours before the onset of symptoms. These contacts go into quarantine:

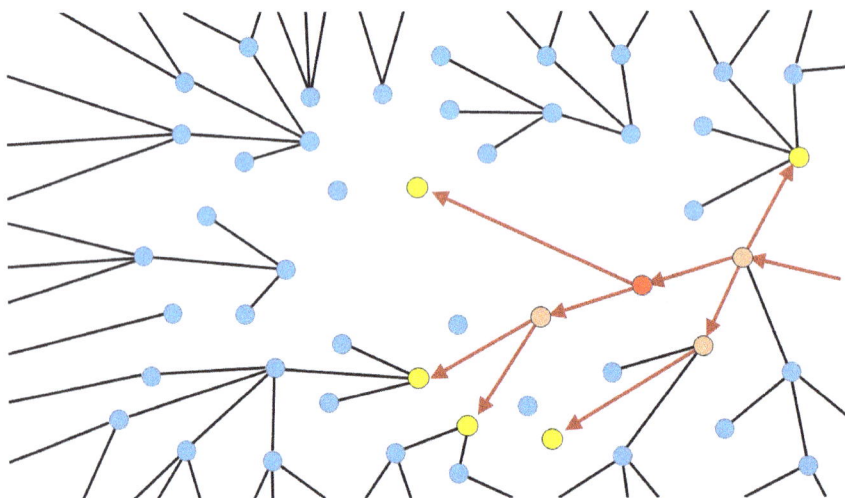

Fig. 19.5   Symon's recent close contacts go into quarantine.

Bob: Why don't Layla and Lane go into quarantine?

Alice: That's because I have assumed that they would have had contact with Symon only after he developed symptoms. They will not be identified during the contact tracing.

Cindy: And why did Ingham not go into quarantine?

Alice: The transmission from Ingham to Symon would typically have happened more than 48 hours before the onset of Symon's symptoms, and Ingham would not have been identified as Symon's close contact. Right now, I am only talking about forward contact tracing.

Let's look at what might happen over the next few days:

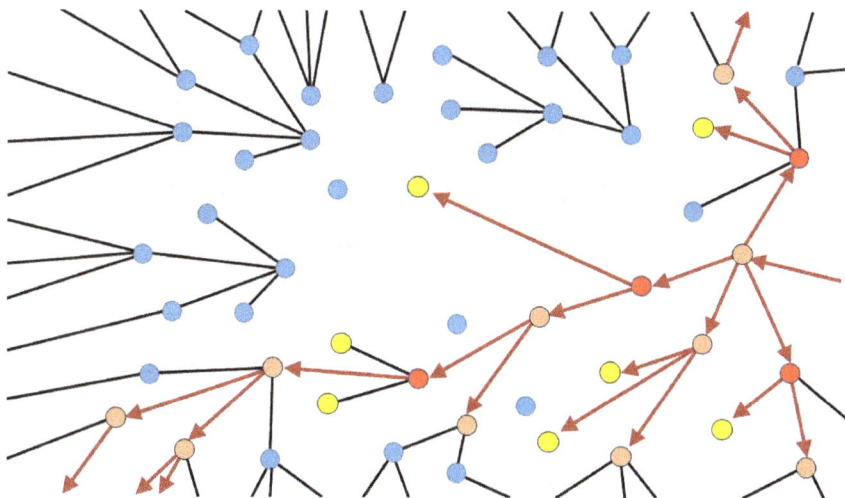

Fig. 19.6   Sylvia, Sierra, and Sigmund also developed symptoms.

We can see that three more patients developed symptoms.

In my next picture, I'll assume that the one on the left—let's call her Sylvia—took a test, that the contact tracing was successful, and her recent contacts went into quarantine. But I also assume that the two on the right—let's call them Sierra and Sigmund—only went into isolation:

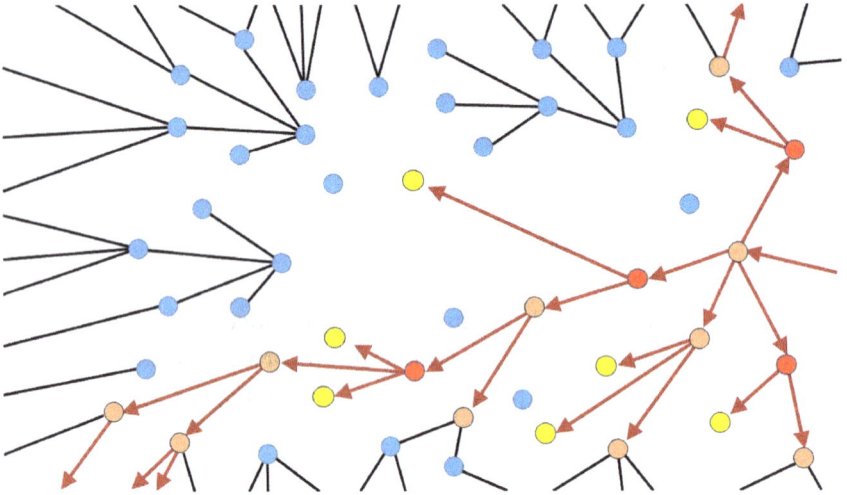

Fig. 19.7   Sylvia's recent close contacts went into quarantine.

Cindy: Why would Sierra and Sigmund only go into isolation?

Alice: This may happen for a number of reasons. There may be a shortage of tests or they may be unwilling to take one. Then they would not even get tested.

They may get tested, but the test results may be false negatives. Or they may need to wait too long for the test results so that contact tracing would have no effect.

Bob: Also, with a shortage of contact tracers, perhaps not all cases can be investigated.

Alice: Good point, Bob! And even if there is a case investigation, not all relevant contacts might be identified during the interview or not all of them could be reached by the contact tracer.

Frank: Welcome to the real world!

Alice: When the outbreak has run its course, most infections on the left of my picture would have been prevented by the forward contact tracing. The isolation of symptomatic patients would also have prevented a few transmissions on the right, but most of them would still have occurred, as in the following picture:

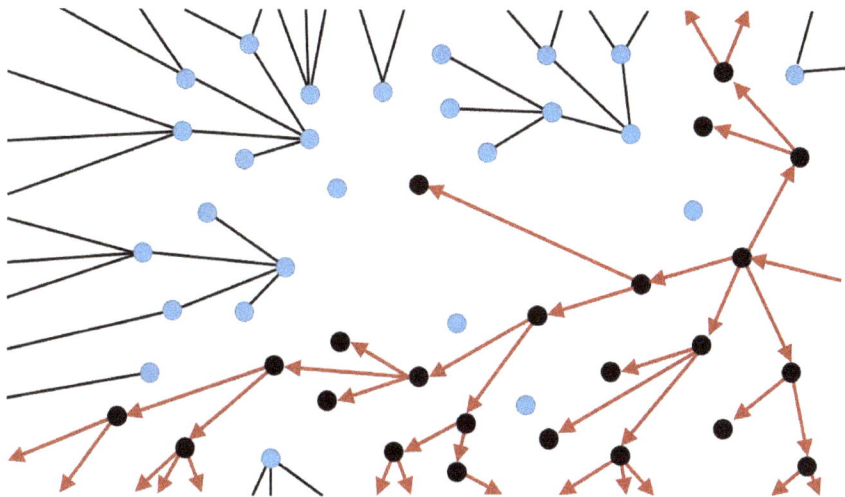

Fig. 19.8 Transmissions of the infection with forward contact tracing, isolation, and quarantine.

Bob: Would backward contact tracing have helped with those?

Alice: Let's see what would have happened:

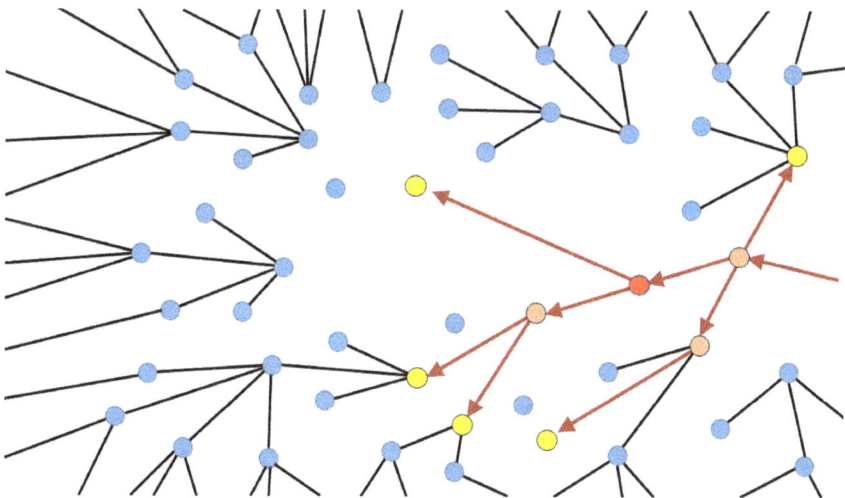

Fig. 19.9 Symon lists Ingham among his close contacts during backward contact tracing and Ingham quarantines himself.

If Symon's case investigation had been done for both forward and backward contact tracing, then Symon would have told the contact tracer about his close contact with Ingham some time back, Ingham would have been notified, and would have quarantined himself. Down the road, with everything else as in the previous example, this would prevent the chains of transmissions in the lower right of the picture:

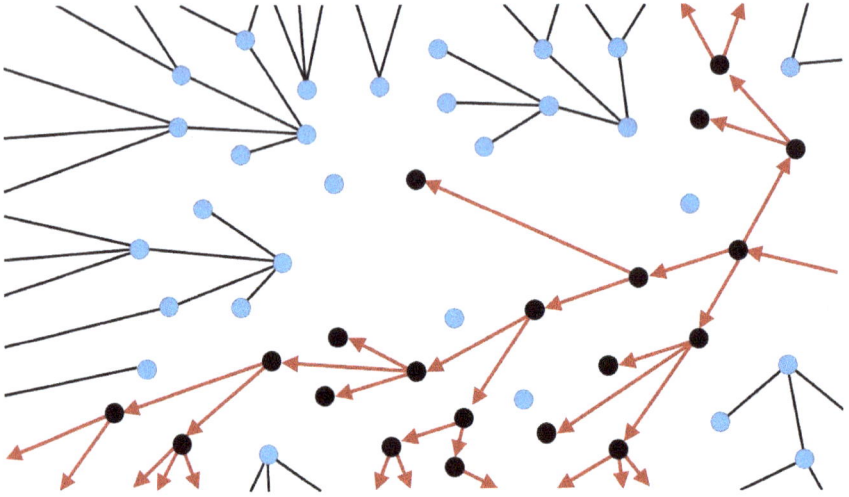

Fig. 19.10   Transmissions of the infection with forward and backward contact tracing, isolation, and quarantine.

Bob: But doing both forward and backward contact tracing would be much more expensive. Many people might be unnecessarily quarantined. And all this for finding one more infectious person.

On your picture, it does not look like many more infections can be prevented in this way. I wonder whether it's worth the additional expenses.

Alice: I agree with you that in fighting against Covid-19 we need to use our limited resources as effectively as possible. It may not appear from my example that backward contact tracing helps all that much, but some studies have shown that it can be very effective.[103]

Cindy: Should the close contacts of Covid-19 patients be tested?

Alice: That's an important question. So far, we have assumed that only people with symptoms take tests. The CDC currently recommends that the close contacts of confirmed cases also get tested. I will show you that this is very effective.

Let me start from our second last picture. I will assume both forward and backward contact tracing in my example. But the effect of testing close contacts is similar if only forward contact tracing is done.

In my example, once Symon shows symptoms, he will get tested, and all his close contacts, including Ingham, will then be identified through forward and backward contact tracing. They would be advised to get tested in addition to going into quarantine. It is important that this be done quickly. Here Symon's two infected and asymptomatic contacts would receive a positive result, and their close contacts would also be quarantined. As in the following picture:

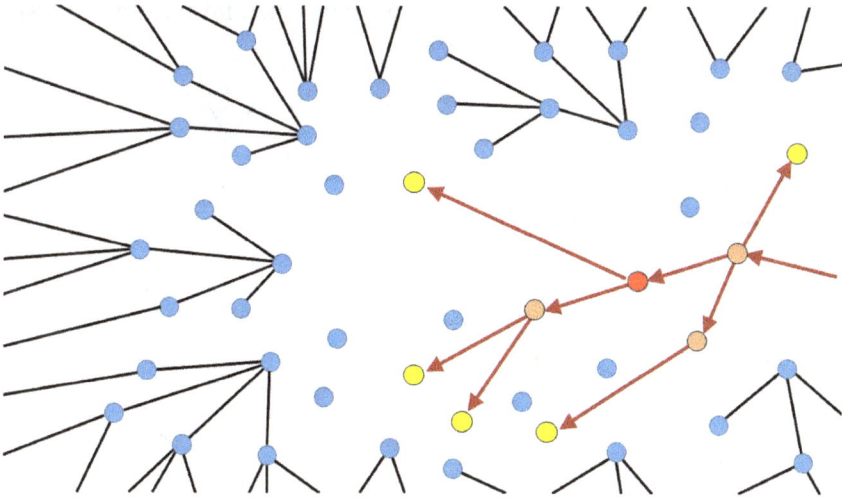

Fig. 19.11 All of Symon's close contacts get tested. Those who are infected undergo contact tracing, and their close contacts will also go into quarantine.

At this point, all chains of transmission have been cut in my example. All people who remain susceptible in this picture will escape infection.

Cindy: This looks a lot less gruesome than what we had in the previous example. I'm so glad that our CDC made this recommendation that close contacts be tested!

Alice: We can only hope that the CDC will stick to it.[104]

Bob: I think testing all close contacts will not always work as well as in your example. I can see though why it would be very effective.

But your last picture shows quarantines also for people who were not actually infected. They may not be able to go to work and lose income. Some might risk losing their jobs.

Frank: And sitting alone at home for a couple of weeks can drive a person crazy. If they get tested as part of the contact-tracing strategy, they should at least be released from quarantine if the test comes back negative.

Alice: Your idea seems very natural, Frank. But it is problematic.

Let's see what might happen if persons with such false negative tests are released from their quarantines:

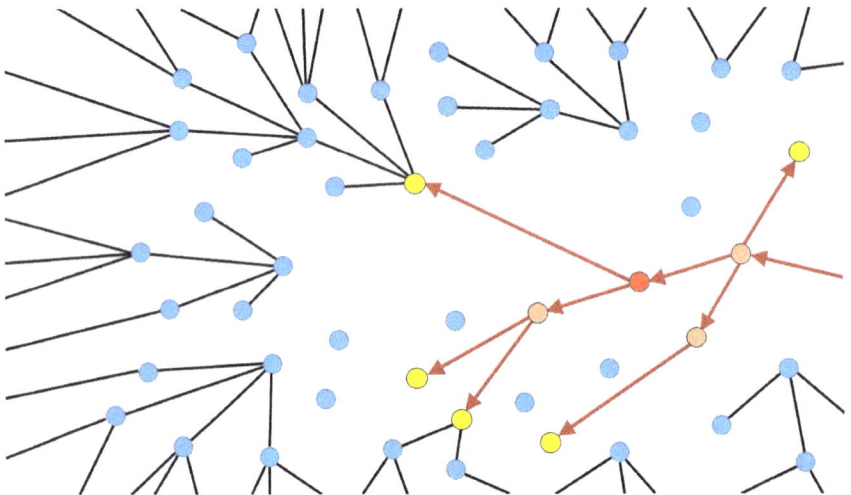

Fig. 19.12   Elaine and Eduardo are released early from quarantine.

In this example, I have assumed that the tests for the exposed person in the upper middle, let's call her Elaine, and the exposed person in the lower middle, let's call him Eduardo, were false negative. For all other tests, I have assumed that they came back positive.

Frank: Two false negative tests among the few quarantined people in your example? How likely would this be?

Alice: Quite likely, actually. Testing close contacts will usually be most effective when it is done as soon as a contact is identified. But if the exposure occurred very recently, the virus particles may not yet have multiplied enough in the contact's body for the test to detect them. In this case, the test will come back false negative.

If Elaine and Eduardo were both released from quarantine after testing negative, they would then spread the virus further:

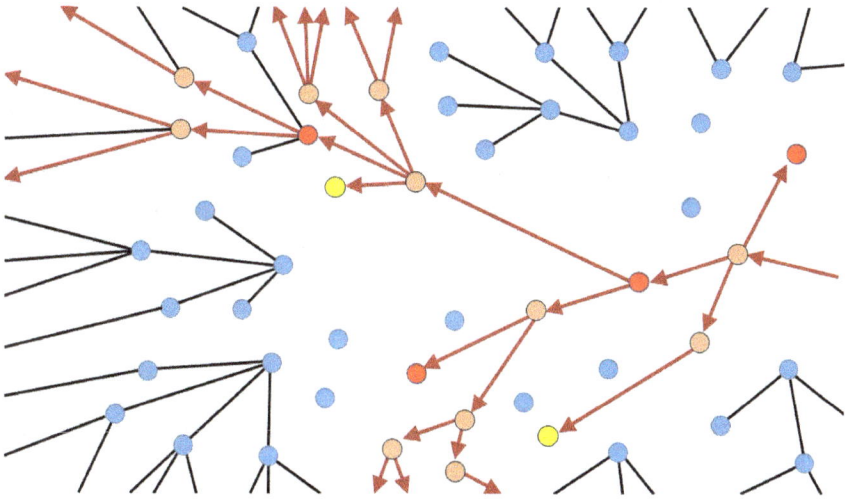

Fig. 19.13   Chains of transmissions have been propagated by Elaine and Eduardo.

In my next picture for this example, one of the people infected by Elaine, let's call her Shayanne, has developed symptoms. She will go into quarantine. This will prevent some new transmissions, but won't cut all chains that take the infection outside of this population in the upper left and lower middle of the picture:

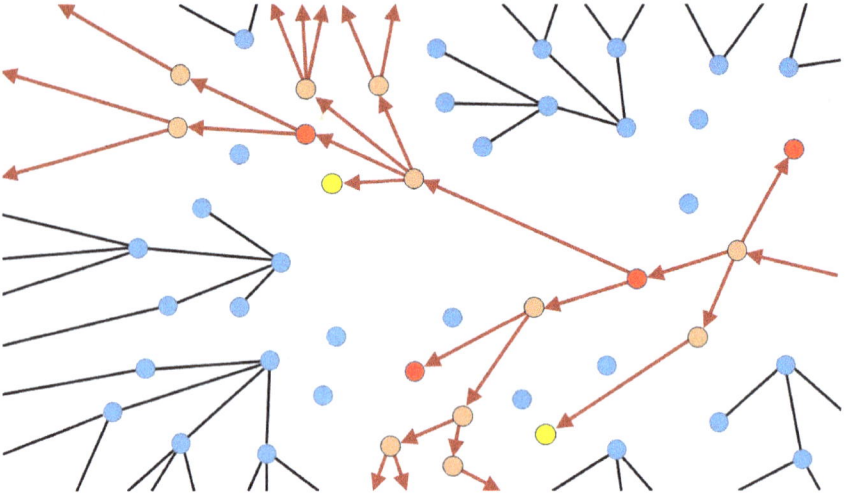

Fig. 19.14   Shayanne goes into quarantine.

Bob: Elaine and Eduardo were only in the exposed state when they got tested. Did you want to show in your example they had been infected only very recently and the test was not sensitive enough to already show an infection?

Alice: Yes, this is what I wanted to show. It will happen frequently when a test is taken too early.

Frank: OK, false negatives of tests given too early may be a problem. So how about waiting a few days longer before contacts are being tested?

Alice: Then it may be too late for cutting the chains of transmissions that have been started by those who are already infectious when they are identified as close contacts.

Cindy: Perhaps each closed contact should get tested twice: right away, and then maybe 5–7 days later?

Alice: The Robert Koch Institute, the German counterpart of the CDC, makes exactly this recommendation for their country.[105] If the second test comes back positive after the first one was false negative, it triggers a new case investigation and new contact tracing effort. The idea here is to find as many cases as possible.

Frank: So, will contacts who test negative twice then be released from quarantine in Germany?

Alice: Actually, no.

Frank: Why not?

Alice: It seems to me that the Robert Koch Institute prefers to be overly cautious rather than accept a small risk of some chains of infections being propagated by people with two false negative tests. We need to keep in mind that the numbers of daily new cases in Germany are currently very low. This also makes the cost of perhaps somewhat excessive quarantines very low on the scale of the entire country. By being super cautious, the Robert Koch Institute hopes to keep these numbers as low as they are.

Bob: I see. By having low numbers to begin with, they can spend more resources on each single case. If this keeps the numbers down, the overall cost will then also be low. And they may need fewer restrictions on the economy.

Alice: Yes, I believe this is how their reasoning goes. If we had as few cases per million in the U.S. as they do, we could perhaps take the same approach. But with our numbers being as high as they are, this may not be feasible.

Bob: So, our numbers are likely to stay high for much longer because they are so high right now and we may not have the testing and contact tracing capacity per case that would bring them down more. What a Catch-22!

Cindy: And many more people will suffer and die because of this. What a shame!

Alice: Yes, it's a terrible situation, and it makes me very sad. I wish our country would have done a lot better. It was possible.

Today I have shown you how some options for contact tracing and testing work. At least in principle. In the real world, the situation is more complicated than in my pictures.

Scientists study how effective various options are. The CDC and similar institutions around the world translate the findings of the research into specific recommendations. They also need to take into account how much testing and contact tracing can be done with the available resources. As the situation on the ground changes and as we gradually learn more about how Covid-19 actually spreads, the particular policy recommendations may change as well.

Endnotes

[99] See [1] for information on the shortage of contact tracers in the U.S. in early August. Updates on the numbers of contact tracers in the U.S. can be found at [2].

[100] See [3] for the complete definition of the CDC.

[101] Based on first-hand knowledge of the author who participated in such discussions.

[102] A variety of digital contact tracing tools is available worldwide. Adoption rates significantly differ from country to country; see, for example, [4]. While most of the available technology is based on voluntary adoption, South Korea used phones and credit card data to trace prior movements of confirmed cases and find their contacts. Where they walked before they fell ill was broadcast to the cell phones of everyone who was nearby [5]. This approach appears to have significantly contributed to the country's success in quickly bringing its outbreak in early spring under control.

[103] For example, a model published in [6] predicts that across ranges of parameter values consistent with dynamics of SARS-CoV-2, backward tracing is expected to identify a primary case generating 3–10 times more infections than average, typically increasing the proportion of subsequent cases averted by a factor of 2–3.

[104] On August 24, 2020, shortly after this conversation took place, the CDC dropped the recommendation that close contacts of confirmed Covid-19 cases be tested [7]. This change appears to have been made in response to political pressure and provoked an outcry in the scientific community [8]. By September 18, 2020, the

CDC again was recommending that close contacts be tested even if they remained asymptomatic [9].

[105] Based on information obtained from [10] and [11] on August 27, 2020. The numbers of cases in Germany have gone up in the meantime, and the policy appears to have changed as a result.

References

[1] Simmons-Duffins S. Coronavirus cases are surging. The contact tracing workforce is not. National Public Radio 2020 Aug 7. [cited 2020 Dec 14]. https://www.npr.org/sections/health-shots/2020/08/07/899954832/coronavirus-cases-are-surging-the-contact-tracing-workforce-is-not

[2] Johns Hopkins University of Medicine. Coronavirus Resource Center. Contact tracing: Center for Health Security/NPR state survey. [cited 2020 Dec 14]. https://coronavirus.jhu.edu/contact-tracing/state-survey-results

[3] Centers for Disease Control and Prevention. COVID-19. Contact tracing: Frequently asked questions. [updated 2020 Oct 21; cited 2021 Jan 4]. https://www.cdc.gov/coronavirus/2019-ncov/php/contact-tracing-faq.html

[4] Statista. Adoption of government endorsed COVID-19 contact tracing apps in selected countries as of July 2020. [cited 2020 Dec 14]. https://www.statista.com/statistics/1134669/share-populations-adopted-covid-contact-tracing-apps-countries/

[5] McNeil Jr DG. The virus can be stopped, but only with harsh steps, experts say. The New York Times 2020 Mar 22. [updated 2020 Mar 25; cited 2020 Dec 14]. https://www.nytimes.com/2020/03/22/health/coronavirus-restrictions-us.html

[6] Endo A, Centre for the Mathematical Modelling of Infectious Diseases COVID-19 Working Group, Leclerc QJ, Knight GM, Medley GF, Atkins KE, Funk S, Kucharski AJ. Implication of backward contact tracing in the presence of overdispersed transmission in COVID-19 outbreaks. Wellcome Open Res. 2020 Oct 13. [cited 2020 Jan 4]; 5:239.

`https://www.ncbi.nlm.nih.gov/pmc/articles/`
`PMC7610176/` DOI: 10.12688/wellcomeopenres.16344.1

[7] Gumbrecht J, Fox M, Michael Nedelman M. Updated CDC guidelines now say people exposed to coronavirus may not need to be tested. CNN 2020 Aug 26. [cited 2020 Dec 14]. `https://www.cnn.com/2020/08/26/health/`
`cdc-guidelines-coronavirus-testing/index.html`

[8] Stolberg SG. Top U.S. officials told C.D.C. to soften coronavirus testing guidelines. The New York Times 2020 Aug 26. [updated 2020 Sep 2; cited 2020 Dec 14].
`https://www.nytimes.com/2020/08/26/us/politics/`
`coronavirus-testing-trump-cdc.html`

[9] Gumbrecht J, Fox M, Howard J. CDC updates, again, guidelines on testing people without coronavirus symptoms. CNN 2020 Sep 18. [cited 2020 Dec 14].
`https://www.cnn.com/2020/09/18/health/covid-testing-`
`guidance-update-cdc-bn/index.html`

[10] Robert Koch Institute. Coronavirus SARS-CoV-2. Nationale Teststrategie–wer wird in Deutschland auf das Vorliegen einer SARS-CoV-2 Infektion getestet? [cited 2020 Aug 27].
`https://www.rki.de/DE/Content/InfAZ/N/Neuartiges_`
`Coronavirus/Teststrategie/Nat-`
`Teststrat.html?nn=13490888`

[11] Robert Koch Institute. Coronavirus SARS-CoV-2. Kontaktpersonen-Nachverfolgung bei Infektionen durch SARS-CoV-2. [cited 2020 Aug 27].
`https://www.rki.de/DE/Content/InfAZ/N/Neuartiges_`
`Coronavirus/Kontaktperson/Management.html#`
`doc13516162bodyText3`

Chapter 20

How can we safely socialize?

Alice, Bob, Cindy, and Frank meet on August 18, 2020. The preventive measures against the spread of Covid-19 have drastically altered social life and are affecting people's mental health and well-being. With many people confined to their own homes during much of the day, there has been a worldwide surge of domestic violence. In the U.S., symptoms of depression are three times more prevalent than before the pandemic. In Japan—a country that has been very successful fighting Covid-19—after an initial decrease at the beginning of the pandemic, suicide rates are increasing over the summer.[106]

Frank: I can see now why this social distancing makes sense. But wearing a mask and staying six feet apart when I'm with good friends? Give me a break!

Bob: Well, I think with friends we still want to be careful. But within our family, with people who live in the same household? This would be impractical. On the other hand, what if an elderly person who is especially at risk lives in the household? Should the others then keep a distance from that person?

Cindy: But grandma needs a hug once in a while! And how about me and my boyfriend? We have been together for almost two years. We want to be intimate, but I am so scared that one of us might catch coronavirus from the other. That would be so awful!

Alice: You all brought up important questions. There are rules and guidelines for what to do in public. But in our private lives, we need to exercise common sense and make our own decisions.

Today I want to talk about an important concept that will help us in deciding wisely.

Bob: But don't make it too abstract.

Alice: Let's start with households. As you said, it's simply impractical for people to socially distance inside their own home. So we need to think about ourselves and the family members who live with us as a unit. If one of us gets Covid-19, then there is a high likelihood that our entire family will become infected. We need to accept that we are all in this together.

Cindy: So how can I then protect my family, especially grandma?

Alice: The best way of keeping our entire family safe is to strictly adhere to social distancing and mask wearing when we meet people from outside our own homes. And wash our hands thoroughly as soon as we get home.

Then we don't need to stay away from other members of our household. It is also the best way to care for grandma. If she lives with us, let's not keep a distance from her; this would only make her feel isolated. She does need a hug once in a while. We all do.

Bob: But what if a member of the household had a close contact with an infected person?

Alice: Then this member of the household should quarantine her- or himself in a separate room and maintain only absolutely minimal contact with others for the recommended time. We discussed this earlier when we talked about isolation and quarantine.

There is no guarantee that this quarantine will prevent the spread of Covid-19 to others in the same household. Some transmissions may already have happened before the close contact became known. But there is a reasonable chance that it will work and protect the entire family.

Cindy: And how about me and my boyfriend? We are very close, but we don't live together.

Alice: The same principle applies when we are with our romantic partner. We humans need intimacy, including sexual intimacy. Think about you and your partner as forming a unit, even if you don't live in the same household. If one of you contracts Covid-19, the partner probably will also catch it. You are in this together.

The best way to protect each other is not to reduce intimacy with your partner, but to socially distance from everybody else. Spend *more* time alone with your partner. Either your relationship will grow stronger, or you will find out that you are not meant for each other.

Frank: But we also need a group of friends. Not everybody has a partner. Even those in stable relationships want to meet with other people once it a while. And not only with their friends. College isn't only about taking classes, it's also about meeting new people!

Alice: I agree. The time in college offers great opportunities for broadening our horizons: Meeting new people, listening to their ideas, and having interesting discussions with them. Would these new acquaintances be the close friends you want to hang out with on a Saturday evening when you are relaxing, Frank?

Frank: Not exactly. Some of them may become close friends later. But not right away. I was thinking mostly about getting together with my old buddies, relaxing over a beer at my place and not worrying about those damn masks and keeping six feet apart.

Alice: Let us think about it this way: We all have people in our immediate social circles. These are sometimes called social bubbles, and I like this expression.[107]

Such a social bubble may be a household, a couple in an intimate relationship, or a group of close friends. When we meet with people within our social bubbles, we don't want to wear protective masks; neither social masks nor cloth masks. We want to relax, be completely ourselves, and feel close to them. It would be unnatural to practice social distancing and to wear masks when we are interacting *only* with other people in our social bubbles.

These are also the people we care about most. So here is what we can do to protect all of them: Let us each think really carefully about who is in our social bubbles and who isn't. Make sure we only let people into our social bubbles who care about each other and whom we can trust. Then discuss protection against Covid-19 with the other members of the bubble and try to reach an agreement.

Bob: Seems you want us to say: "We want to be close to each other, so we will not socially distance when among ourselves. If one of us gets Covid-19, then probably all of us will catch it. We are in this together. So, in order to protect all of us, we will meticulously practice social distancing with all others who are not in our group."

Alice: Yes, something like this. Each of us needs to say it in our own words.

Bob: I have my doubts whether people could reach such an agreement and would keep their promises.

Alice: Whether or not one's close friends and family members would behave responsibly outside of the bubble is a complicated and very personal question. I cannot answer it for you; each of us will need to use our own judgment. Mutual trust is key.

That's why you need to make conscious decisions about who is and who isn't in your bubble. Keep it very small; not more than 4–5 people, I would say.[108] Then spend more time with people in your social bubbles. Spend less time with people outside of them. Practice social distancing and wear masks when you do. This will protect your partners, close friends, and family members. It will allow you to be close to them without putting them into too much danger.

If a member of a social bubble gets sick, all members of it should quarantine themselves for two weeks. In the case of a household, the one who shows symptoms should also immediately isolated him- or herself in a separate room.

Frank: Even if all of this were possible, how would it keep us safe?

Alice: Very good question, Frank! Nothing will keep us 100% safe from Covid-19 infections. But let us consider the What-If scenario of restricting our close contacts to our social bubbles and explore why it would keep us reasonably safe.

Let me show you a picture of a population of 25 people, each of whom belongs to a social bubble—a household, a couple of partners, or a social group of close friends. These bubbles are shown as ellipses:

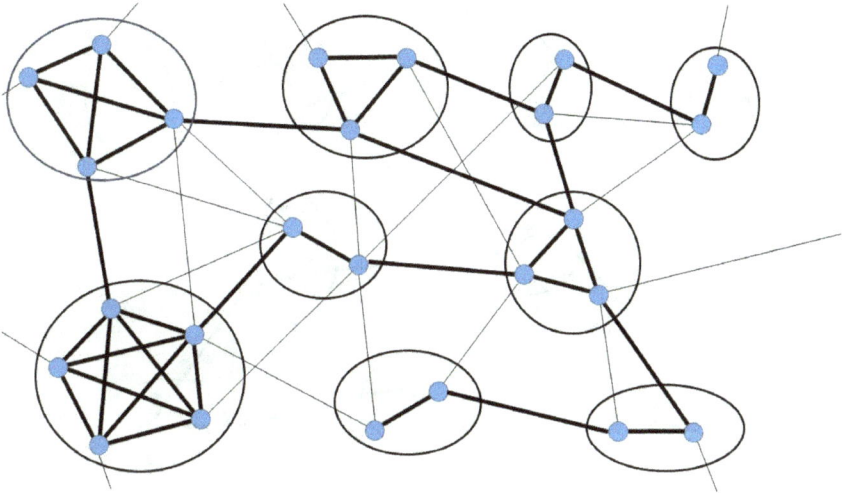

Fig. 20.1 Social bubbles and some contacts in a population of 25 people who don't practice social distancing.

As we discussed earlier, there will normally be lots of contacts between members of the population and with other people outside of it. Most will be low-intensity, some will be high-intensity. I have shown here most of the high-intensity contacts over some time interval, and a few low-intensity contacts.

As we discussed, people normally interact a lot within their social bubbles. In my picture, I have assumed that each member of each social bubble had high-intensity contacts with all other members of the same social bubble. As before, I have drawn these contacts as thick lines.

Cindy: But there are also high-intensity contacts between people from different bubbles!

Alice: Right! The picture shows the contacts without any social distancing. Like in normal times, pre-Covid-19.

Now assume one member of this population, let's call him Ingham again, becomes infected through a contact with somebody outside of the population. This would most often happen through a high-intensity contact, but occasionally also through a low-intensity contact, as in my second picture:

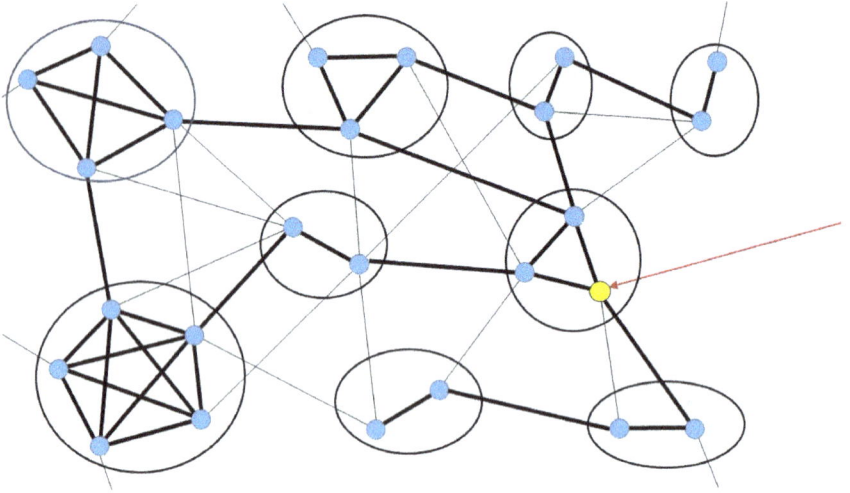

Fig. 20.2   Ingham becomes infected by somebody outside the population.

My next picture shows how the infection might spread through this population when nobody follows recommendations about social distancing, isolation, and quarantine:

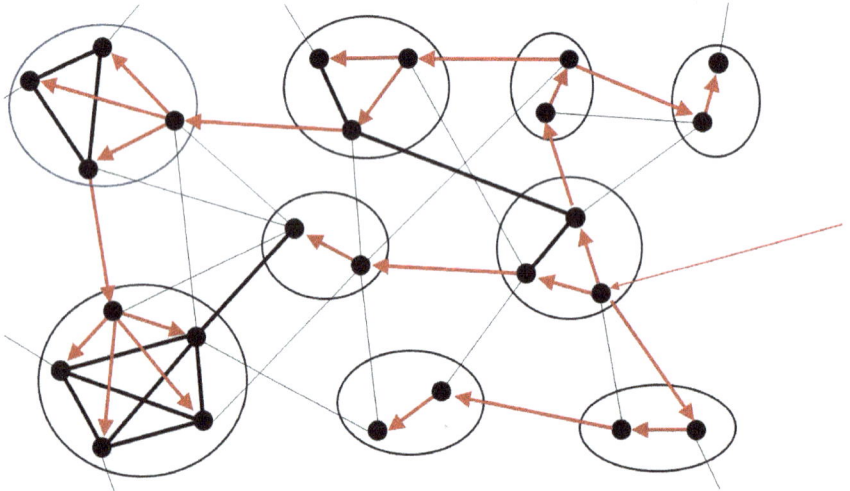

Fig. 20.3   Spread of the outbreak started by Ingham without social distancing or quarantining.

Not all high-intensity contacts between infectious and susceptible persons will be effective and lead to transmissions. But many of them will be, especially the contacts within the social bubbles.

Cindy: All members of the population became infected. This is terrible. They should at least have followed the recommendations for isolation and quarantine!

Alice: Now let's see what might happen if people were quarantining and isolating themselves as recommended by the CDC. I will again assume that nobody practiced social distancing outside their bubbles as long as they had no information of any of their close contacts being infected.

The next picture shows the first steps of the spread of the infection. I assumed that Ingham, our index case, remained asymptomatic. In this situation, nobody went into quarantine so far:

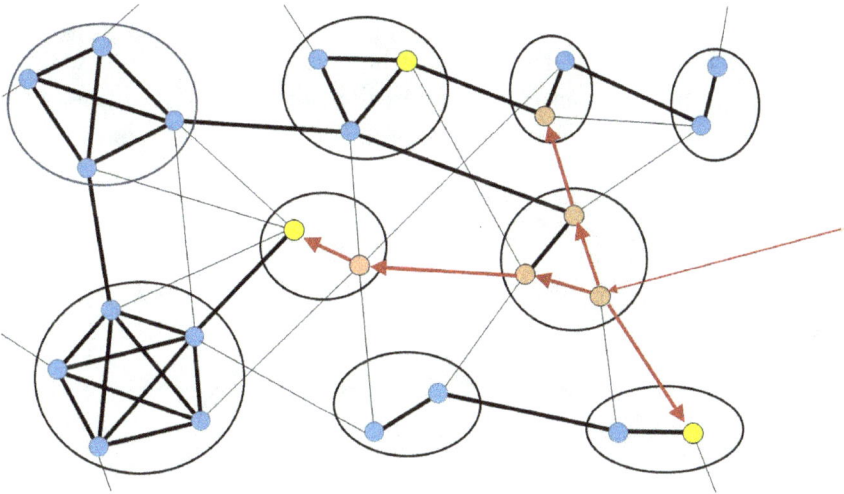

Fig. 20.4 The first steps in the spread of the infection. Nobody went into isolation or quarantine so far.

Asymptomatic cases are shown again in pink salmon color. Later one of them may develop symptoms; let's call him Symon again. He is shown in a bright red in my next picture, and all members of his bubble will quarantine themselves:

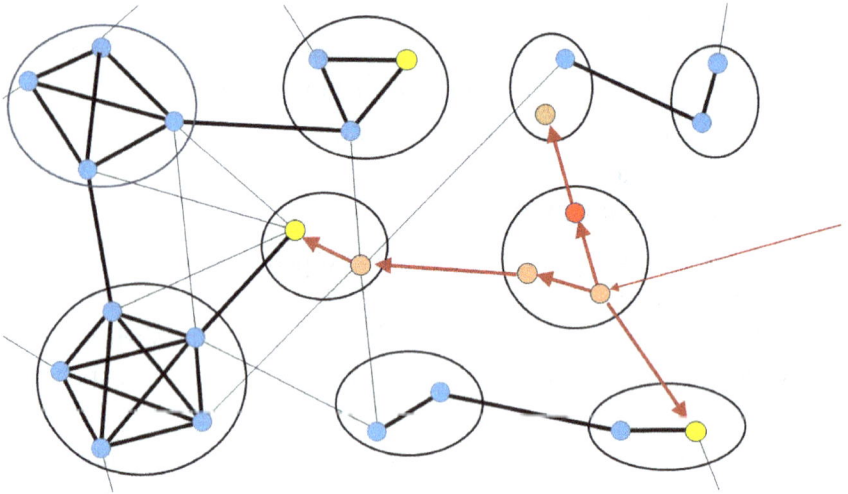

Fig. 20.5   Symon developed symptoms and his close contacts quarantined themselves.

If Symon takes a test, the person who was infected by him will be notified through contact tracing and will also go into quarantine. But the infection will spread further:

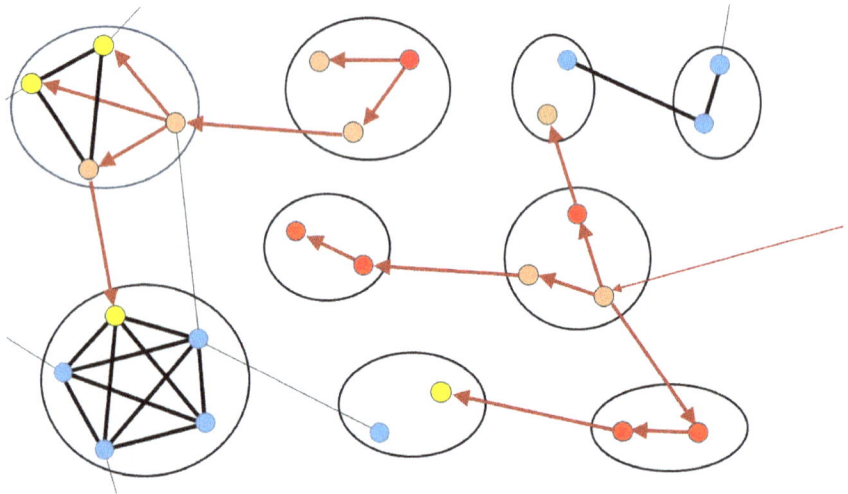

Fig. 20.6   Next steps in the spread of the infection. More people became symptomatic or tested positive and isolated themselves, while their close contacts went into quarantine.

Bob: Is that because in Fig. 20.5 of your example, it had already spread beyond the members of Symon's close contacts that are now in quarantine?

Alice: Yes. Over time, more cases will become symptomatic, which will trigger more isolations and quarantines.

Cindy: Let me see whether I got this right. I will look at the infected person in the middle bubble in the lowest row of your last picture (Fig. 20.6). Can I call her Ellen?

Alice: Sure.

Cindy: So Ellen has learned that she had a close contact with somebody who is now infected and has quarantined herself. She has cut the close contact with her partner for a while. Since so far she is only in the exposed state and not infectious, she has not yet infected her partner, who is now safe.

Alice: Right! This is what I wanted to show in this picture.

Frank: Wait a sec! People would normally alert others in the same social bubble when they start having symptoms. But Ellen got infected through a close contact with somebody outside of her bubble. So it is not clear whether she would actually have learned about that person's illness.

Alice: Very important point, Frank! For close contacts with infected people outside of our social bubbles, we would normally learn about the possible exposure only through testing and contact tracing.

In my pictures, I have assumed that all symptomatic people take tests and all the ones who had close contacts with them that connect different bubbles are alerted through contact tracing. In real life, this will not always work out.

Bob: When I look at the pictures in this example, I see that all four people who remained protected so far were spared infection thanks to contact tracing at some step in the chains of transmissions. I guess this shows how important testing and contact tracing are, and how important it is that test results come back quickly.

Alice: Good point, Bob!

Ingham will eventually recover, but the infection will spread further in the bubbles on the left:

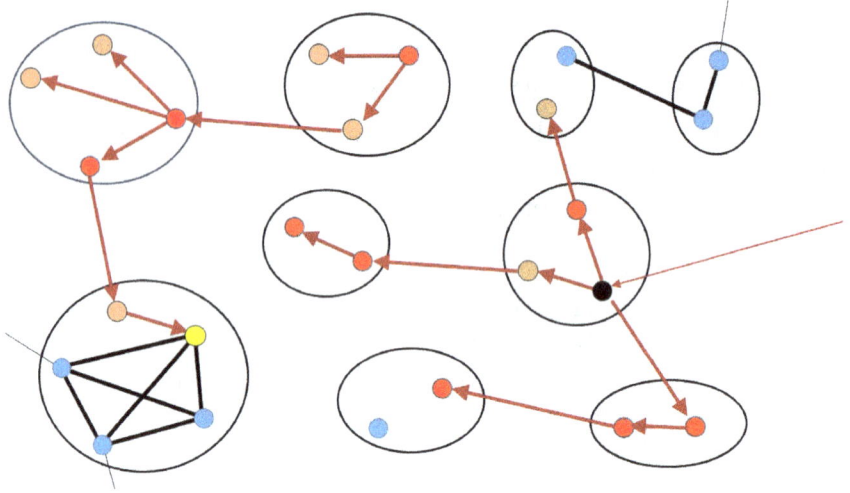

Fig. 20.7   Ingham recovers while new infections spread.

Let's think of the bubble in the lower left corner as a household and call the infectious person in this family Carlos. When Carlos learns through contact tracing about his potential exposure, he will quarantine himself in a separate room.

But in our example, Carlos has already transmitted the infection to another member of this household; call her Gabriela. When Carlos develops symptoms, all family members will socially distance. But the infection may have already spread further within this household.

Cindy: So, if there is an especially vulnerable member of this household, like Carlos' grandma, she may become infected!

Alice: If only Carlos—the household member who got notified of the contact—goes into quarantine, there is no control over how the infection might spread among other people in the family. In my example on the next picture, only one household member was spared infection, and we don't know whether this was Carlos' grandma:

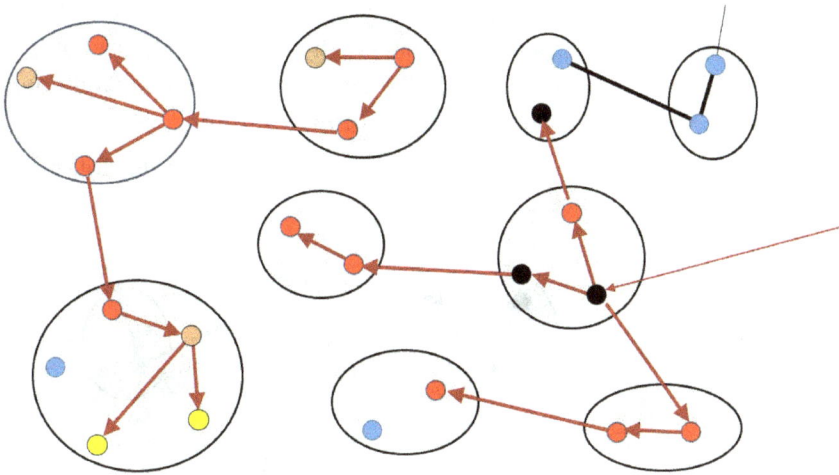

Fig. 20.8   Gabriela has infected others in her family.

But if Carlos' grandma quarantines herself as soon as Carlos does, there is a better chance that she will escape infection:

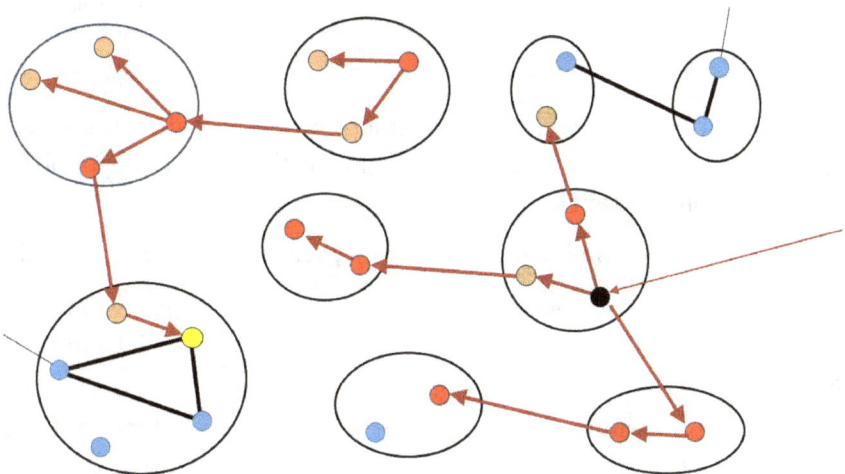

Fig. 20.9   Both Carlos and his grandma go into quarantine.

Quarantining all family members may be impractical. However, if there is an especially vulnerable person living in the household, it would be advisable to also isolate this person from all other members of the household while one of them is in quarantine.

In this modified version of our example, we will get the following outcome:

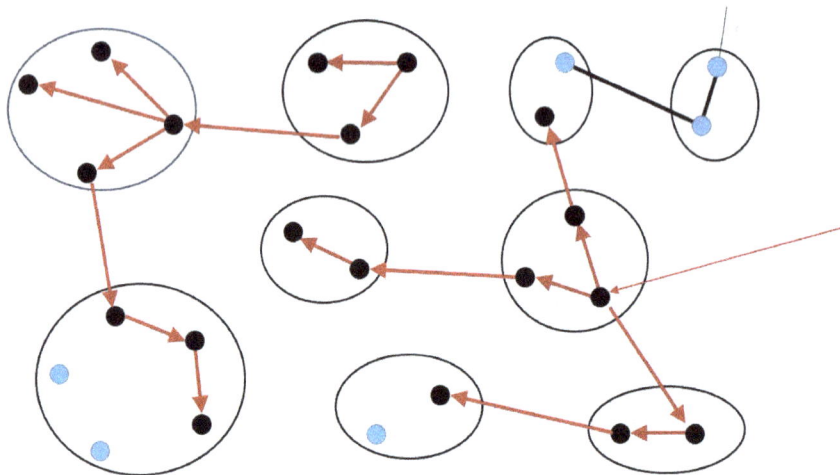

Fig. 20.10   Spread of the outbreak started by Ingham with quarantining but no social distancing.

We can see that quarantines of contacts identified through contact tracing or through direct communication within the social bubbles helped to some extent.

Cindy: But still 19 of the 25 people in your example got infected!

Alice: This is because so far, we have assumed that people will maintain all their normal social contacts outside of their social bubbles, as in our first picture (Fig. 20.1).

But now let's assume that people cut unnecessary contacts outside their social bubbles and turn the high-intensity contacts between different bubbles into low-intensity contacts by wearing masks and practicing social distancing:

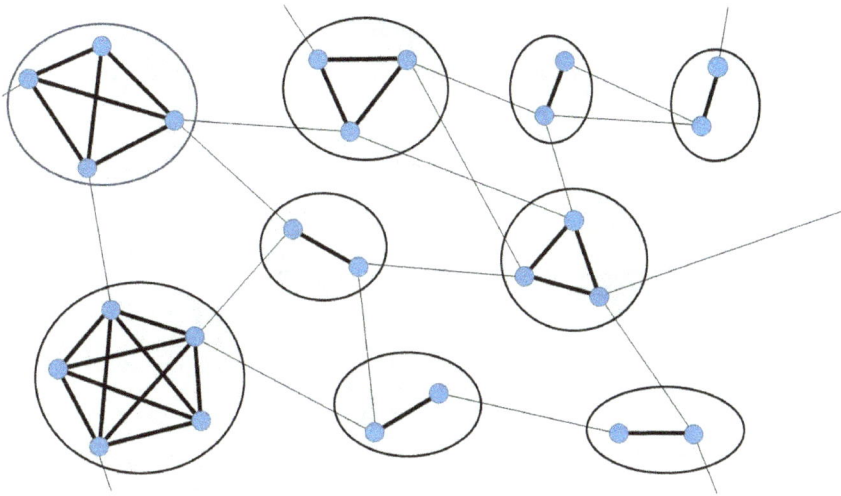

Fig. 20.11 Social bubbles and some contacts in a population of 25 people who practice social distancing outside their bubbles.

Bob: Couldn't then an infection still enter a bubble through a low-intensity outside contact? Like this:

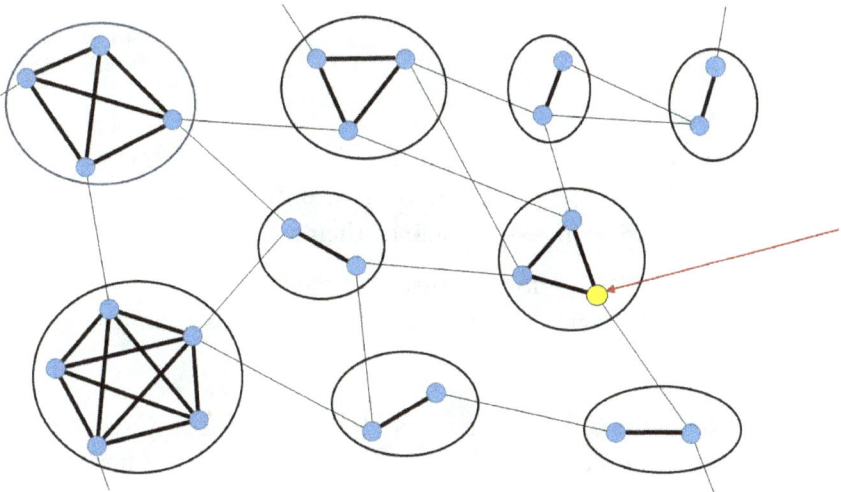

Fig. 20.12 Ingham becomes infected by somebody outside the population.

Alice: Yes, this will occasionally happen.

Cindy: And wouldn't the infection then spread inside the bubble as before?

Alice: Yes, but most likely not beyond the people inside this particular social bubble:

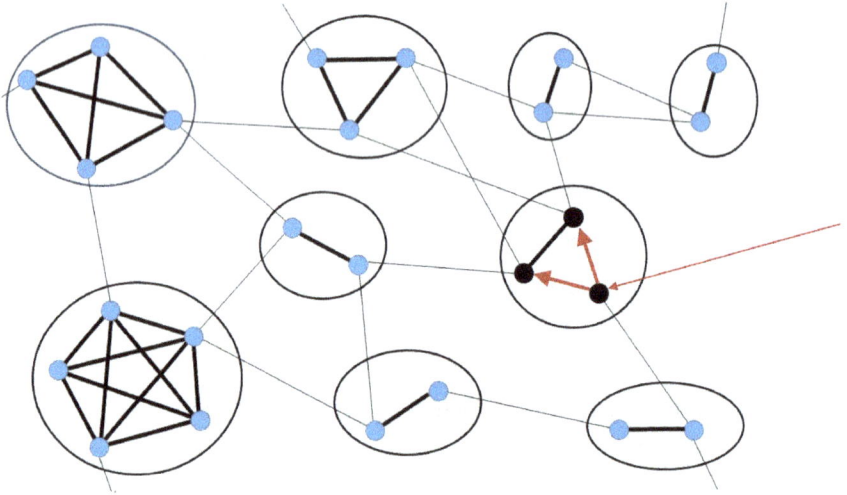

Fig. 20.13 Spread of the outbreak started by one index case with social distancing outside the bubbles.

We can see how people in all other bubbles have protected themselves, their close friends, and their families by practicing social distancing and wearing masks outside of their bubbles.

Cindy: I still feel sorry for the three people in this bubble. But this outcome is much, much better than in the previous examples.

Bob: Neat!

Frank: Too neat, if you ask me. In all these pictures, there was no overlap between different social bubbles. But in reality, there would be. Each of us is normally a member of several social bubbles. Even romantic couples will sometimes take a break from each other and hang out with their other friends. And all of us have social bubbles at home in addition to the ones at college. Especially our families.

Alice: Very important point, Frank! To illustrate how bubbles can prevent the spread of an infection, I've shown you examples for the simplest case when the bubbles don't overlap.

But you are right: Most people would naturally be in several social bubbles. As long as each of us keeps the number of these bubbles small, the same principle still works, although not quite as well as when there is no overlap.

Cindy: So how many different bubbles can a person have and still be safe?

Alice: There are no official guidelines for this. Each person's situation is slightly different, and we need to use common sense. The fewer bubbles, the better. But I think that up to 3 bubbles per person might still keep everybody reasonably safe.[109]

Frank: Why? Then the virus could spread from bubble to bubble through close contacts.

Alice: True. But the principle still can work because we interact with the people from different bubbles at different times.

Let's look at the example of two people in a romantic relationship; call them Joe and Marilyn. They see each other every day, but on Friday night they take a break. Marilyn meets with her three best friends for dinner, and Joe hangs out with his two best buddies for a few beers. Once every few weeks, both go home and visit their families. Each of them spends time in a closely knit household of five.

Cindy: So Marilyn and Joe have 3 social bubbles each?

Alice: Right. My next picture will show this social structure, with Marilyn's bubbles on the left, and Joe's on the right

Notice that the members of each bubble practice social distancing outside of their bubbles, but will typically also belong to several bubbles, some of which are partially shown in the picture:

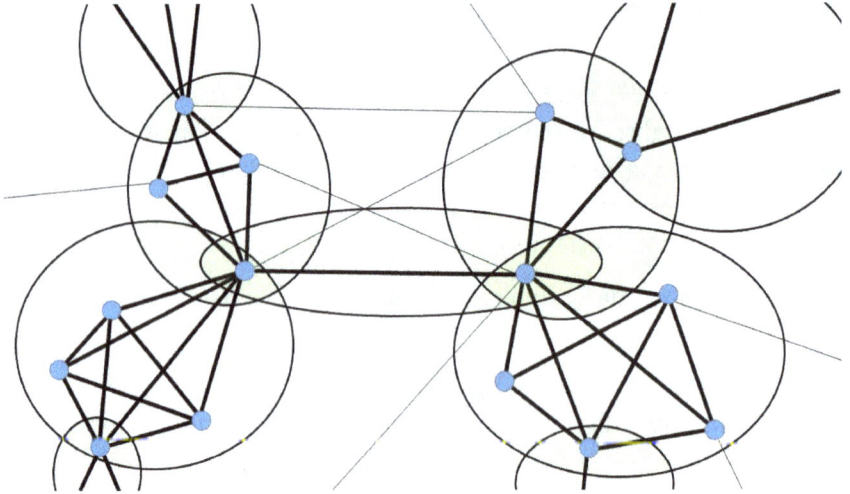

Fig. 20.14 Marilyn's social bubbles are shown on the left, Joe's social bubbles are shown on the right.

Now assume Joe gets infected on a Monday through contact with somebody outside his social bubbles:

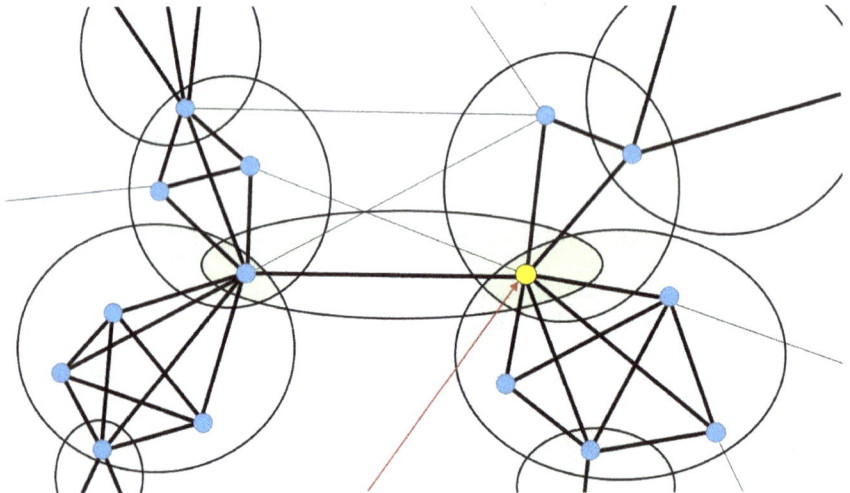

Fig. 20.15 Joe becomes exposed on a Monday.

By Friday, he may have become infectious and transmitted the virus
to Marilyn, but he may still be asymptomatic. On Friday night,
when he meets with his buddies, he will most likely infect them. But
Marilyn is still not infectious at this time and will not infect her
friends over dinner:

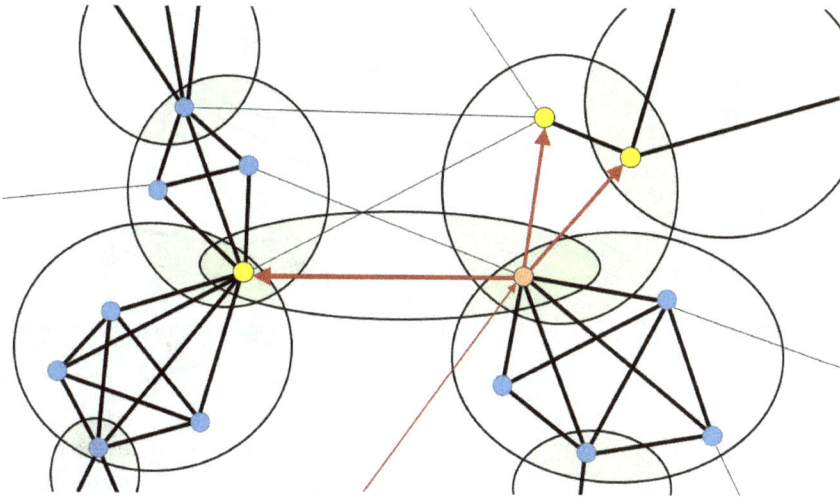

Fig. 20.16   Joe infects his buddies on Friday, but Marilyn is still not infectious.

On Sunday, Joe may have taken a test after developing symptoms,
and learned about his infection. He will tell Marilyn and his buddies
about his infection. They will quarantine themselves.

Bob: Should Joe's family at home also go into quarantine?

Alice: Not if it has been at least two weeks since his last visit.

Bob: Marilyn may be infectious by then. Could she already have
infected other people?

Alice: In my example, she did not interact with her other social bubbles over those two days; and she is unlikely to have infected someone
else through a low-intensity contact. Similarly, Joe's two buddies will
still not be infectious by the time they quarantine themselves. In this
example, the infection will not spread beyond two social bubbles:

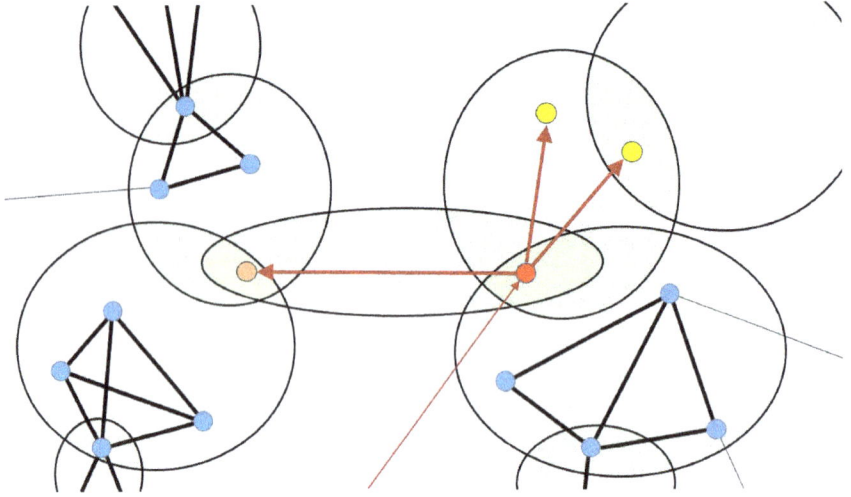

Fig. 20.17   On Sunday, Joe isolates himself. Marilyn and Joe's buddies go into quarantine.

If on that Friday night Joe and Marilyn had gone to a large party without social distancing and wearing masks instead of relaxing with close friends in their social bubbles, the picture might look like this:

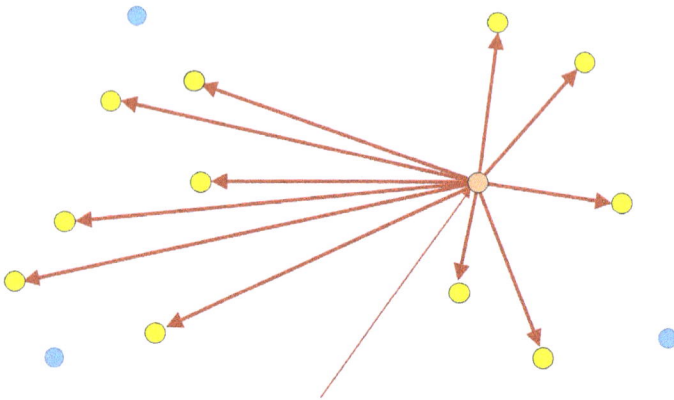

Fig. 20.18   Joe and Marilyn attended a large party without social distancing on Friday night.

Cindy: This would have been terrible! But I still feel sorry for Marilyn, Joe, and his buddies even in the example where they stay in their social bubbles.

Alice: Every Covid-19 infection is unfortunate. But we cannot give up social life altogether.

Cindy: Then we should spend more time in our social bubbles.

Bob: And strictly practice social distancing outside of them. This will keep our partners, close friends, and families reasonably safe. And we can fully enjoy their company.

Frank: Let me say this much: When it comes to socializing in the time of corona, so far I had only been hearing "Don't, don't, don't!" Of course people will not comply if they only hear "Don't!" Thanks, Alice, for your sensible explanation of how it can be done safely. Truly appreciate it.

Endnotes

[106] A Wikipedia article [1] gives useful pointers to references on increased domestic violence during the Covid-19 pandemic in over 30 countries around the world. For a study of symptoms of depression in the U.S., see [2]. Suicide rates in Japan during the pandemic were investigated in [3].

[107] Social bubbles are sometimes also called "social pods." Also, the literature usually makes a distinction between households and social bubbles. Here households are treated as examples of social bubbles, which should make it more transparent how they contribute to limiting the spread of Covid-19.

[108] It should be emphasized that Alice is giving a personal opinion here that is based on common sense. While there is some research that supports effectiveness of social bubbles in limiting the spread of Covid-19 [4,5], there is also skepticism on whether the concept can work in practice [6]. In the U.S., there are no official recommendations of the CDC or the federal government on forming social bubbles [6]. New Zealand, a country that has

been extremely successful in controlling Covid-19, encourages social bubbles [7], and there is also support for social bubbles by regional governments elsewhere. The guidelines for the Canadian province of Ontario specify that a social bubble may contain up to 10 people, but that there can be no overlap between different bubbles [8]. In the U.K., there are separate rules for England, Scotland, Wales, and Northern Ireland. Their common feature is allowing two separate households to form one bubble [9].

[109] Again, it needs to be emphasized that Alice is giving a personal opinion here. It is based on common sense and to some extent supported by theoretical research [5]. But it does not concur with existing public health recommendations (see previous item).

References

[1] Wikipedia: The free encyclopedia. Wikimedia Foundation, Inc. Impact of the COVID-19 pandemic on domestic violence. [cited 2020 Dec 13]. `https://en.wikipedia.org/wiki/Impact_of_the_COVID-19_pandemic_on_domestic_violence`

[2] Ettman CK, Abdalla SM, Cohen GH, Sampson L, Vivier PM, Galea S. Prevalence of depression symptoms in US adults before and during the COVID-19 pandemic. JAMA Netw Open 2020 Sep 2. [cited 2020 Dec 13]; 3(9):e2019686. `https://jamanetwork.com/journals/jamanetworkopen/fullarticle/2770146` DOI:10.1001/jamanetworkopen.2020.19686

[3] Ueda M, Nordström R, Matsubayashi T. Suicide and mental health during the COVID-19 pandemic in Japan. medRxiv 2020 Dec 20. [cited 2021 Jan 4]. `https://www.medrxiv.org/content/10.1101/2020.10.06.20207530v5` DOI: 10.1101/2020.10.06.20207530

[4] Leng T, White C, Hilton J, Kucharski A, Pellis L, Stage H, et al. The effectiveness of social bubbles as part of a Covid-19 lockdown exit strategy, a modelling study [version 1; peer review: 1 approved]. Wellcome Open Res. 2020 Sep 10. [cited 2021 Jan

4]; 5:213. https://wellcomeopenresearch.org/articles/5-213/v1 DOI: 10.12688/wellcomeopenres.16164.1

[5] Block P, Hoffman M, Raabe IJ, Beam Dowd J, Rahal C, Kashyap R, et al. Social network-based distancing strategies to flatten the COVID-19 curve in a post-lockdown world. Nat Hum Behav. 2020 Jun 4. [cited 2021 Jan 4]; 588(4)588–596. https://www.nature.com/articles/s41562-020-0898-6 DOI: 10.1038/s41562-020-0898-6

[6] Gutman R. Sorry to burst your quarantine bubble. Pod means something different to everyone, and that's a problem. The Atlantic 2020 Nov 30. [cited 2020 Dec 13]. https://www.theatlantic.com/health/archive/2020/11/pandemic-pod-bubble-concept-creep/617207/

[7] Olmstead M. New Zealand's "bubble concept" is slowly letting people socialize again. Would it work in America? Slate 2020 May 6. [cited 2020 Dec 13]. https://slate.com/news-and-politics/2020/05/new-zealand-quarantine-bubble-concept-america.html

[8] Megan DeLaire. How to bubble: A guide to forming your COVID-19 social circle. toronto.com 2020 Sep 30. [cited 2020 Dec 13]. https://www.toronto.com/news-story/10211656-how-to-bubble-a-guide-to-forming-your-covid-19-social-circle/

[9] Roberts M. Support bubbles: How do they work and who is in yours? BBC News online 2020 November 26. [cited 2020 Dec 13]. https://www.bbc.com/news/health-52637354

Chapter 21

How safe is it to travel?

Alice, Bob, Cindy, and Frank continue their discussion on August 18, 2020. Most people are reluctant to travel during the pandemic, and many popular tourist destinations are inaccessible. In the tourism industry, 120 million jobs are at risk worldwide, with economic damage to this sector likely to exceed over 1 trillion U.S. dollars in 2020 alone [1]. In Europe, many people are taking vacations abroad, though. Greece, a popular destination that had been highly successful at controlling the spread of Covid-19 until mid-summer, saw a more than fourfold increase in the 7-day moving average of daily new infections, from 34 on July 27 to 147 on August 17. Spain, another popular tourist destination, saw an increase of over 130% during the same 3-week period [2].

Cindy: I have another question: Is it safe to travel at all while Covid-19 is still spreading? Especially by airplane? I would be so scared to go on an airplane right now.

Alice: There is an higher risk of becoming infected when we travel. But Covid-19 may be with us for many more months or even years. We cannot give up living a life while the outbreak lasts. So we need to think about the risk in a rational way.

We need to keep in mind that there is some risk of contracting Covid-19 during everyday activities, regardless of where we are. It is usually very small, but not entirely zero. When we travel, while we actually move from one place to another, the risk may be higher. Certainly when we travel by plane, bus, or train.

Airplanes do pose a risk, but it seems smaller than most people believe.[110] They have very good air filters that catch almost all virus particles. Many airlines now have policies of keeping the middle seats empty and requiring all passengers to wear masks. If you do take a plane, make sure to use an airline that has such policies and strictly follows them. Take direct flights when possible. Keep the overhead vent open so that the filtered air blows directly onto you. Then you will inhale the filtered air and not the air exhaled by the passenger sitting next to you. Make sure you disinfect your hands a few times during the flight with hand sanitizer and tissues, especially before touching food or your face.

This will not keep you entirely safe, but the flight puts you at somewhat higher risk only for a few hours. That's usually a very short time compared to the entire trip.

Bob: I would travel by myself in my own car. This seems to be the best way to remain safe from Covid-19.

Alice: Yes, when you travel like this, you will probably be less likely to contract Covid-19 than having a car accident. No activity is entirely risk-free. We can make rational decisions only by weighing one risk against another.

When people think about the dangers of traveling, they usually focus on the mode of transportation. But the more important question is why you travel and what you will do in the place you visit.

If you want to spend a week hiking and camping in the wilderness all by yourself or with a close friend, then definitely go! You will take a slightly higher risk during the few hours in airports and on the plane. But during the remainder of the week, you will be a lot safer from Covid-19 than almost anywhere else.

Frank: I can go hiking in the woods with my buddies right where I live. If I could afford going on a vacation, I would want to see the most wonderful places of this planet and meet new people.

Alice: I am all for this in normal times. But with Covid-19 going around, it may be very risky. Popular tourist hotspots tend to be very crowded. Usually, people eat out in restaurants when on vacation. They meet new people in bars. All of these activities carry a high risk for becoming infected. This is the biggest risk associated with travel.

Popular travel destinations in Europe, such as Spain and Greece, have experienced rapid increases in new infections over the last few weeks. These were in large part caused by young people on vacations who partied a lot. When they returned to their home countries, they brought the virus with them.[111]

Cindy: They should have stayed home and kept everybody safe!

Alice: We all need to thoroughly relax once in a while. I don't want to say: "Don't go on vacation." But going on a vacation can be very dangerous, both to yourself and others whom you might infect. If you do decide to travel, think carefully about your destination and what you want to do there.

If you have a choice between going to a popular place on everybody's must-see list or some less popular place off the beaten path, go to the less popular place. It will likely be less crowded. If you have a choice between going on a tour in the hope of meeting many new people or going somewhere secluded with an old friend whom you haven't seen in years, go with your friend. Spend most of the time just with the friend and reconnect.

Either way, practice social distancing on the trip except with your closest travel companions. They will be in your social bubble on the trip. Avoid the crowds as much as possible and have meals outdoors as much as possible.

Cindy: How about visiting our family? Is this also risky?

Alice: A lot less risky than meeting many new people in crowded tourist spots. But not entirely risk-free. Let us think about these risks in terms of social bubbles. We naturally have most of our intense social contacts within our social bubbles, and these bubbles overlap.

Let me draw you a picture that shows some of the social bubbles at college on the left, and those in your home town on the right. Normally there would be no overlap between the social bubbles on campus and the ones at home. I'll not draw any lines for contacts in this picture. We all remember that with responsible decisions about social distancing and wearing masks, infections will rarely spread between bubbles that do not overlap:

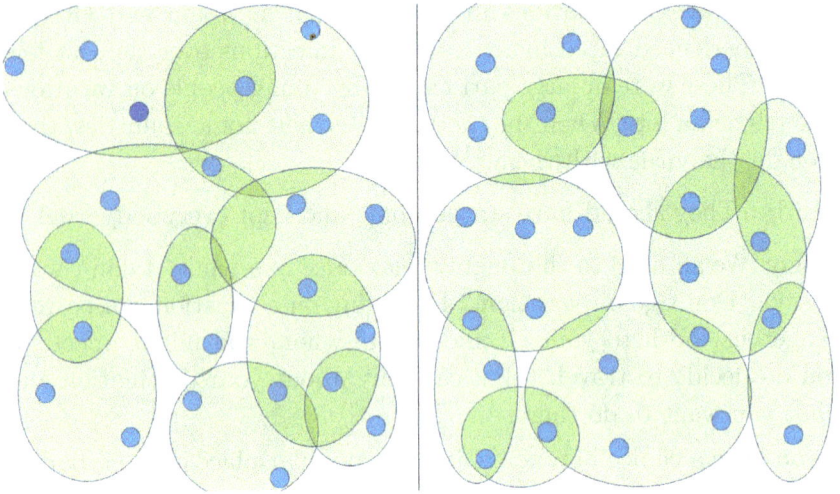

Fig. 21.1   Social bubbles at college and our home town.

But from time to time, an infection through contact with someone outside a social bubble will happen. As in my next picture:

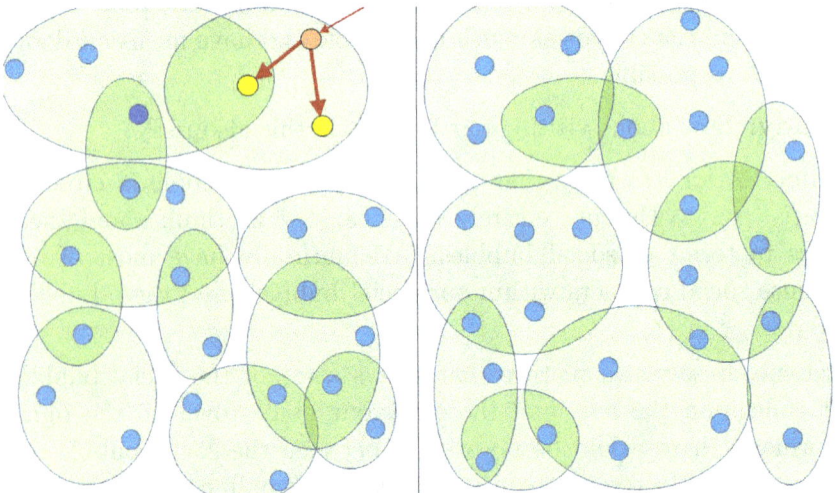

Fig. 21.2   A student got infected.

Infections will quickly spread inside a bubble. They may then enter other bubbles because there is overlap. But since people in different bubbles meet on separate occasions, this will take some time. Eventually, some infected people will become symptomatic and alert the members of their bubbles. With proper quarantining, the spread of the infection can then be confined to a few bubbles. In my first picture (Fig. 21.1), only one other bubble is at immediate high risk.

Now suppose that one of the newly exposed students, call him Travis, travels home. Then one more bubble will contain an infected person, as in the next picture:

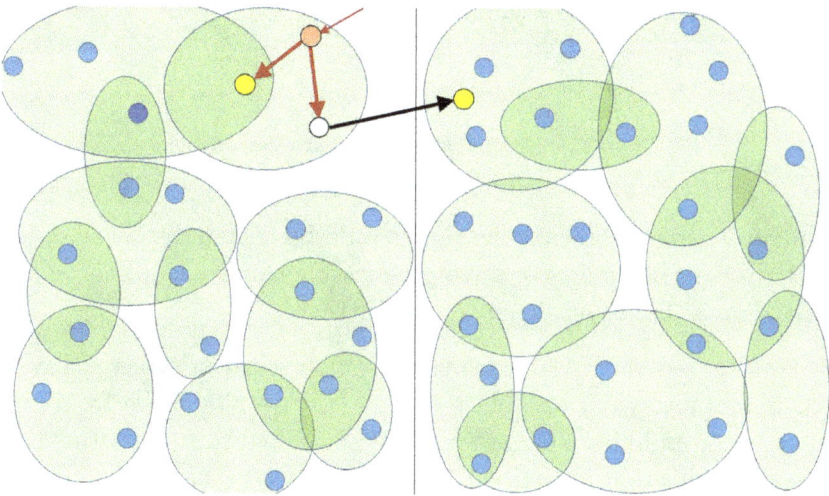

Fig. 21.3   Travis visits his family.

A few days later, the index case may become symptomatic. At this time, further spread can be prevented by quarantine. But even if this works, the infection would have already reached people in additional social bubbles.

Let me share with you one more picture that shows how things may look after Travis' family visit. Without the family visit, at this point in time the infection would have spread to people in 4 social bubbles; with the family visit, it would have reached 6 bubbles total:

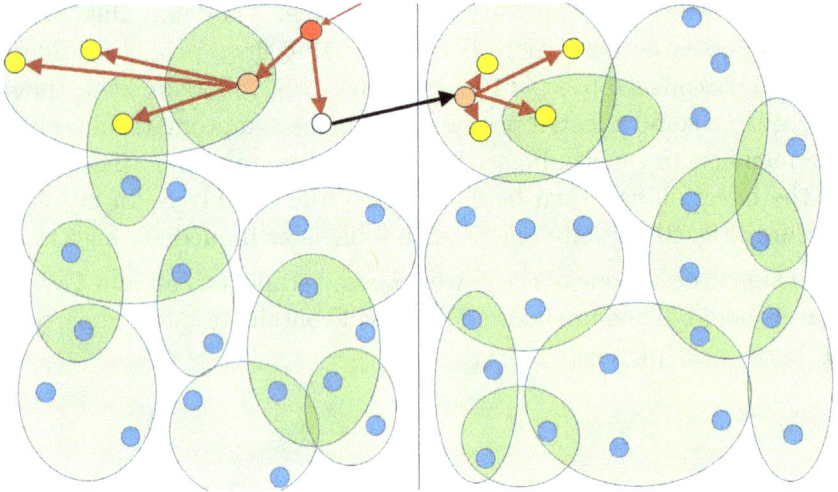

Fig. 21.4 The infection has reached three social bubbles.

Cindy: Travis' bubble on the right would be his family. Some of his relatives may be elderly or have pre-existing conditions. This would make Travis' family visit dangerous for them.

Bob: I can see that. And it would be similar for most types of travel: When we move from one place to another, we also move from one set of social bubbles to another set of social bubbles. And this can spread an infection farther than it would reach otherwise.

Alice: That's correct. I don't recommend giving up travel altogether, but it's dangerous. Avoid unnecessary trips.

If you go on a vacation, think carefully about your destination and what you want to do there. Visit your family, but perhaps less often. During any trip, in the two weeks before you go, and in the two weeks after you return, be super careful with your social contacts.

If you notice any symptoms, or if you had close contact with an infected person shortly before the planned trip, isolate or quarantine yourself, postpone the trip, or cancel it altogether.

This should keep you, your friends, your family, and all of us reasonably safe.

Endnotes

[110] For more detailed information on the the relative risks of traveling by air, see the article [3] in Vox.

[111] Many tourists visiting Greece or Spain came from Germany or the Netherlands. Between July 27 and August 17, the 7-day moving average of daily new infections increased by 110% in Germany, from 556 to 1,169 and by 244% in the Netherlands, from 178 to 613 [2].

References

[1] Richter F. COVID-19 could set the global tourism industry back 20 years. World Economic Forum 2020 Sep 2. [cited 2020 Nov 25]. https://www.weforum.org/agenda/2020/09/pandemic-covid19-tourism-sector-tourism/

[2] Worldometers.info. Dover, Delaware, U.S.A. COVID-19 coronavirus pandemic. [cited 2020 Nov 25].
https://www.worldometers.info/coronavirus/

[3] Belluz B, Resnick B. How risky is air travel in the pandemic? Here's what the science says. Vox 2020 Nov 12. [cited 2020 Nov 25]. https://www.vox.com/21525068/covid-19-airplane-risk-coronavirus-pandemic-airports

Chapter 22

Case numbers are going up, deaths are going down. What to make of it?

Alice, Bob, Cindy, and Frank meet on August 22, 2020. Covid-19 has
already claimed more than 817,000 lives worldwide, but the 7-day moving
average of daily reported deaths have been slightly declining over the last
10 days, from 6,006 on August 11 to 5,781 on August 21. In the U.S., it
has also slightly declined from its second peak of 1,181 on August 4 to
1,027 on August 21 [1].

Bob: A couple of months ago, around June 20, I was talking with
some friends from Arizona and Florida. At that time, the daily
numbers of infections in their states were going up a lot and I thought
that was a very bad sign. But they told me that the numbers of tests
in their states were also increasing, and that this would explain why
more cases were being detected and reported.

Cindy: We already talked about how one can see from changes
in the positivity rate whether or not actual infections increase even
when the number of tests changes.

Bob: I understand this now, but I did not know it back in June.

There is still something from that conversation that bothers me: My
friend from Arizona told me that the reported numbers of deaths
from Covid-19 were staying pretty flat in Arizona, and the guy from
Florida said that they were even trending downward in his state.
Both thought that reported numbers of deaths were much more reliable than test data, and that no action was needed when there was
no increase in the numbers of deaths.

I thought they had a point, because practically all deaths from coronavirus infections are being reported, while only a fraction of people

with infections are tested. But their argument didn't feel quite right. I'm still not sure what to make of the conflicting trends and what I should have replied to my friends.

Alice: We need to remember that all reported numbers give us snapshots of the past. It may take a week from the time of exposure to the time when an infected person gets tested, and then a few more days for the test results to come back and to get recorded. So the reported number of new infections on a given day would tell us about transmissions that might have happened about 10 days earlier.

Frank: That's only if test results come back quickly, within a couple of days. If people have to wait more than a week for their test results, the reported numbers of new cases would show transmissions that happened 3 weeks earlier.

Alice: Important point, Frank! In severe cases that lead to death, the patient typically suffers for a couple of weeks after onset of symptoms before dying.

Cindy: Those last days alone in great pain on the ventilator with no friends and family around for comfort must be so horrible. Just thinking about this makes me cry.

Alice: Yes, Cindy. It is a slow and terrible death. It is heartbreaking to think about what these patients go through. But we need to be aware of what is going on in the hospitals if we want to understand how important it is for each of us to do our part to prevent such suffering.

For our discussion here, we need to realize that, in fatal cases, the average time between exposure and recording of the death is about 1 month. This includes the incubation period, the illness itself, and the time lag between the death and its reporting [2].

So while numbers of reported deaths from Covid-19 for a given day may be fairly accurate,[112] they only give us a picture of transmissions that happened about 1 month earlier.

Cindy: That's about 3 weeks longer than the time lag between the exposure and when the new infection gets reported. Does this mean that if daily numbers of reported new infections will go up, then we should expect daily numbers of reported deaths to go up about 3 weeks later?

Alice: Yes. Around 3 weeks later; it could be a little longer or a little shorter. We would expect a similar time shift for the peaks in these numbers.

Bob: I get it. Did things turn out in Arizona and Florida as predicted?

Alice: We now have data up to August 21, and we can see what happened. Let's see first look at the daily number of reported new infections for Arizona. The trend curve peaked on July 6:

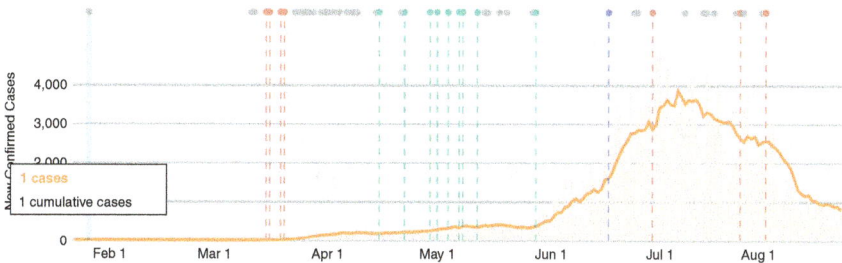

Fig. 22.1 Reported daily new infections in Arizona until August 21 together with closing and opening decisions by the state. The graphs in this chapter were adapted from graphs published by the Coronavirus Resource Center at Johns Hopkins University of Medicine [3, 4].

Cindy: What are the dots and dashed lines in this picture?

Alice: The red ones show the dates when certain restrictions were imposed in this state. The first few of them happened during the gradual start of their lockdown. The green ones show when restrictions were lifted. We can see that Arizona ignored federal guidelines[113] and lifted the lockdown while daily numbers of infections were still increasing.

Frank: I guess they wanted to restart the economy as quickly as possible. Who could blame them?

But it seems to have backfired; they again slapped some restrictions on people a few weeks later, in July and August.

Alice: Now let me show you daily numbers of reported Covid-19 deaths in Arizona:

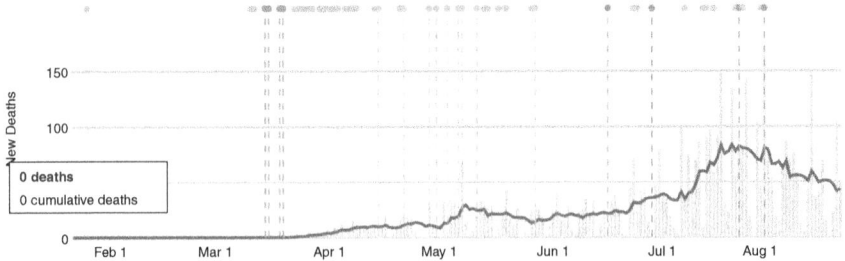

Fig. 22.2   Reported daily deaths from Covid-19 in Arizona until August 21.

You can see that the trend curve for reported deaths peaked later than the trend curve for reported new infections.

Frank: Wait a minute! It peaked on July 18; only 12 days later than the one for reported new cases. This is a much shorter time lag than 3 weeks!

Bob: Could this be because they conducted a lot more tests in the weeks before July 6? If the positivity rate in Arizona peaked earlier than on July 6, then we might get a time lag that is more in line with what Alice and Cindy had predicted.

Alice: Possibly. We will need to look at the graph for testing in Arizona. Let me share it with you (Fig. 22.3).

Frank: The trend curve for Arizona's positivity rate peaked even a few days later than July 6, not a few days earlier. So this doesn't explain why there was so little time lag between the two peaks. The prediction of 3 weeks was definitely off.

Cindy: Perhaps there is another explanation?

Alice: Yes there is, and Frank has already mentioned it.
In our estimate of 3 weeks between the peaks, we had assumed that reported new cases on a given day show transmissions that occurred about 10 days earlier. This would be reasonably accurate if tests

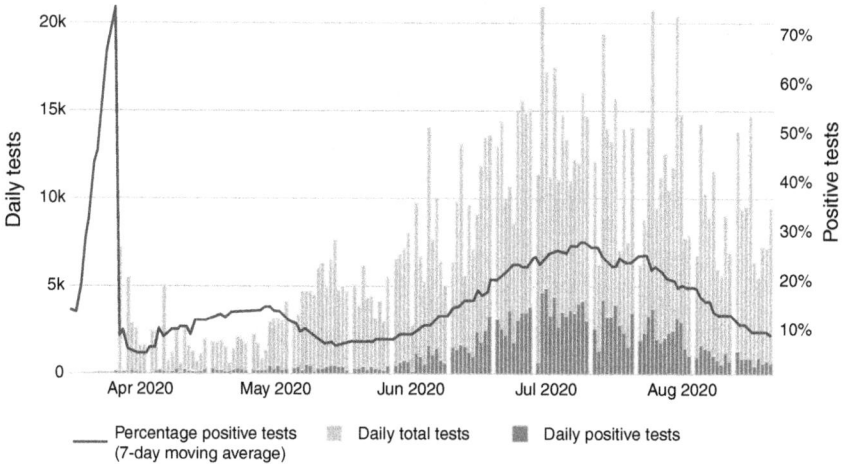

Fig. 22.3 Testing volume and test positivity in Arizona until August 21.

were easily available and their results came back within a couple of days.

But in Arizona, there has been such a shortage of testing capacity that people needed to wait for hours to get tested. This would have discouraged many of them to take a test as soon as they needed one. And they had to wait a long time for their test results [5, 6].

Bob: This made the tests useless. Perhaps this is one reason why Arizona saw such a large increase in the number of new infections.

Frank: Maybe so. In any case, it means that the data on new cases and positivity rate for Arizona in late June really showed transmissions that may have happened 2 to 3 weeks earlier, not 10 days earlier. But the reporting of new deaths from coronavirus would not have been delayed by the shortage tests. So for Arizona, we should have expected a time lag between the two peaks of less than 2 weeks. As we saw in the graphs.

Alice: Right! Now let's look at the data from Florida, where test results came back more quickly than in Arizona. First the daily numbers of reported new infections. In Florida, the trend curve peaked on July 16–17:

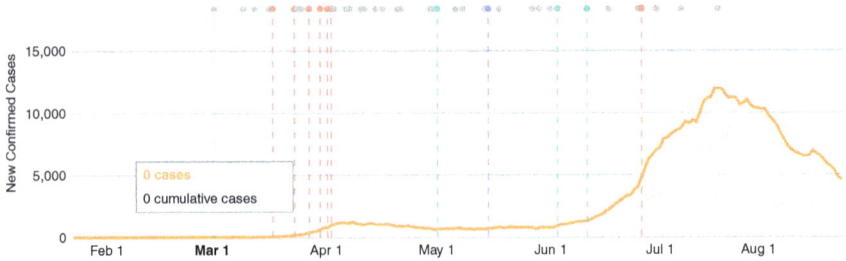

Fig. 22.4   Reported daily new infections in Florida until August 21 together with closing and opening decisions by the state.

The trend curve for reported deaths from Covid-19 peaked on August 5:

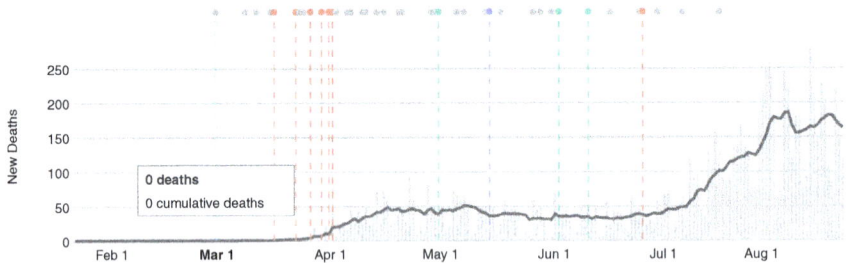

Fig. 22.5   Reported daily deaths from Covid-19 in Florida until August 21.

Cindy: Almost exactly 3 weeks later, as we had predicted!

Bob: But shouldn't we then see a sustained downward trend in the reported numbers of new deaths after August 5? So that the shapes of the two trend curves after the peaks match each other?

Alice: All else being equal, this is what we would expect to see.

Frank: But we don't. There was even a second peak in the number of reported deaths; around August 15 it seems. So all else was not equal. What was going on here, Alice?

Alice: Good question, Frank! What could have caused this mismatch?

Frank: Something about that positivity rate, I guess.

Alice: So let me show you the testing data for Florida:

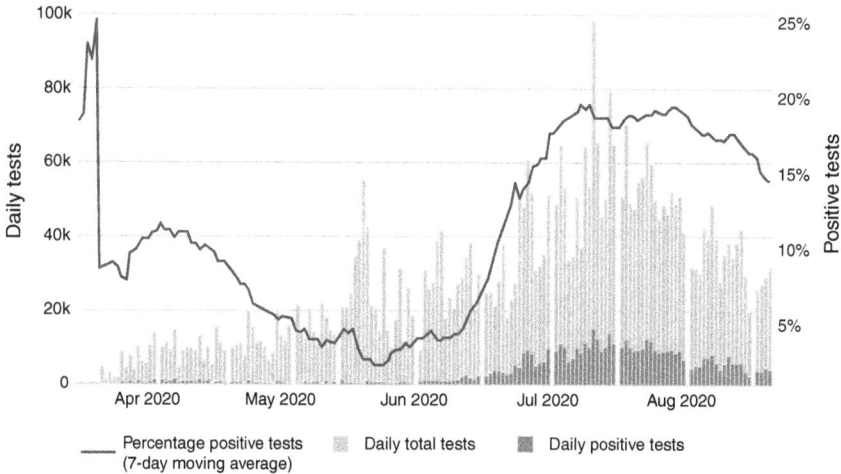

Fig. 22.6   Testing volume and test positivity in Florida until August 21.

Frank: For some strange reason, the numbers of Covid-19 tests in Florida have been sharply trending downward since the state reached the peak of reported daily new infections.

Cindy: The positivity rate went down a little right after mid-July, but then it went up again later that month. Now it is going down, but not nearly as much as the numbers of reported new cases.

Bob: And this pattern is closely matched by the numbers of reported deaths about 20 days later.

Alice: I would expect to see a more sustained downward trend in the number of deaths going into September, but we don't have these data yet.

Bob: Now I know what I should have told my friends from Arizona and Florida:

"You are right that the reported numbers of new deaths are more accurate than the estimates we can get from the reported numbers of new cases. But they start increasing only a few weeks later than reported new infections and become available only after people have already died. I hate to say this, but when actual new infections increase too much, corrective action will need to be taken at some point. If we insist on waiting until the increase shows up in the numbers of deaths, the preventive measures will come too late for many who will get infected in the meantime and may even die. If we want to save lives, we need to act on early warning signs."

Endnotes

112 There is, however, some evidence that deaths from Covid-19 have been underreported in the U.S. [7].

113 See Chapters 13 and 23 for a discussion of some of these guidelines.

References

[1] Worldometers.info. Dover, Delaware, U.S.A. COVID-19 coronavirus pandemic. [cited 2020 Dec 13].
https://www.worldometers.info/coronavirus/

[2] Centers for Disease Control and Prevention. COVID-19 Pandemic Planning Scenarios. 2020 Jul 10. [cited 2020 Oct 17].
https://www.cdc.gov/coronavirus/2019-ncov/hcp/planning-scenarios-archive/planning-scenarios-2020-09-10.pdf

[3] Johns Hopkins University of Medicine. Coronavirus Resource Center. Critical Trends. Impact of opening and closing decisions by state. [cited 2020 Aug 22].
https://coronavirus.jhu.edu/data/state-timeline

[4] Johns Hopkins University of Medicine. Daily state-by-state testing trends. [cited 2020 Aug 22]. https://coronavirus.jhu.edu/testing/individual-states/usa

[5] Martell A. Arizona's main COVID lab running behind as demand for tests soars to twice capacity. Reuters 2020 Jun 23.

[cited 2020 Dec 13]. `https://www.reuters.com/article/us-health-coronavirus-testing-arizona/arizonas-main-covid-lab-running-behind-as-demand-for-tests-soars-to-twice-capacity-idUSKBN23U3C8`

[6] Kliff S. Arizona 'overwhelmed' with demand for tests as U.S. system shows strain. The New York Times, 2020 Jun 25. [cited 2020 Dec 13]. `https://www.nytimes.com/2020/06/25/upshot/virus-testing-shortfall-arizona.html`

[7] Lu D. The true coronavirus toll in the U.S. has already surpassed 200,000. The New York Times 2020 Aug 12. [cited 2020 Oct 17]. `https://www.nytimes.com/interactive/2020/08/12/us/covid-deaths-us.html`

Chapter 23

What if lockdowns had been imposed earlier?

Alice, Bob, Cindy, and Frank meet on August 25, 2020. A number of universities in the U.S. had already fully re-opened for face-to-face instruction, and there were large outbreaks of Covid-19 on several campuses, including more than 500 cases at the University of Alabama in Tuscaloosa and nearly 160 at the University of Missouri in Columbia[114] Ohio University took a more gradual approach. When classes started on August 24, only a few classes in select subjects starting meeting face-to-face, and the Covid-19 infections were closely monitored. Decisions about how many students could return to campus at the end of September in Phase 2 of re-opening were deferred for a couple of weeks.

Alice: Classes started yesterday. I guess all of ours are online for the time being. How are you all doing?

Frank: Totally ticked off, if you really want to know. Online is not the same as taking a real class. My internet connection at home doesn't work half of the time. And I don't have my job in university dining services back, but they still charge tuition.

Cindy: I'm so sorry for you, Frank. They also canceled my internship at the student health center in patient records. But maybe that's for the better. At other universities, there have been large outbreaks right after students came back to campus and threw big parties. With the classes, I don't know yet. My profs are trying really hard, but I'm still confused about how their courses are supposed to work online.

Bob: I'm afraid we will not learn nearly as much as in face-to-face classes. At least we had some advance notice this time. When we were told last semester right after the start of Spring Break that we will not come back, it was a total mess. I had all my books and stuff on campus and suddenly needed to find some quiet space for studying at home. Not easy with three small sibs. I guess back then, the university didn't have much of a choice with the statewide restrictions.[115] But all this came at the worst possible moment. At least they should have told us before Spring Break!

Cindy: I've read that if states gone into lockdowns earlier, many new infections and many deaths could have been avoided.[116] Can you tell us about this, Alice? Is it true?

Bob: Come on Cindy! Even if it were true, the economy would have suffered longer than it already did. Many more people would have lost their jobs.

Frank: Anyway, it didn't happen. Period. So why waste our time talking about it?

Alice: We can study this What-If scenario and see what it might have changed. We may learn something from it that could be useful in the future when the numbers of infections might go up again.

Cindy: Let's do this! What would have happened to the numbers of infections with an earlier lockdown?

Bob: And what would it have done to the economy?

Alice: I will show you a model that can answer your questions.

Cindy: But keep the math simple, please!

Frank: And don't make up stuff along the way!

Alice: All models are based on simplifying assumptions. We need to keep the model transparent if we want to learn from it about what makes a big difference and what doesn't. The assumptions of a model never fully match the situation in the real world, which is always more complicated. But they should match it as closely as possible.

When we want to compare the prediction of a model for answering our question, we need to keep all assumptions and parameters the same, except for the date of the lockdown. Then we will not "make up stuff along the way", to use Frank's expression.

Frank: Sounds reasonable.

Alice: So let's assume that initially we have $R = R_0 = 3$, until the lockdown gets imposed. We will set this date to two different values, one week apart. And we will assume that when the lockdown is imposed, the reproduction number R will gradually decrease over 20 days to $R_\ell = 0.8$ and will remain at this value after the effects of the lockdown have fully kicked in.

We will further assume that the lockdown gets gradually relaxed when we have observed 14 consecutive days of sustained decrease in new infections, as the federal guidelines [1] recommend, and that the reproduction number will then gradually increase to $R_r = 0.95$ over 30 days and stabilize at this value.

Cindy: So you could then predict the weekly numbers of infections from this model, right?

Alice: Yes.

Bob: But how would the model show what the lockdown does to businesses?

Alice: Could we measure the impact on the economy as the number of days the lockdown stays in place?

Bob: Good idea! The longer the lockdown lasts, the harder the economy will be hit.

Alice: To predict this impact more accurately, I will use daily numbers of infections instead of weekly numbers.

Frank: Actual or reported numbers of new infections?

Alice: I will use reported numbers of new infections. That's because decisions about imposing and lifting restrictions can only be made based on reported numbers.

Alice: Let me first assume that the lockdown would be imposed on March 23, and that there were 100 new infections on March 23. That's close to the number that was reported in Ohio on this day.[117]

Let me show you a graph with the predictions of this model for our parameters:

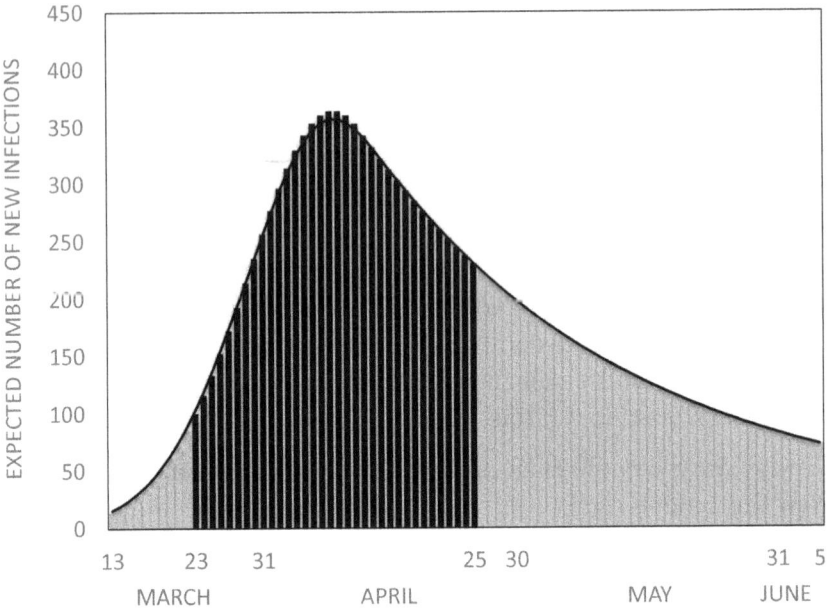

Fig. 23.1 Predictions of the first model with a lockdown on March 23. The days under lockdown are shown in black.

Cindy: So how many people would get infected and how many would die from Covid-19?

Bob: Wouldn't we need to specify a time frame for answering this question?

Alice: For many models, we would need to. But I have assumed that the reproduction number will not exceed $R = 0.95$ at any time after lifting the lockdown. When the reproduction number remains a constant below 1, it is actually possible to calculate the total number of people who would experience infection even if we would need to wait for a vaccine or cure for a very long time. However, details of this calculation are mathematically more difficult than I want to discuss here.[118]

For the parameters in the first scenario, with a lockdown starting on March 23, the model predicts around 42,700 reported infections total. The model itself does not directly predict the number of people dying. We need to make one more assumption, about the mortality from Covid-19. Since we are modeling numbers of reported infections, we can treat it here as the case-fatality rate, the ratio of reported deaths to known infections. If we estimate this ratio based on the numbers for Ohio until yesterday,[119] the model would then predict nearly 1,500 total deaths from Covid-19.

Cindy: It makes me feel horrible to think about all these people dying alone in intensive care units with no relatives allowed to visit!

Alice: Me too. I want to prevent this from happening. That's why I study epidemiology.

Bob: But the lockdown also caused preventable deaths. Many people were scared to see a doctor and did not seek treatment for other illnesses or skipped routine medical exams.

So how about the impact on the economy?

Alice: You can see this from the graph. Remember that the model assumes that re-opening starts when there have been 14 days of sustained decrease in the number of new infections.

Bob: Right! Your graph shows that reopening starts on April 26. The worst impact on the economy would last 34 days under this scenario.

Alice: Exactly!

Alice: Now let me show you the predictions of this model when we assume that the lockdown would be imposed one week earlier, on March 16, and keep all other parameters of the model the same. The graph would then look like this:

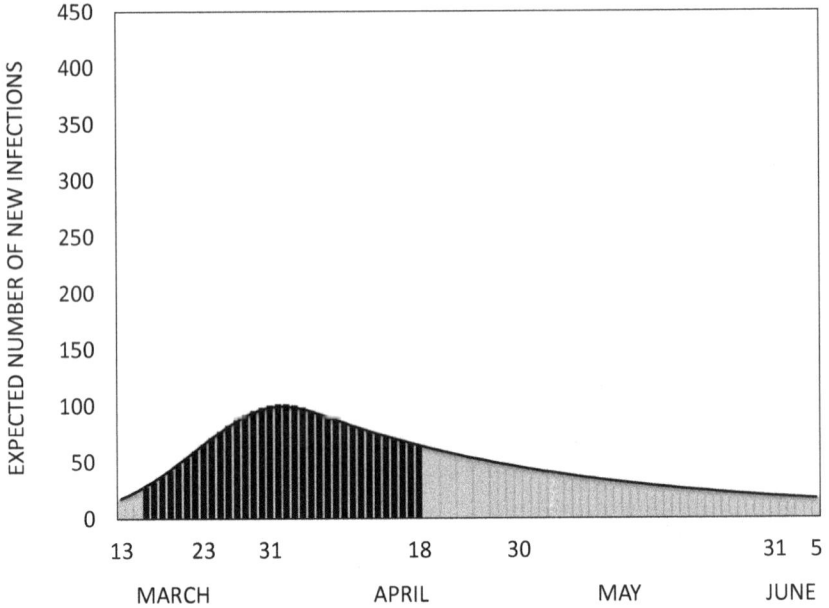

Fig. 23.2   Predictions of the first model with a lockdown on March 16. The days under lockdown are shown in black.

How would the earlier lockdown impact the economy, Bob?

Bob: Well, the lockdown would last from March 16 until April 19. That's again 34 days. Hmm. Not what I had expected. The impact on the economy would be exactly the same if we had gone into lockdown earlier. Neither better and nor worse.

Alice: Exactly! How would the number of people dying from the disease change, Cindy?

Cindy: But Alice, I cannot do all these complicated calculations that you did!

Alice: You don't need to, Cindy. Just compare the heights of the bars in the two graphs:

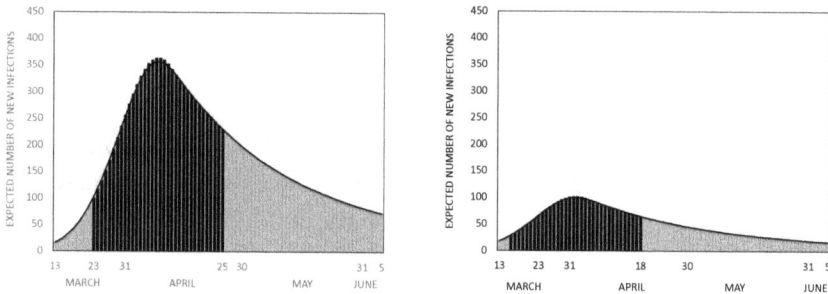

Fig. 23.3 Comparison of the predictions of the first model with two different dates of the lockdown. The days under lockdown are shown in black.

Cindy: In the second graph they are, like, only a third of those in the first graph. Does the model then predict that the number of deaths from Covid-19 would have been cut to about a third—to about 500 from 1,500—with a lockdown that started one week earlier?

Bob: And with essentially no additional cost to the economy?

Alice: Yes. This is what this simple model predicts for our parameters. More detailed and more complicated models arrived at very similar conclusions.[116]

Bob: So why didn't epidemiologists recommend an earlier lockdown back then in March?

Alice: Many did. But scientists can only make recommendations; politicians make the decisions. In any case, our state of Ohio was one of the first to impose a lockdown; most other states waited even longer.[120]

Frank: I still don't buy the predictions of your model. Even for the actual date of the lockdown in Ohio, you said that the model predicts around 42,700 during the entire course of the pandemic. But, until yesterday, we had already more than 115,000 reported infections [2].

And our lockdown ended only on May 1 [3]. I guess that's in the same ballpark as April 26 in your model. But the total number of reported infections is not.

Alice: Are you saying that the assumptions of this model may have been too optimistic for the actual situation in Ohio?

Frank: I guess that is what I meant.

Alice: I agree. But I wanted to show you only a very simple model that makes the effects of an earlier lockdown easy to understand. As I said, more detailed and more realistic models arrived at similar conclusions.

Frank: But we saw some big increase in the numbers of new infections in Ohio and elsewhere starting in late June.[121] This would not be at all as in your model.

Alice: No, it isn't. What do you think, which of the assumptions of my model was no longer true when that increase in June started?

Frank: The assumption that $R \leq 0.95$ at all times after the lockdown. The reproduction number must have crept up above 1 at some time before June 20. I remember that we talked about this.

Alice: Right. The assumption that we can keep the reproduction number R below 1 after re-opening was crucial for the success of the recommended strategy. Had this worked, the model we just discussed would have been more consistent with the data throughout the entire summer.

Frank: So why didn't the strategy work so well?

Cindy: I think it was because many people were not wearing masks and were not practicing social distancing.

Alice: This was probably the biggest factor. Once the lockdowns in our states had ended, many people falsely believed that the Covid-19 outbreak in the U.S. was practically over and became careless in their behavior. This false sense of security seems to have been the major cause of the increase in late June and early July.

But right now I want to talk about a different factor that also played a role and that we also discussed: If we want to keep the reproduction number below 1 without most of the restrictions that we had during the lockdown, we need to conduct extensive testing and contact tracing.

Bob: This requires that sufficiently many tests and contact tracers are available. We talked about this. When the number of daily infections is too large, we may not have enough resources available for these components of the strategy.

Alice: This seems to have been the case in many states.

Cindy: So the government should have recommended that re-opening be postponed until the daily numbers of new infections had come down enough!

Alice: The federal guidelines did recommend that a robust testing program be place for at-risk healthcare workers [1]. But the program may not have been robust enough for the entire population.

In practical terms we can think about a What-If scenario with an added recommendation that the daily numbers of reported new infections should be low enough when re-opening starts so we can keep up with testing and contact tracing.

Bob: So could we modify your model as follows: By the time the lockdown gets lifted, the daily numbers of new infections should have been decreasing for at least 14 days and should have decreased to, for example, no more than 200 per day?

Alice: Yes, this would be a good way of modifying my model. As you said, the number 200 is only an example. We can use it in our second model and explore the new What-If scenario with this new parameter. We can run the model with two different starting dates for the lockdown and see how the total numbers of infections and the impacts on the economy differ.

Frank: I bet an earlier lockdown will again cut the number of infections and deaths. But with the added condition on when it can be lifted, it will last longer and hurt the economy even more.

But go ahead, Alice, do your number-crunching!

Alice: Here is the graph for the daily new infections with a lockdown imposed on March 23:

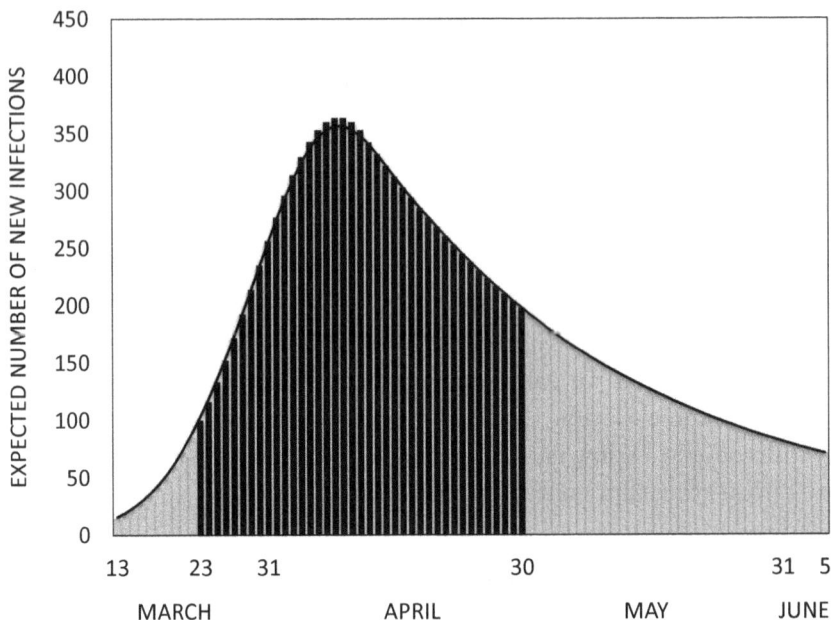

Fig. 23.4   Predictions of the second model with a lockdown on March 23. The days under lockdown are shown in black.

Cindy: The curve goes down faster than in our first model (Fig. 23.1). So there will be fewer infections and fewer deaths than with our first model for the same date of the lockdown.

Alice: Very good observation, Cindy! The difference will be relatively small though. The new model predicts only on the order of 10 fewer deaths than our first one with the same starting date.

Bob: But the lockdown would only end on May 1, as it in fact did in Ohio, and last 39 days instead of 34. This would be a lot worse for the economy than in the first model!

Frank: Told you so!

Alice: In the short run, yes. But in the long run, under the scenario of the first model, it is more likely that the numbers will go up again and that some restrictions may need to be re-imposed. So the long-term economic impact may actually be larger when the lockdown is lifted early, as in our assumptions of the first model.

Frank: Sounds almost like you are talking about a second lockdown. No way!

So, what does the second model predict when the lockdown starts a week earlier, on March 16?

Alice: Here is the graph for the daily new infections:

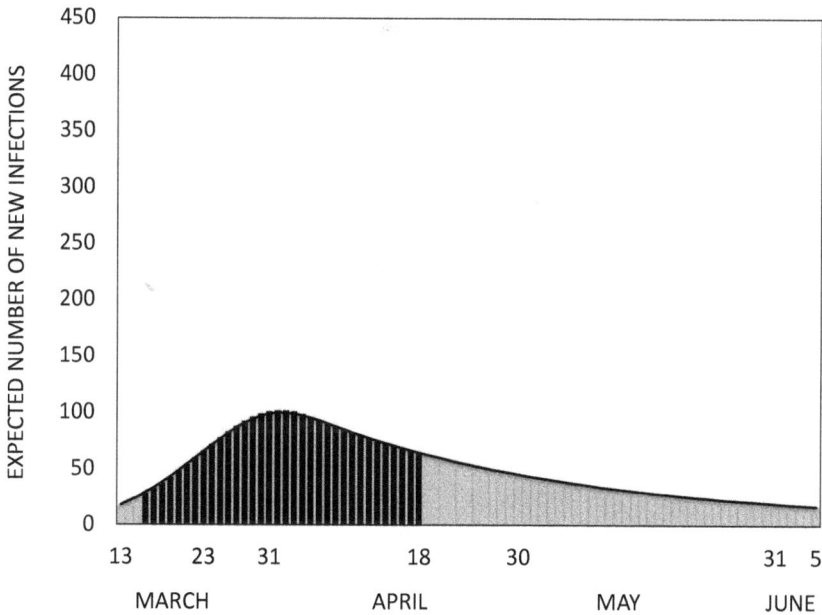

Fig. 23.5 Predictions of the second model with a lockdown on March 16. The days under lockdown are shown in black.

Frank: Wait! We have seen this graph before.

Cindy: That's the one with the much smaller number of total infections and deaths, right?

Alice: Exactly. The number of daily new infections in this model with the earlier lockdown would never have been even close to 200.

So, the lockdown could already have been lifted after the 14 days of sustained decrease of new infections.

Bob: The economic impact would still be the same as before.

Alice: Yes. The short-term economic impact would be the same as in our first model, and smaller than in the second model with the lockdown starting on March 23.

Frank: And the long-term economic impact might have been much smaller because new restrictions on business would have been avoided. We didn't have such new restrictions in Ohio recently, but in other states they again closed bars and other businesses in the summer.[121] They might have avoided that with earlier lockdowns.

Alice: You said it, Frank!

Endnotes

[114] Quoted from the article [4] in the Washington Post. The New York Times continuously tracks Covid-19 outbreaks on College and University campuses in the U.S. [5].

[115] Ohio Governor DeWine declared a state of emergency on March 9, right at the start of Spring Break at Ohio University. On March 12, he announced that all schools will be closed for three weeks beginning on Monday, March 16 [3].

[116] For example, a study by Pei et al. [6] showed that nationwide around 55% of reported infections and deaths as of May 3, 2020 could have been avoided if the same control measures had been implemented just one week earlier. A nontechnical description of this study can be found in the article [7] of the New York Times.

[117] According to the New York Times [8], the number of cases reported in Ohio was 104 on March 22 and 93 on March 23, 2020.

[118] Assuming a serial interval of 7 days and $R = 0.95$, the simple model that is described here would predict a daily decrease of reported cases by a factor of approximately 0.993. If there are n reported cases on the first day when R reaches 0.95, the model then predicts that the total number of reported infections from

that day on will be given by the sum of the geometric series $\sum_{t=0}^{\infty} n\,0.993^t = \frac{n}{1-0.993} \approx 143\,n$. This observation underlies the estimates of the total number of infections that Alice quotes for the models described in this chapter.

[119] Based on 115,768 total cases and 3,999 total deaths reported for Ohio prior to August 25, 2020 [2], Alice estimated the case-fatality rate as approximately 0.0345 and then obtained the estimates of the total deaths from Covid-19 for this model by multiplying this rate by her estimate of total reported infections. This gives 1,475 predicted deaths. She rounded this number to 1,500 as more precise predictions are meaningless for this type of models.

[120] A Wikipedia page [9] gives a table that shows when the lockdowns in U.S. states started and some of the restrictions that were put in place.

[121] See Chapter 18.

References

[1] U.S. Federal Government and Centers for Disease Control and Prevention. Opening Up America Again 2020 Apr 16. [cited 2020 Dec 17]. https://www.whitehouse.gov/openingamerica/

[2] Worldometers.info. Dover, Delaware, U.S.A. COVID-19 coronavirus pandemic. [cited 2020 Oct 31].
https://www.worldometers.info/coronavirus/

[3] Johns Hopkins University of Medicine. Coronavirus Resource Center. Critical Trends. Impact of opening and closing decisions by state. [cited 2020 Dec 21].
https://coronavirus.jhu.edu/data/state-timeline

[4] Knowles H. Universities sound alarm as coronavirus cases emerge just days into classes—530 at one campus. The Washington Post August 26, 2020. [cited 2020 Dec16].
https://www.washingtonpost.com/education/2020/08/25/college-coronavirus-cases/

[5] The New York Times. Tracking the Coronavirus at U.S. Colleges and Universities. [cited 2020 Dec 16].
https://www.nytimes.com/interactive/2020/us/covid-college-cases-tracker.html

[6] Pei S, Kandula S, Shaman J. Differential effects of intervention timing on COVID-19 spread in the United States. Science Advances 2020 Dec 4. [cited 2021 Jan 4]; 6(49):eabd6370. https://advances.sciencemag.org/content/6/49/eabd6370.full DOI: 10.1126/sciadv.abd6370

[7] Glanz J, Robertson, C. Lockdown delays cost at least 36,000 llves, data show. The New York Times 2020 May 20. [updated 2020 May 22; cited 2020 Dec 17]. https://www.nytimes.com/2020/05/20/us/coronavirus-distancing-deaths.html

[8] The New York Times. Covid in the U.S.: Latest map and case count. [cited 2020 Dec 17]. https://www.nytimes.com/interactive/2020/us/coronavirus-us-cases.html

[9] Wikipedia: The free encyclopedia. Wikimedia Foundation, Inc. U.S. state and local government responses to the COVID-19 pandemic. [cited 2020 Dec 21].
https://en.wikipedia.org/wiki/U.S._state_and_local_government_responses_to_the_COVID-19_pandemic

Chapter 24

Could we have safely avoided a lockdown altogether?

Alice, Bob, Cindy, and Frank continue their meeting on August 25, 2020. The lockdowns in early spring 2020 caused a huge economic downturn worldwide and major economic indicators declined. The Hang Seng index of Hong Kong dropped by 27%, from 29,065 on January 16 to 21,696 on March 22; the FTSE index of the London Stock Exchange dropped by more than 34% from 7,622 on January 14 to 4,993 on March 23; and the Dow Jones Industrial Average of the New York Stock Exchange dropped by 37% from 29,551 on February 12 to 18,592 on March 23. By late August, stocks had partially rebounded. The Dow Jones index already reached 28,308 on August 24, 2020; close to its value in early January.

Bob: I have another question about the model you just showed us. After the lockdown ended, new infections still kept decreasing.

Alice: Yes, this model assumes that even after re-opening has been fully phased in, the reproduction number R stays below 1.

Cindy: And that this could be achieved with some restrictions on large gatherings, especially indoors, social distancing, wearing masks, frequent hand-washing, extensive testing, contact tracing, and quarantines for infected people, right?

Alice: Right. Businesses would continue to operate, at least at reduced capacity, kids would go back to school, students would go back to universities. And we could all lead reasonably normal lives.

And infections would continue to decrease after the lockdown ended, like in this graph:

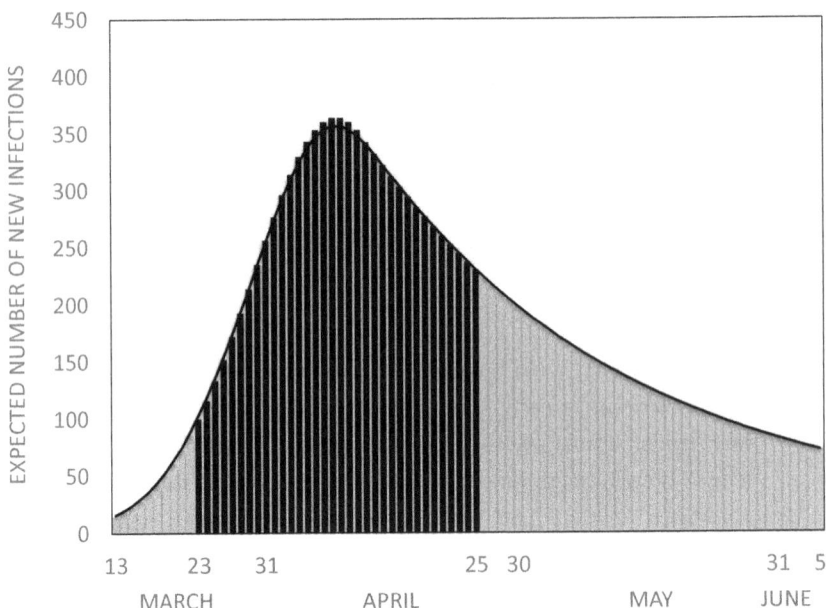

Fig. 24.1   A model with $R = 0.95$ after re-opening. The days of the lockdown are shown in black.

Frank: But there was a large second peak earlier this summer. So it didn't work out as in your model.

Alice: Unfortunately, in many states it didn't. But there are some states, like Connecticut, where this plan has been working so far.[122]

And is has been working in other countries. One example is Italy. In March, Italy had a terrible number of infections, hospitalizations, and deaths that overwhelmed its healthcare system.[16] But the country brought down these infections a lot, and they continued to decline after re-opening.

Italy imposed its lockdown in stages and phased it out very gradually. But we can take March 9 as the start of the lockdown and May 17 as its end; this is when the most significant restrictions were imposed and then lifted.[123] Until the beginning of July, the picture in Italy looked very similar to the graph for the predictions of my model:

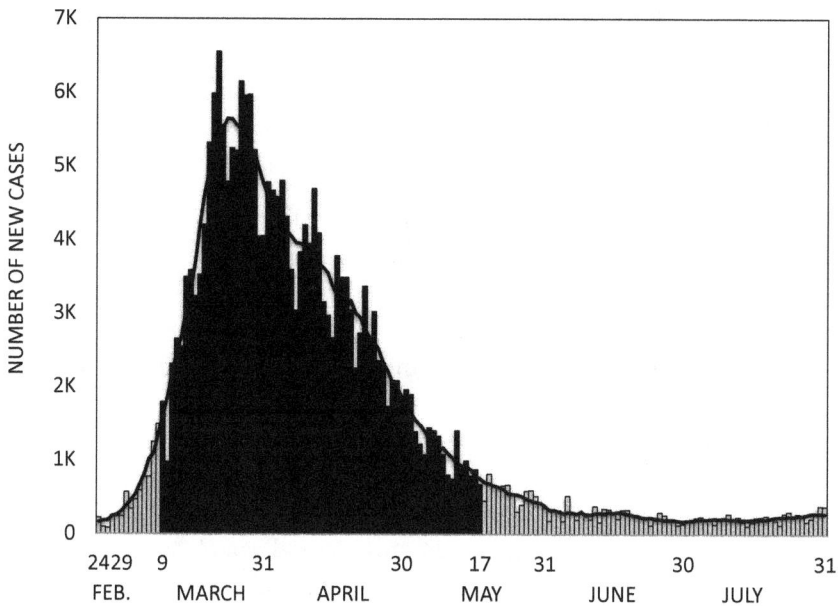

Fig. 24.2 Daily new reported infections in Italy. The days of the lockdown are shown in black. Based on data published by the Italian Ministry of Health [1].

The curve has been pretty flat since then, with slight ups and downs. But so far the strategy seems to be working in Italy.

Bob: So you are telling us that the combination of control measures that remain in place after re-opening could be sufficient to keep the reproduction number R below 1 and prevent the numbers of infections from going up. With far fewer restrictions than under lockdown and without messing up the economy.

Alice: Yes. This is what epidemiologists hope for. All over the world.

Bob: But if this can work, why did then most countries and most of our states impose lockdowns? Why could we not have kept the spread of Covid-19 under control with only these milder control measures right from the start?

Frank: That's something, Bob! If wearing masks, social distancing, testing, and contact tracing are sufficient to keep the number of infections down, we should have been doing just that. Without these lockdowns that sent the economy into a tailspin and practically imprisoned people in their homes for weeks and weeks!

Alice: In fact, not all countries and not all states in the U.S. imposed full lockdowns.[124] It's a very interesting question how well this worked and whether lockdowns could have been avoided in more places. I expect that it will be discussed a lot in the years and decades to come. If you want, we can get ahead of this discussion and study a What-If scenario for it.

Bob: Yes, I'd like to see how this might have worked in Ohio.

Alice: Let's first specify the assumptions. As before, we will assume that the reproduction number R stays equal to $R_0 = 3$ until the control measures are adopted. To make the calculations easier, let's go back to time steps of weeks, as in some of our earlier conversations, and assume that the control measures will decrease the reproduction number from $R_0 = 3$ to $R_r = 0.96$.

Let's assume that this decrease happens gradually, over a period of 8 weeks.

Bob: Why would this take so long?

Alice: Closing businesses or issuing a stay-at-home order can be implemented overnight. We have already seen that even then it takes a while before their full effect shows up in the numbers of new infections.[125] But here we are talking about social distancing, wearing masks, and frequent hand-washing. It takes some time to educate people about how important these things are.

Cindy: Even now, more than five months later, many people still don't understand why we all need to do this!

Alice: Right. It would take a while to convince people to do all of this. And back in March, there was a big shortage of commercially available masks. Surgical and N95 masks are most effective. But in March, we barely had enough of them to protect our doctors and nurses [2]. It took a while to ramp up their production so that they could become available for everybody.

Bob: Wasn't the same also true for tests?

Alice: Yes. The very first tests in the U.S. became available only at the beginning of March, and there were some glitches [3]. But for keeping reproduction numbers low, a lot of tests are needed, and it would take a while to produce sufficiently many of them. Similarly for contact tracing. This requires recruiting and training sufficiently many contact tracers.

Frank: Still, 8 weeks seem a lot of time for all of this.

Alice: The What-If scenario we are discussing here is more speculative than the others we studied. I chose 8 weeks only as an example to illustrate a principle. With commitment of sufficient resources to testing and contact tracing and effective messaging by the government, it might take less time.[126]

Frank: OK, let's go with 8 weeks. What does your model then predict?

Alice: First I need to tell you about my other assumptions. To keep the numbers simple, let's say that in Week 3 we would have had new 500 infections, which is in the same ballpark as the reported number in Ohio during the week right before the lockdown.[127] With my parameters, we can treat these predictions as a rough model for Ohio. We will again model reported infections.

Bob: Will they again reach a peak and then continue to decrease, as in your previous model?

Alice: Yes. If we have to wait for a vaccine for a very long time and make the same assumptions about mortality as we did earlier today, we might then see on the order of 1.3 million total reported infections and 45,000 deaths from Covid-19 in our state.[128]

Cindy: This sounds so awful!

Alice: It would be even worse than that. On my next graph, I will show you the predictions of this model for the numbers of new infections in Weeks 1 through 15:

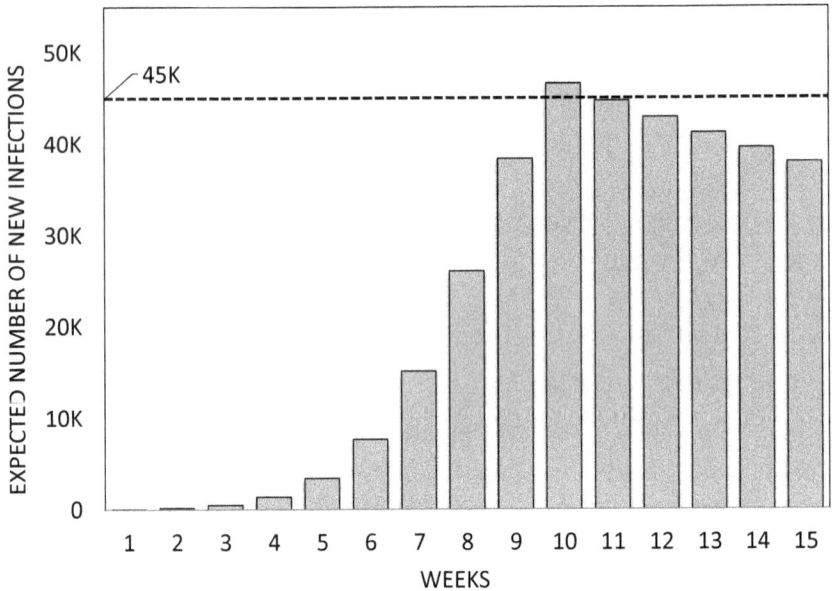

Fig. 24.3   Predictions of the model with control measures starting in Week 4.

Under our very optimistic assumptions we had made when we talked about the basic reproduction number,[129] the state of Ohio would run out of available hospital beds when the reported weekly new infections cross the threshold of 45,000. In this model, it would happen in Week 10.

Bob: I hate to say this, but if this model is the best we could have done without a lockdown, the lockdown was necessary.

Frank: If the model really shows the best options without a lockdown. A big if. I think the state could have done better.

Bob: How?

Frank: We talked about this earlier today. Had they started with those milder restrictions a week or two earlier, reported infections would not have crossed this threshold.

Alice: This is an interesting conjecture. Let me show you the graph for the version of this model where control measures start in Week 3 instead of Week 4:

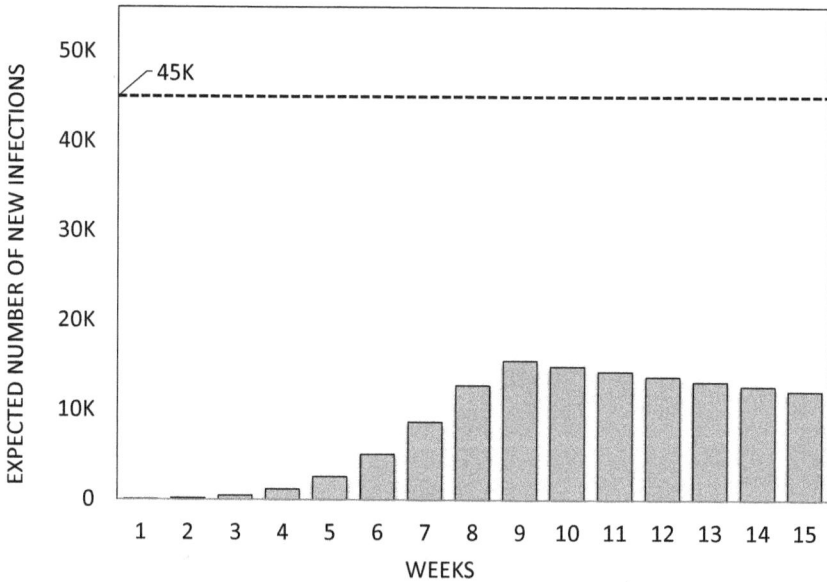

Fig. 24.4   Predictions of the model with control measures starting in Week 3.

Now the model predicts that the total number of reported cases in Ohio would be on the order of 430,000 infections and 15,000 deaths.[130] The maximum number of weekly infections would be predicted as around 15,500.

Bob: A lot fewer than our threshold of 45,000. So the state should have gone this route.

Alice: Possibly, but it would have been risky. There were many unknown factors back in March, and there still are. The numbers would have changed roughly following the pattern predicted by the model, but might easily have been off by a factor of 2 or 3. And we calculated the threshold under very optimistic assumptions. Even in this scenario, our healthcare system in Ohio might already have become overwhelmed.[48]

Frank: So they should have started these control measures two weeks earlier.

Alice: Let me show you the graph for these modified assumptions:

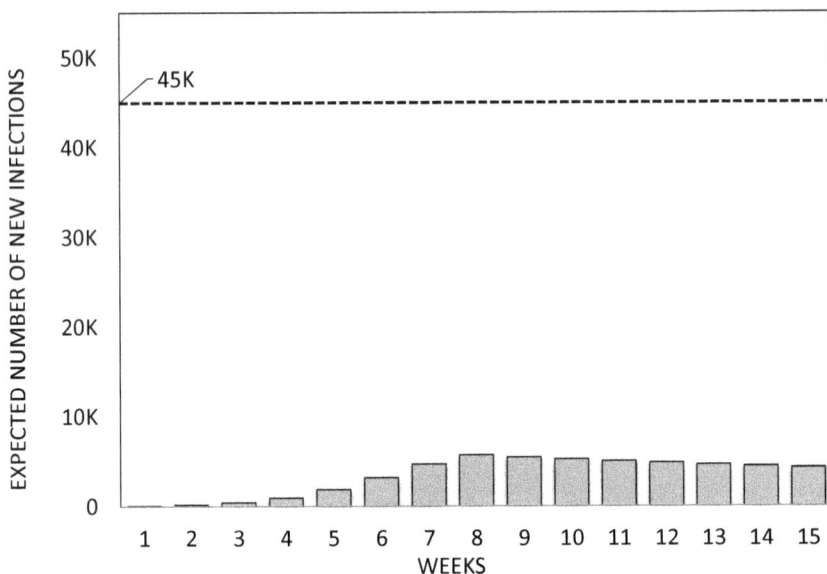

Fig. 24.5 Predictions of the model with control measures starting in Week 2.

The model predicts that the total number of reported cases in Ohio would be on the order of 140,000 infections and 5,000 deaths. The maximum number of weekly infections would be around 5,200.[130]

Cindy: These are still such horribly large numbers!

Bob: Yes, Cindy. But the number of people who lost their jobs because of the lockdown was also horribly large. Without the lockdown, most people would have kept them. And the maximum number of predicted weekly infections is actually lower than the numbers reported for the worst week of the lockdown of Ohio.[131]

Frank: So why did the state not go this route?

Alice: Actually, our governor deserves great credit for making an attempt to avoid a full lockdown by acting early. A state of emergency was declared in Ohio on March 9, exactly two weeks before the lockdown, and some restrictions were put in place over those two weeks.[115] Unfortunately, they did not work well enough to avoid the lockdown.

Bob: Why not?

Alice: There were a number of reasons. Covid-19 is a new infection. In March, we did not yet understand it well enough to know which control measures would be most effective. Also, a strategy such as in our model requires certain conditions that were not satisfied in March.

Frank: Are you talking about availability of masks, of sufficiently many tests, and sufficiently many people trained to do contact tracing?

Alice: I have already built these factors into my model by assuming a gradual reduction of reproduction numbers over 8 weeks.

But it is not sufficient that masks are available. People actually need to wear them when social distancing is not an option, practice social distancing whenever possible, wash their hands often and thoroughly, and avoid touching their faces.

Frank: Yeah, yeah! Epidemiologists have been telling us these things for months now. People are sick and tired of hearing it. Why couldn't they have made the same pitch in March?

Alice: In early March, there were not enough masks available for everybody, so we wanted to make sure the most effective ones would go to those most at risk, especially healthcare workers. And there was not yet clear scientific evidence how much protection against Covid-19 transmission masks actually provide.[132]

Epidemiologists did recommend social distancing and frequent handwashing already back in early March. But it was very difficult to get this message across.

Frank: I guess nobody likes to be told what to do by those know-it-all epidemiologists!

Cindy: All people should follow these recommendations!

Alice: But the fact is that many do not. Scientists need to base their predictions and recommendations on how real people behave, not on wishful thinking. On March 9, when Ohio declared the state of emergency, there were only 3 confirmed cases in our state. Epidemiologists knew what was going on, not because they are smarter than others, but because of years of scientific training and studying other infectious diseases.

But practically nobody in Ohio actually knew any infected person, and the pictures of makeshift hospitals and deaths in Italy that we saw on TV seemed to come from far away. How likely is it that in such a situation people could have been convinced to wear those masks, even if they had been widely available, and to practice social distancing?

Frank: Wouldn't have convinced me, I'll admit.

Alice: Thank you, Frank, for being honest about it. When the outbreak in Ohio was still practically invisible, people would have followed these recommendations only if they trusted scientists. This level of trust in science that just wasn't there and still isn't. Far from it [4].

And people would have needed to understand the reasons why scientists recommend these behavior changes, why they are important for preventing damage to our health and our economy. Nobody likes to be told what to do and what not to do. But I believe most people would decide to do the right thing if they clearly understood what's at stake and why they are being asked to put up with these inconveniences.

I am only a student of epidemiology and cannot reach very many people. But I can try to explain here in my chat room how things work, what is important for all of us to do, and why it is important. Then each of us will be able to make informed decisions.

Endnotes

[122] See Chapters 18 and 28 for more information on Connecticut.

[123] On March 9, the Italian government extended all measures previously applied only in the so-called "red zones" to the whole country. Starting from May 18, most businesses could reopen, and free movement was granted to all citizens within their region [5].

[124] A Wikipedia article [6] gives a list of countries and U.S. states that did not impose lockdowns. The article [7] of the New York Times discusses the long-term economic impact in Iowa, one of these states.

[125] This was briefly discussed in Chapter 11.

[126] For example, the first Covid-19 case in South Korea was confirmed on January 20. The country mounted a rapid response based on massive testing together with extensive contact tracing, but without a lockdown [8]. The first significant peak of the 7-day moving average of daily reported cases peaked already on March 4, and steeply declined thereafter [9].

[127] Worldometer [9] shows a 7-day moving average of 56 daily infections for March 23, which corresponds to 392 infections for the week.

[128] See the endnotes of Chapter 23 for a description of the same method for performing these calculations. [118,119]

[129] See Chapter 9.

[130] With a reproduction number $R = R_0 = 3$, this model predicts a threefold increase of cases per week, so the number infections and deaths that are expected in the long run would decreases roughly by a factor of 3 if control measures are implemented one week earlier.

[131] During the lockdown, the 7-day moving average of daily reported cases in Ohio reached its highest value of 904 cases on April 22, which corresponds to 6,328 cases for the week [9].

[132] A Nature news feature [10] describes some research on the effectiveness of masks against the spread of Covid-19.

References

[1] Github Inc. Dati COVID-19 Italia. [cited 2020 Jul 5]. https://raw.githubusercontent.com/pcm-dpc/COVID-19/master/dati-andamento-nazionale/dpc-covid19-ita-andamento-nazionale.csv

[2] Miroff N. U.S. cities have acute shortages of masks, test kits,

ventilators as they face coronavirus threat. The Washington Post, 2020 Mar 27. [cited 2020 Dec 21].
`https://www.washingtonpost.com/national/coronavirus-mayors-mask-equipment-shortage/2020/03/27/fc2a45a4-701f-11ea-96a0-df4c5d9284af_story.html`

[3] Leonhardt D, Leatherby L. The unique U.S. failure to control the virus. The New York Times 2020 Aug 6. [updated 2020 Aug 8; cited 2020 Dec 21]. `https://www.nytimes.com/2020/08/06/us/coronavirus-us.html`

[4] Howard J, Stracqualursi V. Fauci warns of 'anti-science bias' being a problem in US. CNN Politics 2020 Jun 18 [cited 2020 Dec 6]. `https://edition.cnn.com/2020/06/18/politics/anthony-fauci-coronavirus-anti-science-bias/index.html`

[5] Wikipedia: The free encyclopedia. Wikimedia Foundation, Inc. COVID-19 pandemic in Italy. [cited 2020 Dec 6]. `https://en.wikipedia.org/wiki/COVID-19_pandemic_in_Italy`

[6] Wikipedia: The free encyclopedia. Wikimedia Foundation, Inc. COVID-19 pandemic lockdowns. [cited 2020 Dec 21]. `https://en.wikipedia.org/wiki/COVID-19_pandemic_lockdowns`

[7] Casselman B, Tankersley J. Iowa Never Locked Down. Its Economy Is Struggling Anyway. The New York Times 2020 Oct 22 [updated 2020 Nov 3; cited 2020 Dec 21].
`https://www.nytimes.com/2020/10/22/business/economy/economy-coronavirus-lockdown-iowa.html`

[8] Wikipedia: The free encyclopedia. Wikimedia Foundation, Inc. COVID-19 pandemic in South Korea. [cited 2020 Dec 21].
`https://en.wikipedia.org/wiki/COVID-19_pandemic_in_South_Korea`

[9] Worldometers.info. Dover, Delaware, U.S.A. COVID-19 coronavirus pandemic. [cited 2020 Dec 21].
`https://www.worldometers.info/coronavirus/`

[10] Peeples L. Face masks: what the data say. Nature 2020 Oct 6. [cited 2020 Dec 21]; 586(7828):186–189.
`https://www.nature.com/articles/d41586-020-02801-8`
DOI: 10.1038/d41586-020-02801-8

Chapter 25

What is logarithmic scaling?

Alice and Cindy meet on August 30, 2020. The worldwide 7-day moving average of reported daily new Covid-19 infections had been fairly constant, on the order of 260,000, throughout the preceding month. But some countries that had brought the pandemic under control earlier in the year, such as South Korea and Spain, experienced large surges of cases in August. In South Korea, the 7-day moving average increased from 34 on August 11 to 343 on August 29. Many websites offer visual tools for tracking the development of the outbreak, including graphs that use logarithmic scaling.

Cindy: Hi Alice! I have a stupid question. On those graphs with the numbers of cases, sometimes it says "logarithmic". I don't know what this means. I'm so terrible at math. Can you tell me while the others are not here yet?

Alice: Don't worry, Cindy. There are no stupid questions. Yours is a very good one.

Are you talking about graphs like this one (Fig. 25.1), from Worldometer?

Cindy: Yes. This is what I meant. It says "linear" and "logarithmic" in the upper left corner. What do these tabs mean?

Alice: Let's start with "linear." Right now, the graph displays the data with linear scaling. This just means that on the vertical axis the actual numbers are marked in equal increments.

For this graph, they are the numbers of total reported Covid-19 infections worldwide. The trend curve then shows how these numbers changed over time, which is marked on the horizontal axis.

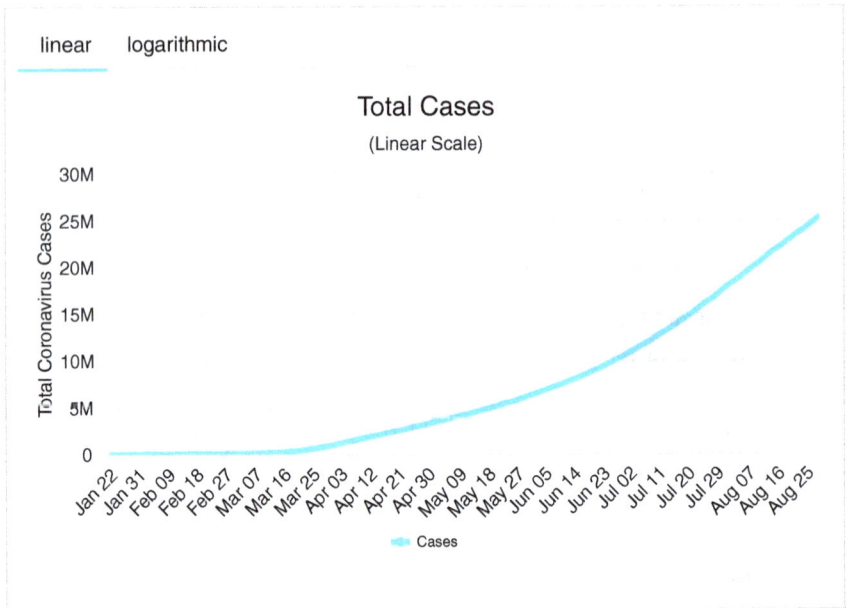

Fig. 25.1   Total reported Covid-19 cases worldwide until August 29, 2020 with linear scaling. The graphs in this chapter are adapted from Worldometers.info [1].

Cindy: So does "linear scaling" then simply mean that the data are displayed in the usual way?

Alice: Yes. That's all there is to it.

What can you tell from this graph about the change of the total numbers of reported cases over time?

Cindy: The curve bends upward for the second half of March. Would this be like exponential increase?

Alice: It could be. But not all curves that increase and bend upward indicate exponential increase. It's not clear from this graph that the numbers grew roughly exponentially in late March.

Cindy: For April, the graph almost looks like a straight line. This wouldn't be exponential increase, would it?

Alice: Not if the line is really straight. If the line still bends up, even slightly, it could also be exponential increase. But at this resolution, we couldn't make out whether or not there still is a slight upward bend.

Cindy: There was another upward bend later, in June. I think this could also mean exponential increase. But maybe not.

Then the curve becomes almost a straight line again. But I cannot make out when, exactly, the line starts and stops bending upward.

Alice: Right. I cannot make it out either.

And what happened in February?

Cindy: It looks like there were no cases. Or at most a few.

But wait! The lowest tick mark on the vertical axis says 5M; that's 5 million, right? So maybe not so few. I can't tell from the graph.

If only they had stretched the vertical axis and put the lowest tick mark differently, like 5 thousand perhaps. But this may be too low. Then the other numbers, for April and later, would no longer fit in the picture. So I don't know.

Alice: Right. The graph gives us some information, but leaves a lot of questions unanswered. Logarithmic scaling allows us to visually display answers to some of them.

To understand how logarithmic scaling works, we first need to talk a little about logarithms. There are many different types of logarithms. Let's talk here about decimal logarithms, or logarithms to base 10. These are the easiest to understand.[133]

Formally, if y is a positive real number, then the decimal logarithm of y, sometimes denoted by $\log y$ or $\log_{10} y$, is the number x such that if we raise 10 to the power x, we get y. That is, $10^x = y$.

Cindy: I've seen this definition in precalculus. But it totally confused me. I'm so terrible at math!!

Alice: It confused me too when I saw it for the first time. Let's try to understand it with some examples.

$10^1 = 10$. So when we let $y = 10$, then we would have $10^x = y$ for $x = 1$. From the formal definition, we then get $\log 10 = 1$. And $10^2 = 100$, so for $y = 100$ we would have $\log 100 = 2$.

Cindy: And for $y = 1,000$ we would get $\log 1,000 = 3$, because $10^3 = 1,000$. Is this how it works?

Alice: Exactly!

Cindy: Then $\log 10,000 = 4$, $\log 100,000 = 5$, and ...

But I don't like writing all these zeros.

Can I write $\log 1k = 3$, $\log 10k = 4$, $\log 100k = 5$, $\log 1M = 6$, $\log 10M = 7$, $\log 100M = 8$?

Alice: We would not write like this in a research paper. But here we are talking about data visualization. So this is fine.

Now try to mark the numbers that you mentioned, from 1k to 100M, on a sheet of paper to scale. Start from 100M.

Cindy: But how could I do this? 100M would be way up, 10M would already be close to the lower margin, 1M practically right next to the lower margin, and then all the other numbers, 100k and lower, would all be practically in the same place. Please don't make fun of me, Alice! I know that I'm terrible at math ...

Alice: You are not. You have perfectly described the problem we run into when we try to draw these numbers to scale. To linear scale, to say it more precisely.

How would you mark the decimal logarithms of these numbers on your sheet of paper?

Cindy: That's easy! I would simply put down equally spaced tick marks: Number 8 on top, that's for $\log 100M$; then number 7, that's $\log 10M$; all the way down to number 3, that's $\log 1k$. Now the tick marks would no longer be crowded together near the lower margin.

Alice: Very good, Cindy! Did you ever run into this problem before? I mean, that interesting numbers are all crowded together near the lower margin of a picture?

Cindy: Wasn't this, like, with these numbers of infections for February? They were all indistinguishable from 0 because the lowest tick mark was at 5M.

Alice: Yes. Can you think of some way to make them visible, together with all the larger numbers up to the end of August?

Cindy: Could we mark on the vertical axis the logarithms of these numbers instead of the numbers themselves?

Alice: Congratulations, Cindy! You have discovered logarithmic scaling.

Let's click on the tab and see what this trick does to the graph:

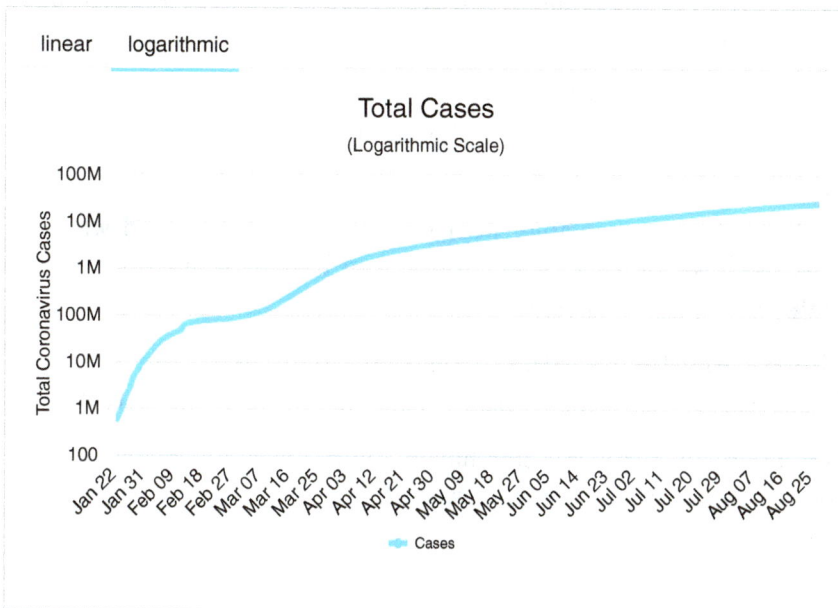

Fig. 25.2 Total reported Covid-19 cases worldwide until August 29, 2020 with logarithmic scaling.

Cindy: Wow! This wasn't difficult at all with your help. Thank you Alice! Now all the numbers show up; I mean, their logarithms do.

But the graph looks kind of strange. It almost levels off near the end of February, and it has this weird kink some time after February 9.

Alice: Until late February, the Covid-19 outbreak was largely confined to China. It was quickly brought under control there before large outbreaks started developing elsewhere. This explains why the curve almost levels off in late February.

On February 12 and 13, China reported large numbers of cases that had been backlogged for a while. Over 14,000 such reports on February 12, and over 5,000 the next day. This explains the kink.

Cindy: I'm curious: Can we see from this graph with logarithmic scaling when there was exponential increase? Or nearly exponential increase at least?

Alice: Yes we can. To see how, let's talk about logarithms a little more. Suppose the number of cases would increase by a factor of 10 every 3 weeks.

Cindy: That's almost like in this graph for the 3 weeks that started on March 7, from around 100 thousand to around 1 million, right?

Alice: Not quite that much, but in this ballpark. Here I want to explain only the principle, with very simple numbers. So when we have 1k cases in week 1, we would then have 10k cases in Week 4, 100k cases in Week 7, and so on.

Cindy: And the logarithms would be 3 in Week 1, 4 in Week 4, 5 in Week 7, and so on. Is this what you are trying to get at, Alice?

Alice: Yes, Cindy. We now have a simple formula for the decimal logarithm of the number y_t in week t:

$$\log y_t = 1 + \frac{1}{3}t.$$

Cindy: Is this like the formula for a straight line with slope $\frac{1}{3}$ that we learned in precalculus?

Alice: You got it, Cindy! Periods with nearly exponential increase will show up as time intervals where the graph with logarithmic scaling looks like an increasing straight line.

Cindy: The first part of the curve, until January 27 or so, looks like a very steep straight line. And the curve looks almost like a straight again in the second half of March. Would that be when there was exponential increase?

Alice: Nearly exponential increase. That is all we can say; the data never fit our simple models exactly. At best, they may fit a model approximately.

When the curve with logarithmic scaling bends downward, we can say that the increase slows down from nearly exponential to what we call sub-exponential increase.

In terms of our earlier discussions, this would happen when the reproduction number R gets smaller over time and the outbreak is gradually being brought under control. We can see from this graph that this was the case in China in the weeks starting at the end of January, when they were under strict lockdown.

Cindy: And the same would be true between mid-March and mid-April for the entire world?

Alice: Yes, that's when many countries all over the world had imposed shelter-in-place orders.

It is not possible to clearly make out from this graph whether there was nearly exponential increase in June. There appears to have been exponential increase with the curve being nearly a straight line for that time period. But the slope is so gentle that it is not really possible to clearly see whether or not it bends or is nearly straight.

Cindy: When we draw a graph with logarithmic scaling and it comes out as a straight line, is the slope like the reproduction number?

Alice: Great question, Cindy! Roughly speaking, a steeper slope would indicate larger reproduction numbers. One can even estimate the reproduction numbers from the slopes.[134]

But such calculations are complicated for this graph, as it shows the total number of all reported cases. At later stages in an outbreak, even when new cases increase exponentially, these new cases would be added to an already large number of previously reported ones. And the graph shows the cases for all countries together, but nearly exponential increase might occur in different countries at different times.

Cindy: In the graph from Worldometer, the slope is steepest during the first week; much steeper than in the second week of March. Does this mean that the reproduction number was highest at this time?

Alice: It would seem so. But when we compare the slopes of different line segments, we need to be aware that they were also influenced by several factors other than reproduction numbers. Let me mention two such factors here.

Covid-19 had been spreading for a while in China before it was recognized as a new disease and before tests became available. Once testing started, it would have been ramped up over the following days. So we need to assume that the increase of the numbers for the first week shows the combined effects of the spread of the disease and of rapidly expanding testing.

Moreover, all case reports for the first week come from the outbreak in a single country, China. As I had already mentioned, the reports of new cases in the second half of March came from many different countries. For individual countries, the slope may have been much steeper during some weeks. But the outbreaks in different countries grew large at slightly different times. The steepest increases would average out with the numbers from other countries, like South Korea, where large outbreaks were already slowing down.

Cindy: Wow! So many things you need to think about in epidemiology. I couldn't keep them all straight in my head. But at least I understand now how logarithmic scaling works and what it is good for. Thank you Alice, for explaining this so clearly!

Endnotes

[133] For $y, b > 0$, the logarithm of y to base b, denoted by $\log_b y$, is the number x such that $b^x = y$. In the literature, the symbol $\log y$ is typically used as an abbreviation of $\log_{10} y$. But depending on the application, it may occasionally also be used for logarithms to a different base. Of great importance in the scientific literature are logarithms to base $e \approx 2.81$. They are called natural logarithms and are usually denoted by $\ln y$.

[134] If time series-data like the ones discussed in this section grow

roughly exponentially so that $y_t \approx y_0 10^{mt}$, then their decimal logarithms form roughly a straight line with $\log y_t \approx \log y_0 + mt$. The slope of this line then gives an estimate of the base of the exponential increase. This fact can be used to derive rough estimates of reproduction numbers from reported time-series data on infections like Covid-19. However, there are a number of pitfalls that may skew these estimates. Some were mentioned by Alice in this section. In particular, if the volume of testing changes over time, reported incidence data will be misleading. Thus estimates of R_t by this method should be based on changes in positivity rates rather than changes in the numbers of reported cases. This approach is used for the estimates reported at the website [2].

References

[1] Worldometers.info. Dover, Delaware, U.S.A. COVID-19 coronavirus pandemic. [cited 2020 Aug 30].
https://www.worldometers.info/coronavirus/

[2] Krieger M, Systrom K, Vladeck T. R_t COVID-19. [cited 2020 Aug 30]. https://rt.live/

Chapter 26

Can we stop the pandemic by achieving herd immunity?

Bob and Frank join the meeting of August 30, 2020. Most governments around the world temporarily closed educational institutions in an attempt to contain the spread of the COVID-19 pandemic. On April 1, 2020, almost 1.5 billion of learners at all levels of education were affected and there were 172 country-wide closures. At the end of August, there are still 32 country-wide school closures and almost 700 million learners are affected.[135]

Bob: Sorry for being late. Just got out of class.

Frank: Same here.

Alice: No problem. Welcome back, all. How did your first week of classes go?

Bob: Not too bad. My profs have all clearly laid out how they will teach their classes. Putting all these materials online must have been a lot of work for them over the summer. But each of my classes uses a different platform: Some meet regularly using Teams, some use Blackboard, another one uses Top Hat. This is very confusing. And there were technical glitches. I think I'll learn something, but not as much as in face-to-face classes.

Cindy: I miss real classes so much! Talking to other students, asking questions in class. In some of my courses, we meet online for discussions in small groups, and I like them. But in other courses, it's just: Read the materials that are posted online and submit the assignments. This feels so distant.

Frank: Yeah, and they make us pay the same tuition no matter how the class is taught. That's unfair. Some of my engineering classes are supposed to have a lab with hands-on experiments. They still haven't figured out how they will be taught.

Bob: I'm most worried about my little sibs. The youngest is only eight. How can they expect kids of that age to sit down and study at home where all the toys are? It was a disaster in the spring. Some teachers were tech-savvy and put cute stuff on the web; others were totally unprepared for the sudden move online.

There has been a lot of back-and-forth whether in the fall the kids will have their classes online, face-to-face, or hybrid. I hope they will teach face-to-face as much as possible, but nobody knows what's going to happen if cases increase again or too many teachers get sick.[136]

Frank: I think instead of messing up our education, they should have gone for herd immunity. Let the infection spread until enough people have gotten infected and recovered with immunity, and be done with it. We haven't discussed this option yet.

Alice: Let's talk about that today. There are a lot of misunderstandings about how it works. We will need to sort them out slowly.

Cindy: Yes, please explain it slowly! Especially if it's so difficult to understand.

Alice: The key concept is the herd immunity threshold. For an infection like Covid-19, with R_0 estimated to be between 2.5 and 3, it would be reached when between 60% and 70% of all people are no longer susceptible.

So far, we have been assuming that R_0 is equal to 3; let's stick with this number for simplicity. In this case, the herd immunity threshold would be equal to two thirds, or about 67% of the population.[137]

Bob: I always thought that this percentage would be for the people who are already immune to infection. But "no longer susceptible" would mean that 67% are in the exposed, infectious, or removed state.

Alice: This is one of the common misunderstandings about herd immunity. The threshold is only for the percentage of people who are in one of the three states that you mentioned, Bob. We will see later how this matters.

But it's easier to understand how herd immunity works if we think of a population where a little more than 2 in 3 people have already reached the removed state and can no longer be infected or infect others. Let me assume this in my first pictures.

Let's again look at a population of 50 people, and assume that 34 of them have developed immunity to infection, while the others remain susceptible:

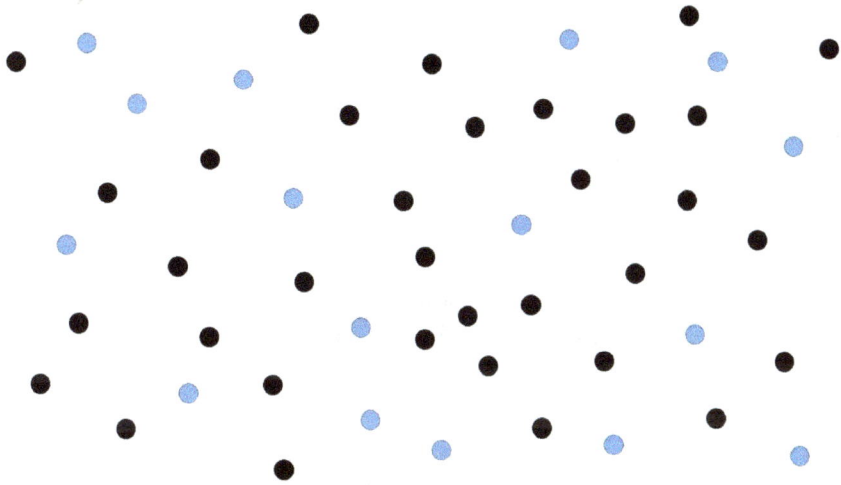

Fig. 26.1 A small population with herd immunity: 68% removed and 32% susceptible individuals.

Now assume one of the 16 susceptible people, let's call him Ingham again, got infected through a contact with somebody outside of this population and became infectious after a few days. I'll show this in my next picture (Fig. 26.2).

Recall from our previous conversations that for $R_0 = 3$, the index case will have on average effective contacts with 3 other people while being infectious.

Cindy: An effective contact is one that would lead to a transmission if it's between an infectious and a susceptible person, right?

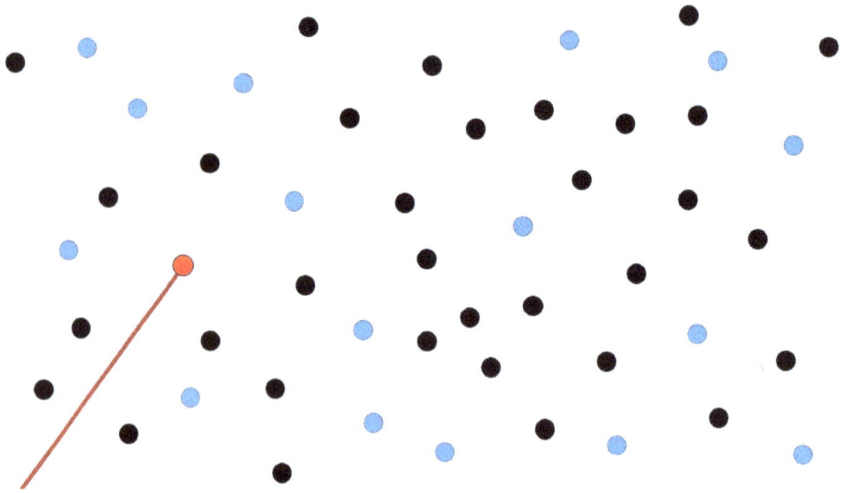

Fig. 26.2   Ingham became infected through an outside contact.

Alice: Right. So let's assume that Ingham makes effective contacts with 3 randomly chosen people in this population:

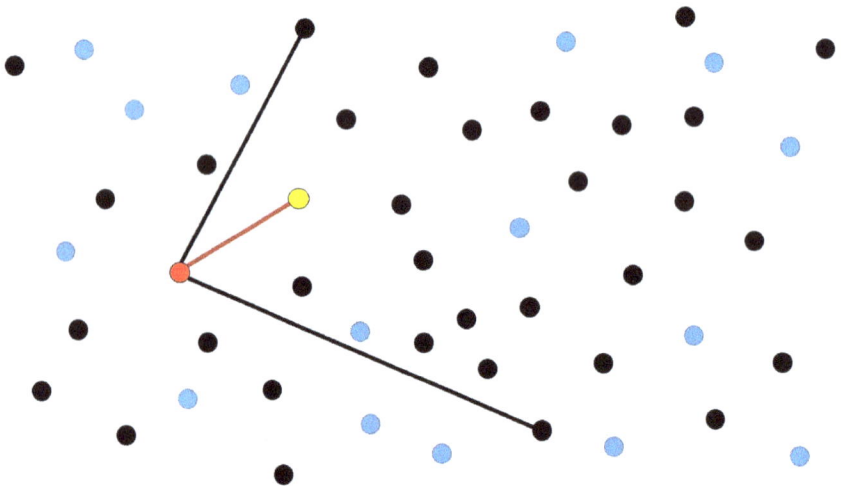

Fig. 26.3   Ingham has effective contacts with 3 people and infects Emily.

Only one person got exposed, let's call here Emily again. The other 2 contacts were with people who were already immune.

Bob: Oh, I see! Yes! We would expect that about 2 out of 3 effective contacts are with people who are no longer susceptible. Those will not lead to new infections.

Alice: Yes. On average, only about 1 out of 3 effective contacts would be with susceptible persons and lead to transmissions of the virus.

Ingham will eventually recover with immunity, and Emily will have effective contacts with about 3 people before recovering. The number 3 is only an average; let's assume in our example that the actual number will be 4.

We'd expect that about 2/3 of 4, that is, 2.67 of these 4 effective contacts will be with people who are no longer susceptible. Let's assume in our example that 3 of Emily's effective contacts were with individuals in the removed state. Then again only 1 of her 4 effective contacts will lead to a new infection:

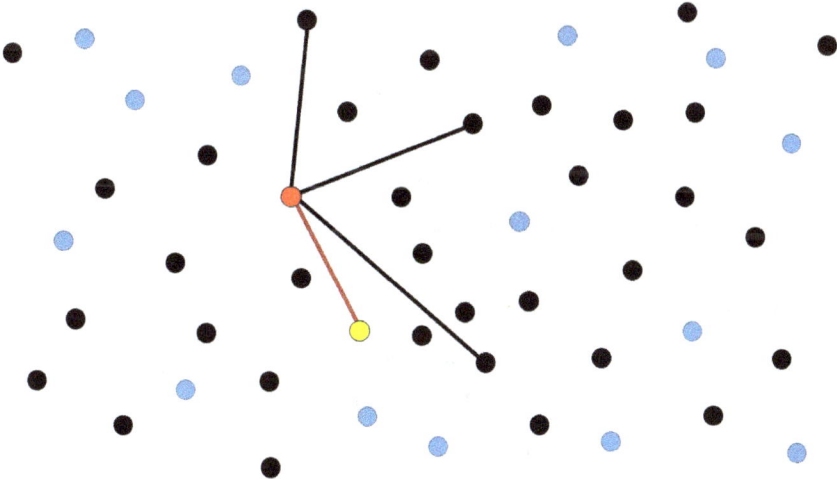

Fig. 26.4 Emily has infected Nova. Her other effective contacts did not lead to transmissions.

Emily will eventually recover. The newly exposed person, let's call her Nova, will become infectious after a few days and may have effective contacts with 2 people before recovering. Recall that the number 3 is only an average. About two thirds of Nova's 2 effective contacts will be with people who are no longer susceptible. Let's assume in our example that this will be the case for both effective contacts:

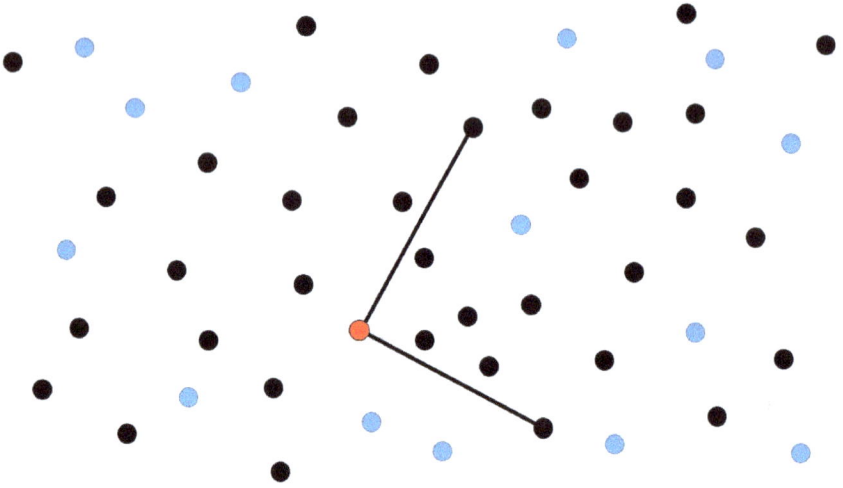

Fig. 26.5   Nova has effective contacts with 2 people, neither of whom is susceptible.

Bob: Then the chain of transmission stops.

Alice: Right. The outbreak started by Ingham has run it course. It was confined to one short chain of transmissions that I'll show you in my next picture (Fig. 26.6).

Cindy: Wouldn't this be almost like in our earlier discussion about the effect of the basic reproduction number R_0 when $R_0 < 1$?

Alice: Exactly! With $R_0 = 3$, each infectious individual makes on average effective contacts with other 3 people before becoming removed. But when more than two thirds of the population are no longer susceptible, on average less than 1 of these contacts would be with someone who is no longer susceptible. So, the average number of new infections caused by an infectious individual would be less than 1.

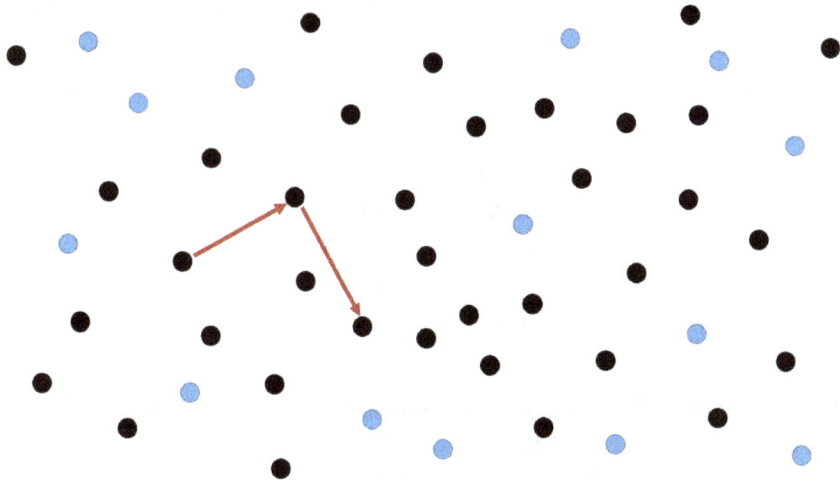

Fig. 26.6 The chain of transmissions in the outbreak started by Ingham.

Bob: In other words, above the herd immunity threshold, the reproduction number R is less than 1. Even without control measures.

Alice: Very well said, Bob! This is true when the proportion of people who are no longer susceptible is above the herd immunity threshold.

In our discussion so far, we have looked only at a population where initially the number of removed individuals exceeds the herd immunity threshold, while all others are still susceptible. In this case, new infections can only occur through contacts with somebody outside of the population, and the chains of transmission started by them will quickly fizzle out. Each such chain will stay short and will not affect many people. So the people who are still susceptible will not be totally protected, but will remain relatively safe.

Frank: Why don't we simply get to that point as quickly as possible, without any of those control measures that destroy jobs and mess up people's lives?

Cindy: But if we were to do nothing to slow down the spread of the virus, our healthcare system would become overwhelmed. We would run out of hospital beds and then have to turn away people with severe Covid-19 infections. Many of them would die unnecessarily!

Bob: Yes, Cindy, we talked about this. So we need to at least slow down the spread.

I'm wondering though whether we could reach herd immunity gradually, with some control measures that don't hurt the economy too much: social distancing, wearing masks, frequent hand-washing, testing, isolation of confirmed cases, and quarantining their contacts. Once we get to herd immunity, all of us could lead normal lives again.

Cindy: But Bob, if for herd immunity two thirds of the population need to become infected, then on the scale of the whole U.S. this would mean about 221 million people! And I recall from our meeting at the end of June that around 1.6 million people would die from Covid-19 in the U.S. We cannot let this happen!

Bob: I think if we want to go for herd immunity, we would need to take extra precautions to protect people who are at especially high risk.

Cindy: But we cannot shut up our grandparents in their own rooms for a year or longer! This would be so cruel. More than anything else, they want to see and hug their grandchildren.

Alice: The strategy of ending the Covid-19 outbreak by achieving herd immunity has actually been tried in the U.K. and in Sweden. We also talked about this when we first met in June.

Sweden is still following the route that Bob had suggested, trying to slow the spread with relatively mild restrictions and to protect especially vulnerable people. In particular, the Swedes did not close schools. But they are still very far from achieving herd immunity, and their number of deaths from Covid-19 per capita is among the 10 highest in the world.[8]

Frank: So there are problems with this strategy. But it seems to be an option.

Alice: That's actually not clear. One big issue is how long immunity against the infection lasts. When people lose immunity after some time and become susceptible again, herd immunity may never be achieved. Epidemiologists worry that immunity after recovery from Covid-19 may only be temporary. Covid-19 has not been around long enough for collecting much data. But a paper just came out about the first documented case of re-infection with Covid-19.[29] It seems unlikely that immunity will last forever.

Frank: Well, there is just one documented case so far. What if immunity were permanent in the vast majority of patients who recovered? Going for herd immunity should then be a realistic strategy.

Alice: Let's discuss this What-If scenario. Assume that immunity after recovery from Covid-19 remains permanent and that we let the infection spread through the population without control measures. Reported weekly numbers of new infections may then look like in this picture:

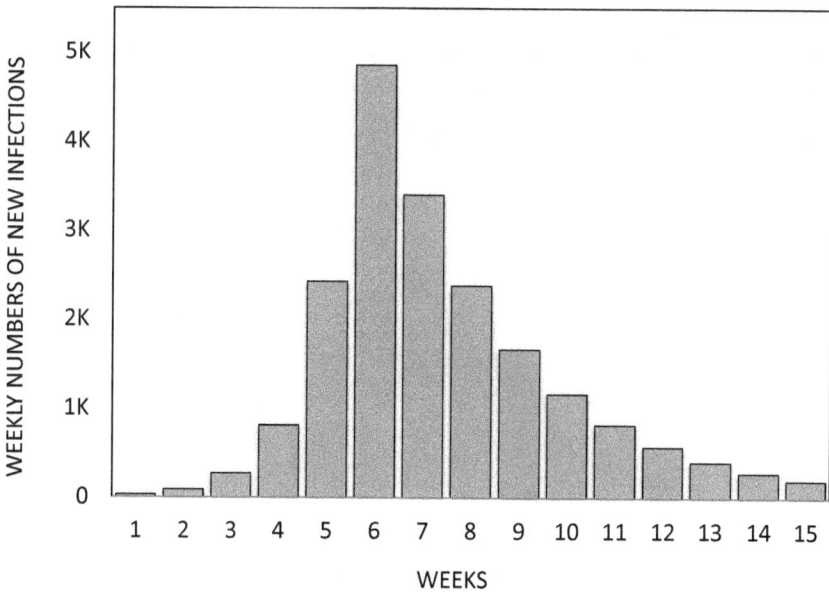

Fig. 26.7 Without control measures, daily new infections peak when the herd immunity threshold is crossed. This happens in Week 6 in the illustration.

The proportion of people who experienced infection will eventually cross the herd immunity threshold. At that time, two thirds of all people will be in the exposed, infectious, or removed states. Then the reproduction number R will fall below 1, and each infectious person will cause on average fewer than 1 new infection. We will then start observing a decrease in the daily numbers of new infections.

Cindy: Does this mean that the daily numbers of new infections will increase until the herd immunity threshold is reached?

Alice: Right! These numbers will reach a peak when the herd immunity threshold is crossed, as in my picture (Fig. 26.7).

Frank: What peak and decrease in the number of new infections? I thought that the transmissions stop when herd immunity is reached.

Alice: This is a common misinterpretation of the effects of herd immunity.

Frank: What's wrong about it?

Alice: When the herd immunity threshold is reached, the states of people in the population would not look like in my first picture (Fig. 26.1), but rather like in this one:

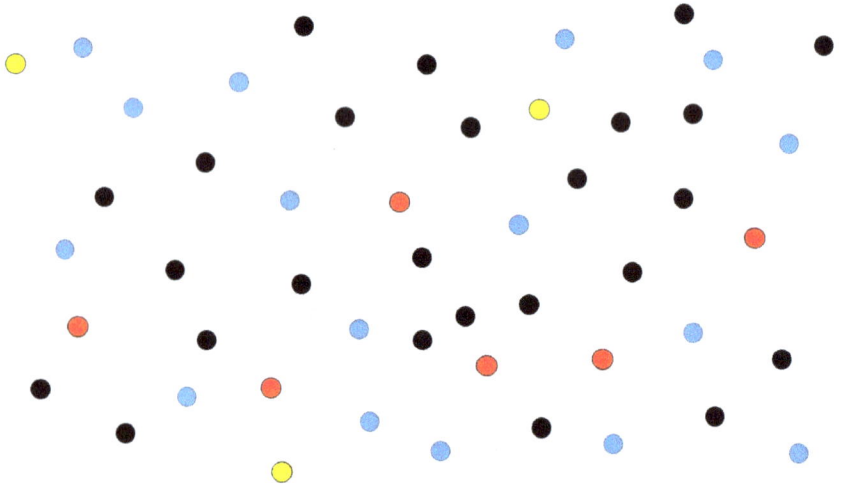

Fig. 26.8   State of a small population when herd immunity threshold is crossed without any control measures.

Frank: Why?

Alice: Let's again assume that each infectious person makes on average effective contacts with $R_0 = 3$ other people before recovering. The populations will reach the herd immunity threshold when two thirds of the population are in either the exposed, infectious, or removed states and the other one third of the population will remain susceptible. There will have been a number of fairly recent transmissions, and a large proportion of the population will still be infected.

Infected people will cause further infections, as in my next picture. Fewer than 1 per person on average, but still new infections:

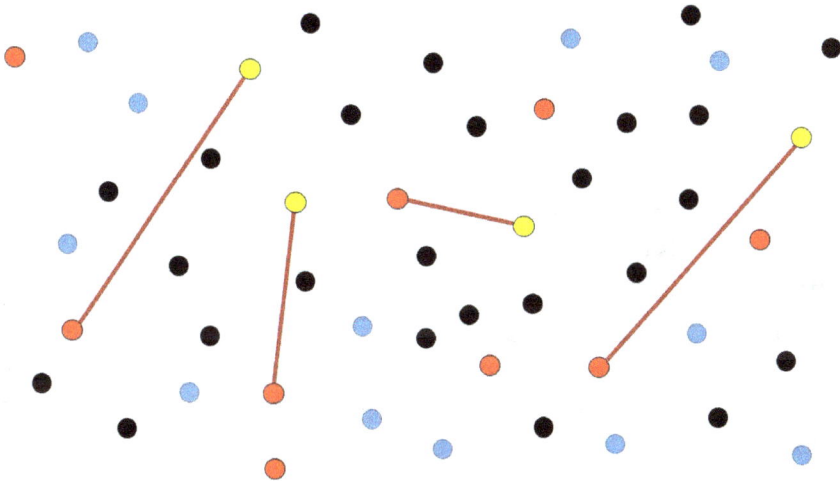

Fig. 26.9   Some transmissions still occur after the herd immunity threshold is crossed.

Eventually those infectious individuals will reach the removed state. But the newly exposed individuals will become infectious and cause some additional infections, as in my next picture (Fig. 26.10).

This process will go on for a while before all new infections stop.

Bob: So, if no control measures whatsoever are taken, more people will experience infection than the minimal percentage needed for herd immunity.

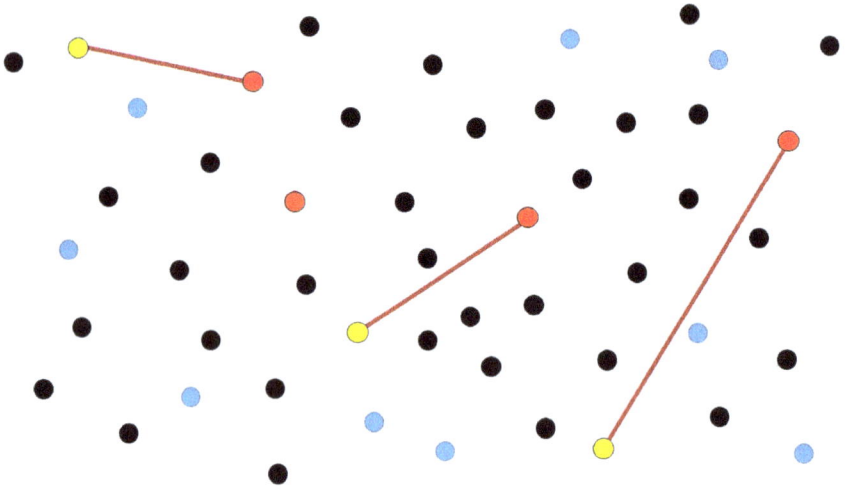

Fig. 26.10   More new infections occur.

Alice: Many more will become infected. This so-called overshoot phenomenon is often overlooked when people talk about herd immunity.

For a value $R_0 = 3$ that we had assumed in our examples, around 94% of all people might experience infection. But herd immunity is already achieved at around 67%. So our models predict that an additional 27% of all people would experience infection as a result of the overshoot.[60] For a population of 50 people, 94% would look like in my next picture (Fig. 26.11).

Cindy: Almost everybody would catch coronavirus. We cannot let this happen!

Bob: So this would be the scenario when we just let the infection spread through the population without any control measures. But what if we do something to slow down the spread and try reaching herd immunity more gradually?

Alice: Then at the time the herd immunity threshold is crossed, there also would be infectious people around, but relatively fewer than without control measures.

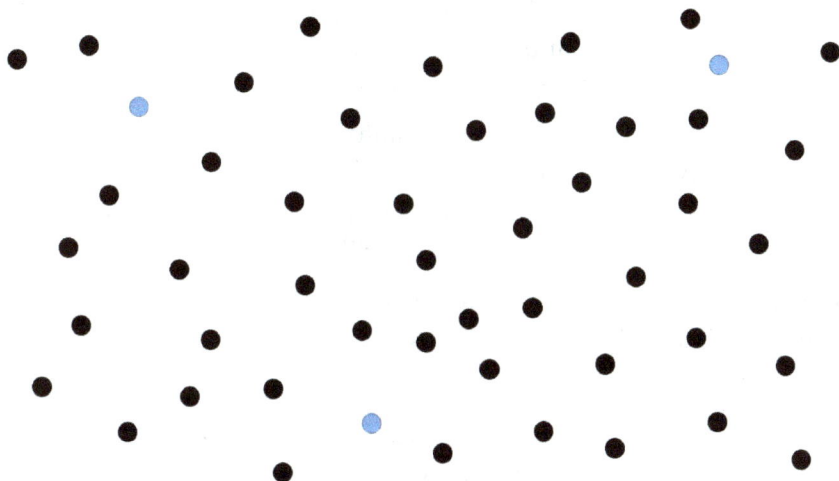

Fig. 26.11 State of the population at the end of an outbreak when no control measures are taken.

With some control measures for slowing down the spread until herd immunity is reached, the state of the population might look more like this:

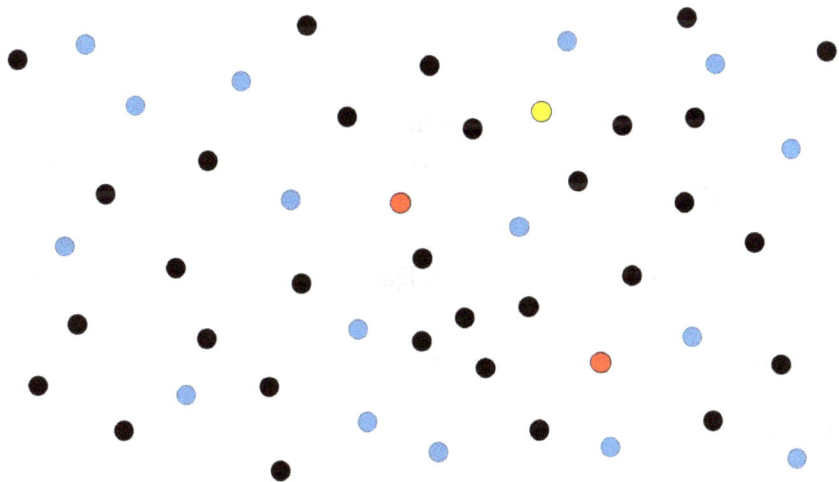

Fig. 26.12 State of a small population when herd immunity threshold is crossed while control measures have slowed the spread.

Some chains of transmissions would still propagate, but not as many as in our previous scenario. There would still be an overshoot, though not as big as without any control measures whatsoever.

Frank: Hmm. Going for herd immunity by letting people catch the infection may not work as well as I had thought.

But could there be a way of putting 67% of all people into the removed state without them getting sick?

Cindy: Where "removed state" means that they are immune from becoming infected and cannot infect others, right?

Alice: Right.

Cindy: Isn't vaccination doing what Frank was asking about? I mean, giving vaccinated people immunity from becoming infected without them having to suffer through the disease?

Alice: Exactly! You have explained the purpose of vaccination very well.

Bob: Can we take a short break and then talk about Covid-19 vaccines?

Alice: Sure.

Endnotes

[135] The UNESCO website has an interactive map that shows how the numbers and percentages of learners affected by school closures changed over time [1].

[136] Bob's lines here are loosely based on private communications with parents in the Cincinnati area, David Gerberry and Jennifer Robbins of Xavier University.

[137] In general, the herd immunity threshold is equal to $1 - 1/R_0$.

References

[1] UNESCO. COVID-19. Education: From disruption to recovery. [cited 2020 Dec 19].
https://en.unesco.org/covid19/educationresponse

Chapter 27

How could vaccination help?

Alice, Bob, Cindy, and Frank continue their meeting on August 30, 2020. Vaccines are widely expected to help end the Covid-19 pandemic. Already in early April, almost 80 companies and institutes in 19 countries were working on developing vaccines against the disease [1]. China had started to vaccinate health care workers with experimental vaccines in July [2], and Russia granted emergency approval for a Covid-19 vaccine on August 11, 2020 [3]. On May 15, the US government announced federal funding for a fast-track program called Operation Warp Speed [4], with the goals of placing diverse vaccine candidates in clinical trials by fall 2020, and manufacturing 300 million doses of a licensed vaccine by January 2021.

Bob: Cindy mentioned that vaccinations give people immunity from becoming infected. How, exactly, does this work?

Alice: Vaccines introduce molecules of viruses into the body. The details of how this can be done are quite complicated, and I don't want to discuss them right now.[138]

These molecules are called antigens. The immune system will recognize them as alien invaders that potentially pose a danger, regardless of whether they sit on the surfaces of real virus particles or are introduced by a vaccine. It will then try to defend the organism by destroying the invaders.

One part of it, called the innate immune system, provides readily available defenses against all sorts of invaders and will spring into action immediately. It can easily deal with a few virus particles. This is why it takes a fairly large number of them to cause an actual infection.

But if there are too many invaders, the innate immune system cannot deal with them all by itself and will activate the adaptive or acquired immune system. This other part of the immune system will learn how to produce antibodies that bind specifically to particular antigens and initiate their destruction. These antibodies provide much stronger defenses against particular viruses than the all-purpose response of the innate immune system.

Vaccines work by introducing enough antigens into the body so that this learning process will produce sufficiently many antibodies. While the antibodies hang around and the acquired immune system retains a memory of how to produce them, these strong defenses will be readily available when real virus particles enter the body. Then the vaccinated person will be immune from infection.

Bob: But learning takes some time, as we all know.

Alice: Yes. That's why in real infections most people get sick for a while before recovering. When the virus particles multiply more rapidly than the innate immune system can destroy them, the adaptive immune system learns by trial and error how to produce the right antibodies against the particular invaders. Once it has figured out the correct recipe, it will ramp up their production until it can destroy virus particles fast enough. After recovery, the antibodies and the memory of how to produce them will still be around and give the patient immunity from re-infection, at least for some time.

The learning process also takes time after vaccination, and it may take even longer than after an actual infection. Nobody becomes immune immediately after receiving a shot of vaccine.

And the immune system's memory may also get a little rusty over time. So it may be necessary to give a second dose of the vaccine, called a booster shot, to fully prepare the immune system for dealing with the real challenge.

Frank: Sounds like a review session before the test. Anyway, some time after that review session, vaccinated people will be in the removed state without suffering through an infection.

Alice: That's exactly how epidemiologists think about vaccinations. Recall that "removed state" means that the person can no longer become infected and can no longer infect others. After the effects of the vaccine fully kick in, a vaccinated individual may no longer become part of a chain of disease transmissions.

Bob: The infection could still spread among unvaccinated people though.

Cindy: But if sufficiently many people get vaccinated, we will achieve herd immunity. Then all of us will be reasonably safe from infection. Both those people who got vaccinated, and those who did not.

Alice: Very important point, Cindy! By vaccinating someone, we aim to cut all chains of transmission that this person otherwise might propagate. By vaccinating sufficiently many people, but not necessarily all of them, we would protect each of us.

Frank: So why not simply wait until we get vaccines, vaccinate enough people, and be done with this pandemic?

Bob: And why are we still waiting? In Russia, they are already vaccinating people!

Alice: When vaccines become available, it will be much easier to get the pandemic under control. Approval of the first vaccines in the U.S. is only expected a few months from now.[139] But we cannot wait that long.

Let's hope the vaccines that are currently under development are found to be safe and effective, and let's fast-forward to the time when they will have been approved. Even then, transmissions of Covid-19 will not immediately stop.

Frank: Why not?

Cindy: Alice just told us: It takes a while after vaccination before immunity fully develops.

Alice: Yes. And there are several other reasons.

We already discussed how herd immunity works: When it is reached, there will still be infectious people around. This is true also when herd immunity is achieved by vaccinations during an ongoing epidemic. These infectious individuals will start new chains of transmissions. With herd immunity and a reproduction number below 1, these chains will fizzle out and the number of new infections will decrease. But it will take time before all new infections stop.

The more infected people there will be at the time, the longer this process will take. In the U.S., we currently have very large numbers of infections. If we want to return to a reasonably normal life as quickly as possible after a successful vaccination campaign, we need to bring these numbers down and keep them down.

Cindy: So, in the meantime, we need to keep up social distancing, wearing masks, and frequently washing our hands.

Bob: As well as testing and contact tracing.

Alice: Right. Now recall that, for Covid-19, with a basic reproduction number R_0 possibly as high as 3, herd immunity would require that we vaccinate at least two thirds of the population. On the scale of the entire U.S., this translates into more than 220 million people.

When vaccines become available, we will not be able to vaccinate 220 million people within a few days. Even if we had that many doses of vaccine, we would not have enough health care workers to administer them so quickly.

Frank: So who should get vaccinated first?

Cindy: I think people who are most at risk of dying from the disease. Older people and people with pre-existing conditions.

Bob: But I think it should be people most at risk for becoming infected, especially healthcare personnel and people who work in crowded environments like meat-processing plants.

Frank: I agree more with Cindy here. As long as those who work in meat-processing plants and in hospitals are young and healthy, they have little to fear from becoming infected.

Alice: You have perfectly described the dilemma we will be facing.[140] Our instinct is to first protect those immediately at risk. But by first vaccinating those people whose professions require them to have many intense contacts with other people, we can cut as many potential chains of transmission as possible. If we target the first available doses of vaccine in this way, each of these doses will also indirectly protect the largest possible number of other people, including those at the highest risk of developing complications from the infection or dying from it.

Frank: I can see why some people might want to jump the line and get vaccinated as quickly as possible. For my part, I'll be more than happy to skip the vaccination altogether. I'm young and healthy, so I'm not worried about catching coronavirus in the first place.

Alice: As Cindy had said earlier, vaccinating one person also protects others. And for achieving herd immunity, at least two thirds of us need to decide to get vaccinated.

I get that you are not overly concerned about contracting Covid-19 yourself, Frank. But let's assume that your grandma is in the high-risk group and cannot get vaccinated for medical reasons. If you happen to be infectious and asymptomatic, so that you don't even know that you have Covid-19, you might transmit the disease to her when you visit. I know you would want to prevent this. Would you then rather decide to get vaccinated and protect both yourself and her? Or would you rather stop visiting her?

Frank: I guess grandpa would want me to get vaccinated in such a case. So I would, to honor his memory. But the point is moot; grandma is in good health and there is no reason she should not get the vaccine herself.

Alice: Well, would you then decide to get vaccinated to protect a good friend and his grandma, who might be in a situation like I just described?

Frank: Hmm. That's a tough question. I'd need to think more about it, quite honestly. But my friend's grandma could become infected also through another chain of transmission, one that doesn't involve me. So it would be better if my friend got vaccinated. As you said, as long as enough people get vaccinated, we all will be protected. It doesn't need to be me.

Alice: Thank you, Frank, for being so honest. It doesn't have to be you. But if more than 1 in 3 of us will decide not to get vaccinated because it would suffice if enough other people volunteer, we will not achieve herd immunity. Covid-19 infections will continue to spread. Many more people will become infected, suffer through the disease, and even die. The economy will still not be able to return to normal functioning. Literally all of us will suffer the consequences.

Bob: Getting vaccinated would be the rational choice for all of us. To protect people's health and get the economy going again. Wouldn't you agree with that, Frank?

Frank: Only if the vaccines don't have side effects that may be worse than Covid-19. I don't buy those claims that vaccines are really safe.

Alice: Safety of vaccines is a great concern. Scientists do everything possible to ensure that they don't have nasty side effects. Before a vaccine is given to millions of people, it first needs to be thoroughly tested on large groups of volunteers. These volunteers then need to be carefully monitored over an extended period of time in order to find out how well the vaccine actually works and whether it may cause side effects. Scientists insist on strict procedures, called protocols, for conducting these tests and the monitoring. The process normally takes several years. They confirm the safety of a vaccine and approve its use only after they have clear evidence that it actually works and does not cause side effects beyond mild discomfort over a few days.

Even though all vaccines that are currently in use against other diseases have gone through a multi-year testing process and are carefully monitored for effectiveness and side effects on a continuing basis, many people remain skeptical about their safety. In the case of vaccines that have been tested for years and used for decades, this skepticism is entirely based on misinformation about the scientific evidence. But it has already done a lot of damage. For example, several recent outbreaks of measles in the U.S. were caused by too many people refusing vaccination. They were entirely preventable [5].

Frank: If it has been tested for years and really did not cause any harm, I might be convinced to get vaccinated. But these vaccines against coronavirus are being developed at "warp speed", over several months, not years [4]. So how can we know they are safe?

Alice: This is an important and difficult question. Scientists are insisting on the established protocols for ensuring effectiveness and safety. If these protocols are meticulously followed and volunteers are monitored over several months, I would be confident that at least there are no significant short-term side effects. Long-term side effects appear to be unlikely, but we would still not have solid data to rule those out.

We have another dilemma here: On the one hand, we want to have Covid-19 vaccines available as quickly as possible, so that we can protect people and prevent unnecessary infections, suffering, and deaths. On the other hand, if the testing and approval process gets abbreviated and these vaccines become available too quickly, we might fail to detect some possible side effects. Vaccinating millions of people might then cause these side effects on a very large scale.[141] Bob had mentioned earlier that Russia is already vaccinating people. So is China. I am not sure that these vaccines have been tested long enough to ensure their safety.

Cindy: But you have not answered Frank's question, Alice. Will it be safe for us to get vaccinated?

Alice: I cannot answer this question before the testing will be completed. So we should all carefully study the scientific evidence and the approval process. If established protocols have been meticulously followed, then the vaccines should be safe. But should there be political pressure to cut corners for speeding things up, I myself would not trust the safety of Covid-19 vaccines nearly as much as I trust the safety of other vaccines.[142]

I can only say this: Read what scientists write about the vaccines when they become available. Rely on the opinions of experts on vaccines who have no vested commercial or political interest. Leading scientific journals try their best to filter out biased and misleading claims, but their articles are sometimes difficult to read. Major news outlets present the research in more digestible form. You can rely on those, as long as they quote sources with a solid reputation in the scientific community.

Bob: I guess there will be all sorts of opinions all over the internet. And too few people get vaccinated, we will not be able to control the spread of Covid-19.

Alice: This is a big concern. If all goes well, the vaccines that are being developed should be safe and effective. But I am not optimistic that we will get sufficiently high vaccine uptake—that is, a sufficiently high percentage of people getting vaccinated—for achieving herd immunity. Besides the vaccine skeptics who will refuse any vaccine whatsoever, many others may perceive vaccines against Covid-19 as dangerous because of how fast they are being developed, even if they will be perfectly safe. This perception may discourage too many people from getting vaccinated.[143]

Cindy: Would we then not even get close to achieving herd immunity?

Alice: It might happen. And there are more factors that may lower vaccine uptake: Some people may not get vaccinated out of inertia or because they lack health insurance and cannot afford to pay for the vaccine.

Bob: That problem can be easily solved: Insurance companies should cover the entire cost for all policy holders, and the vaccine should be available for free to those without health insurance.

Frank: Come on, Bob! Why should insurance companies suffer a loss? And why should our taxes pay for vaccinating those without insurance coverage?

Bob: Economic self-interest. Insurance companies will be better off paying for the vaccine than taking the risk of picking up the bill for treatment if one of their clients gets sick. And the U.S. treasury will easily recoup the layout for letting the uninsured get vaccinated. The more people get vaccinated, the more fully the economy will recover and generate more tax revenue. Better to spend a little on vaccines than a lot on unemployment benefits.

Cindy: I like that! Perhaps we can somehow convince two thirds of all people to get vaccinated. Then we will have herd immunity, after some time the pandemic will be over, and life will be back to normal!

Alice: I'd love to agree with you, Cindy. But unfortunately, herd immunity may not last forever, and even a vaccine uptake of 67% may not get us there.

The others: Why not?

Alice: We all know that we may forget what we have already learned. The immune system may have the same problem. We don't know yet how good it will be at remembering its defenses against Covid-19. It may need a reminder once in a while. In other words, we may need to repeatedly vaccinate the same person against Covid-19. It is not currently known how long the effect of vaccines will last and how often we would need to repeat them.[144]

And there is another issue that is often overlooked. Our estimate of the vaccine uptake that is needed for herd immunity was based on the assumption that the vaccine is 100% effective, that it confers perfect immunity. But for many vaccines this is not the case, and it is unlikely to be the case for the Covid-19 vaccines that are under development. They should be more than 50% effective, but it is unlikely that they will be 100% effective.[145]

Bob: What do you mean by less than 100% effective?

Alice: Let me show you some pictures. The first (Fig. 27.1) will be for a 100% effective vaccine.

The black dots represent vaccinated people; the red dots show 2 infectious individuals. With $R_0 = 3$, they may make effective contacts with about 6 other people while they remain infectious. In our example, one third of these effective contacts were with susceptible and two thirds with vaccinated people. With a 100% effective vaccine in this example, none of the 4 contacts with vaccinated people led to a new infection. Only the 2 contacts with unvaccinated people and started of 2 chains of infections, but with R reduced from 3 to a little below 1, we would expect them to quickly fizzle out:

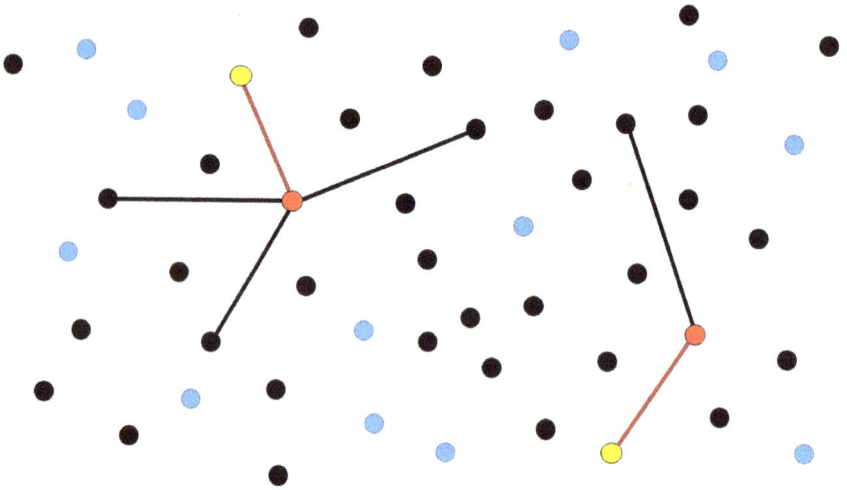

Fig. 27.1   New infections when 68% of the population have 100% immunity.

Now let us look at a similar picture where the vaccination is only 50% effective; shown by the grey dots here:

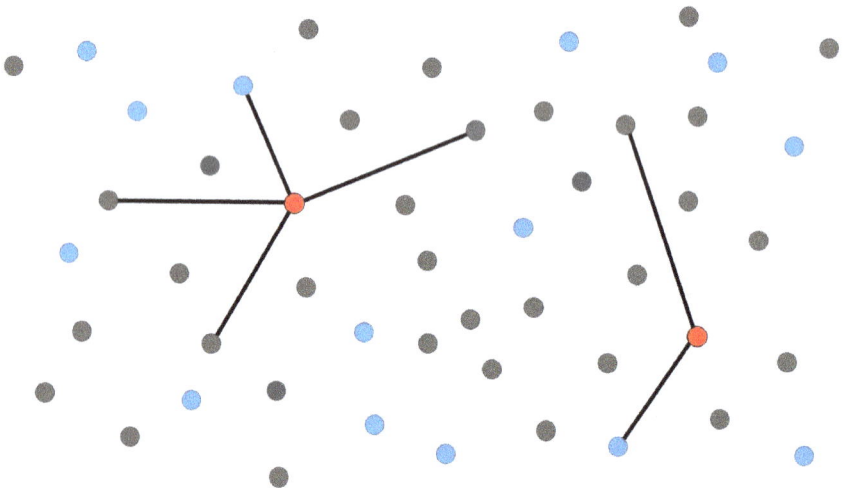

Fig. 27.2   Effective contacts when 68% of the population have 50% immunity.

This picture (Fig. 27.2) shows only the effective contacts. A 50% effective vaccine might not confer total immunity to anybody, but might cut the chances of transmission during an effective contact with an infectious person in half.

In my next picture we see that half of the effective contacts with vaccinated individuals led to transmission, the other half did not:

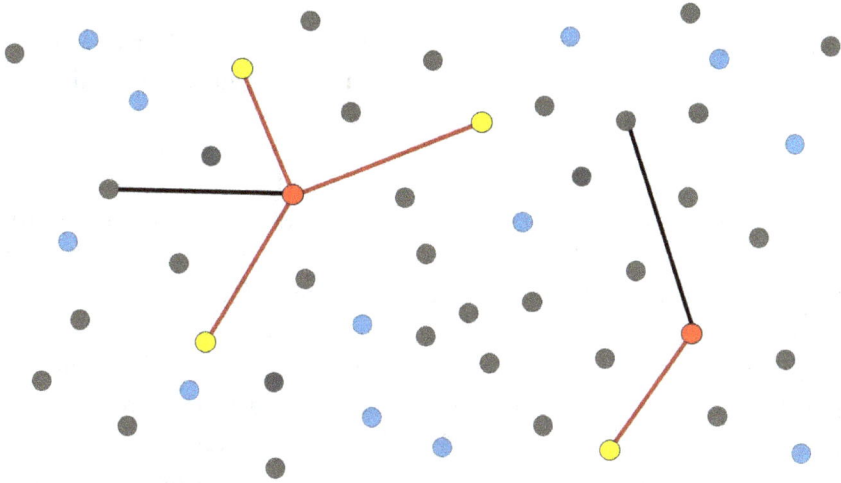

Fig. 27.3   New infections when 68% of the population have 50% immunity.

In this example, the 2 infectious individuals have caused 4 secondary transmissions; on average 2 each. Epidemiologists predict that giving a 50% effective vaccine to two thirds of the population would reduce the reproduction number from $R = 3$ to to $R = 2$.

A vaccine might also be 50% effective if it confers perfect immunity to half of the vaccinated people and has no effect on the other half. The resulting reduction in the reproduction number would be the same: from $R = 3$ to $R = 2$.

Cindy: So, such a vaccine would not help then? You told us that if the reproduction number R is larger than 1, the infection will spread to a large fraction of the population.

Alice: Such a vaccine would not all by itself eradicate the pandemic.

Similarly, a 70% effective vaccine would not eradicate the pandemic, even if it were given to three quarters of the population.[146] Neither would a 100% effective vaccine if less than two thirds of us decide to get vaccinated.

Bob: So, vaccines are no magic bullets after all.

Alice: Not as magic as many people believe. Even after a successful vaccination campaign, some other preventive measures will most likely remain necessary, at least for some time.

But this does not make vaccinations useless. Even partially effective vaccines and less than optimal vaccine uptake will reduce the reproduction number R. Think about it this way: Currently, we have a large number of daily new infections in the U.S., but they are decreasing.[147] With the preventive measures currently in place—social distancing, mask wearing, frequent hand washing, and partial restrictions on how businesses can operate—we seem to have achieved a reduction of R from around 3 to 1. That's where it seems to be right now on the scale of the entire country. In some states, R is still a little higher than 1; in other states, it is currently significantly lower than 1.

After vaccinating a large percentage of our population with an imperfect vaccine and no full herd immunity, we would need to still maintain other preventive measures. But these would need to bring down R only from somewhere between 1 and 2 to below 1, not from close to 3 to below 1. This will be much easier. To completely eradicate the pandemic over time, we may still need to practice social distancing, wear masks in many situations, and frequently wash our hands. But there is hope that we could lift almost all restrictions on the operations of businesses. And we would no longer need to agonize over whether it will be safe for kids to go to school, for us to study on campus, and for everybody to visit relatives or friends who are at high risk for complications. With enough relatively mild preventive measures, this will become reasonably safe.

Endnotes

[138] There are several different methods for introducing viral molecules into the body through vaccinations. Many vaccines contain inactivated viral particles that can no longer cause an infection. Some of the vaccines against Covid-19 belong to a new class of vaccines called mRNA vaccines. They do not introduce viral molecules directly into the body, only genetic material that codes for certain viral proteins, which are then expressed by certain cells in the immune system of vaccinated person. For more details, see [6].

[139] The first Covid-19 vaccine in the U.S. was approved for emergency use on December 11, 2020 [7].

[140] A Politico article [8] gives information on how governments around the world are approaching this problem.

[141] A CNN article [9] discusses potential dangers of premature approval of vaccines.

[142] Documenting political pressure to rush vaccine approval is outside the scope of this book. It should be emphasized that vaccine uptake is influenced by the perception of political pressure, not by how much pressure there actually was and whether or not government agencies like the FDA in fact yielded to it.

[143] A poll conducted by the Kaiser Family Foundation around the time of this conversation found that if a vaccine was approved before Election Day in the U.S. on November 3, 2020, and made freely available to anyone who wanted it, 54% of respondents would not want to get vaccinated [10]. In a similar poll by the Pew Research Center, 49% of respondents said they definitely or probably would not get vaccinated at this time [11]. A subsequent Gallup Poll found that confidence in the vaccine had increased between mid-September and late October [12].

[144] Another potential reason why a vaccination may not give permanent protection is that viruses constantly mutate and can evolve resistance to the vaccine [13].

[145] At the time of this conversation, it was impossible to know how effective Covid-19 vaccines would turn out to be. In general,

effectiveness of vaccines greatly varies. For vaccines against seasonal influenza, for example, estimates range from 19% to 60%, depending on the year [14]. Initial clinical trials of the two vaccine that were recently approved in the U.S. showed effectiveness around 95%; see Chapter 29.

[146] In this scenario, the reproduction number would be reduced to $0.75 \times 0.3 \times 3 + 0.25 \times 3 = 1.38 > 1$.

[147] Over the last three weeks before this conversation, the 7-day moving average of daily reported Covid-19 cases in the U.S. decreased from 56,289 on August 8 to 43,118 on August 29, 2020 [15].

References

[1] Schmidt C. Genetic engineering could make a COVID-19 vaccine in months rather than years. Scientific American 2020 Jun 1. [cited 2020 Dec 15]. `https://www.scientificamerican.com/article/genetic-engineering-could-make-a-covid-19-vaccine-in-months-rather-than-years1/`

[2] Rettner R. China started giving experimental COVID-19 vaccine to medical workers in July. LiveScience. 2020 Aug 24 [cited 2020 Dec 15]. `https://www.livescience.com/china-approved-covid-19-vaccine-emergency-use-medical-workers.html`

[3] Burki TK. The Russian vaccine for COVID-19. The Lancet Resp Med. 2020 Nov 1 [cited 2020 Dec 15]; 8(11), e85–e86. `https://www.thelancet.com/journals/lanres/article/PIIS2213-2600(20)30402-1/fulltext` DOI: 10.1016/S2213-2600(20)30402-1

[4] Federal Government of the United States. Department of Health & Human Services. Trump Administration Announces Framework and Leadership for 'Operation Warp Speed.' 2020 May 15. [cited 2020 Dec 15]. `https://www.hhs.gov/about/news/2020/05/15/trump-administration-announces-framework-and-leadership-for-operation-warp-speed.html`

[5] Centers for Disease Control and Prevention. Measles (Rubeola).

Measles Cases and Outbreaks. [cited 2020 Dec 19].
https://www.cdc.gov/measles/cases-outbreaks.html

[6] Centers of Disease Control and Prevention. COVID-19. Understanding mRNA COVID-19 vaccines. 2020 Dec 18. [cited 2021 Jan 5]. https://www.cdc.gov/coronavirus/2019-ncov/vaccines/different-vaccines/mrna.html

[7] Thomas K, LaFraniere S, Weiland N, Goodnough A, Haberman M. F.D.A. clears Pfizer vaccine, and millions of doses will be shipped right away. The New York Times 2020 Dec 11. [updated 2020 Dec 21; cited 2021 Jan 5]. https://www.nytimes.com/2020/12/11/health/pfizer-vaccine-authorized.html

[8] Heath R, Paun C. Governments around the world weigh thorny question: Who gets the vaccine first? Politico 2020 Nov 27. [cited 2020 Dec 19]. https://www.politico.com/news/2020/11/27/covid-vaccine-world-440807

[9] Christensen J. Past vaccine disasters show why rushing a coronavirus vaccine now would be 'colossally stupid'. CNN 2020 Sep 1. [cited 2020 Dec 19]. https://www.cnn.com/2020/09/01/health/eua-coronavirus-vaccine-history/index.html

[10] Kaiser Family Foundation. Poll: Most Americans worry political pressure will lead to premature approval of a COVID-19 vaccine; half say they would not get a free vaccine approved before Election Day. 2020 Sep 10. [cited 2020 Dec 19]. https://www.kff.org/coronavirus-covid-19/press-release/poll-most-americans-worry-political-pressure-will-lead-to-premature-approval-of-a-covid-19-vaccine-half-say-they-would-not-get-a-free-vaccine-approved-before-election-day/

[11] Tyson A, Johnson C, Funk C. U.S. public now divided over whether to get COVID-19 vaccine. Pew Research Center 2020 Sep 17. [cited 2020 Dec 19]. https://www.pewresearch.org/science/2020/09/17/u-s-public-now-divided-over-whether-to-get-covid-19-vaccine/

[12] Reinhart RJ. More Americans now willing to get COVID-19 vaccine. Gallup 2020 Nov 17. [cited 2020 Dec 19]. https://news.gallup.com/poll/325208/americans-willing-covid-vaccine.aspx

[13] Gorman J, Zimmer C. The virus won't stop evolving when the vaccine arrives. The New York Times 2020 Nov 27. [updated 2020 Dec 2; cited 2020 Dec 19].
https://www.nytimes.com/2020/11/27/science/covid-vaccine-virus-resistance.html

[14] Centers for Disease Control and Prevention. Influenza (Flu). CDC Seasonal Flu Vaccine Effectiveness Studies. [cited 2020 Dec 19]. https://www.cdc.gov/flu/vaccines-work/effectiveness-studies.htm

[15] Worldometers.info. Dover, Delaware, U.S.A. COVID-19 coronavirus pandemic. [cited 2020 Dec 19].
https://www.worldometers.info/coronavirus/

Chapter 28

When were countries and states successful in dealing with COVID-19?

Alice, Bob, Cindy, and Frank meet on September 5, 2020. In total, over 27.4 million cases of Covid-19 infections and 895,000 deaths from the disease have been reported worldwide. In some countries, new infections are decreasing, in others they are on the rise. Over the last 4 weeks—between August 7 and September 4, 2020—in Singapore, the 7-day moving average of daily new infections decreased from around 63 to less than 7 per million people; in France, it increased from about 22 to about 92 per million [1].

Bob: So vaccines are under development, but are still being tested for effectiveness and safety. We don't know yet when they will become widely available and how much they will help. We need to wait and see. In the meantime, we need to rely on social distancing, wearing masks, frequent hand-washing, testing, quarantining, and contact tracing. But is it really possible to control Covid-19 even if we do all of this?

Frank: I bet it isn't.

Alice: There is plenty of evidence that the control measures on Bob's list can keep us reasonably safe even before vaccines become available. Recall that we don't need to prevent all new infections. This would indeed be impossible. In the long run, we only need to prevent enough of them to bring the reproduction number R down below 1 and keep it below 1. And that's possible.

Frank: How do you know?

Alice: Let's visit the website `https://rt.live/`.

Bob: I see that it gives estimates of a number R_t for all our states. I guess that's the reproduction number R and they use the subscript t because it changes over time.

Alice: Exactly. They also call it the effective reproduction rate. That's another name for the reproduction number at a given time t. I will simply use R in our discussions, as we did before.

Bob: How do they estimate these numbers?

Alice: The details are a bit complicated. Let me only say that these estimates can be derived by analyzing how the percentages of positive tests change over time.

Let's look at some of the info that is posted. For today, the website estimates that in 20 of our 50 states, R is below 1

Cindy: This means new infections are going down in these 20 states, right?

Alice: Yes, Cindy. This is what we would predict based on the current estimates of the reproduction numbers. The website also has graphs on how they changed over time.

Let's look at Pennsylvania as an example:

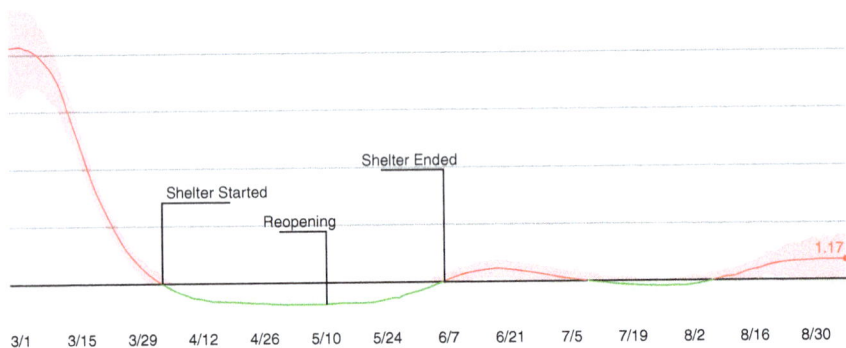

Fig. 28.1   Change of R in Pennsylvania between March 1 and September 4, 2020. The graphs in this chapter were adapted from the website R_t COVID-19 [2].

This state had gradually implemented some restrictions throughout March, including full lockdowns of more and more counties.[148] This brought the reproduction number R down to around 1. During the full lockdown, R then further decreased to about 0.8. Once re-opening began, it crept up to near 1 again. The lockdown ended gradually, around June 7, the date that is shown here. Right after that, there was a bump in R, which went up to around 1.1.

Bob: Did something similar happen also in other states?

Alice: The same general pattern can be seen in almost all states: R was brought down significantly below 1 during the lockdown. But once the lockdown ended, there was a bump that increased R to above 1 again.

Frank: What did you expect? After sitting home alone for many weeks, people wanted to go out, meet friends, have some fun. Have real contact with real people. You told us that more contacts would lead to more transmissions and higher reproduction numbers. And that's why you have those bumps in your graphs.

Bob: I can see that in some states the bumps were a lot bigger than in others. In Nevada, R went up to around 1.4:

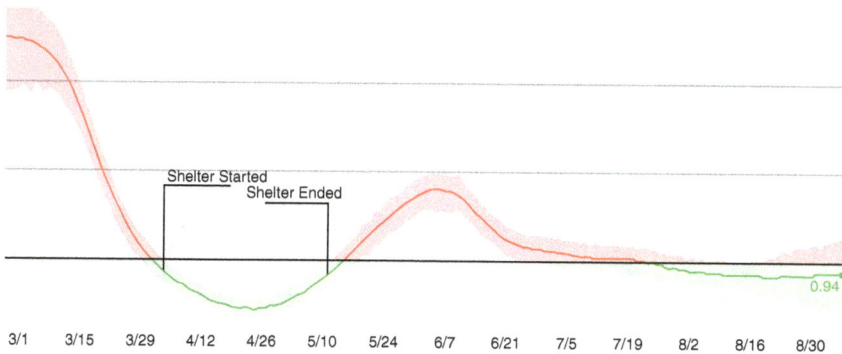

Fig. 28.2 Change of R in Nevada between March 1 and September 4, 2020.

Frank: Seems they partied wildly in Nevada. Doesn't surprise me at all.

Alice: Some bumps were unavoidable. But R did not need to go all the way up above 1 again.

In Connecticut and New Hampshire, the bumps were a lot smaller and R never crept up much above 1 after their lockdowns. Let's look at New Hampshire first:

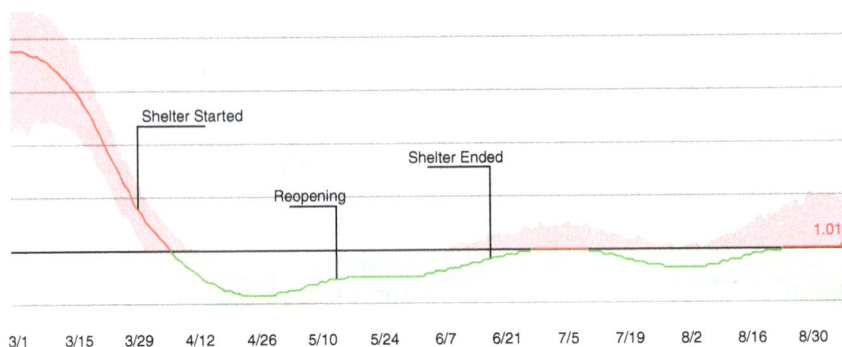

Fig. 28.3   Change of R in New Hampshire between March 1 and September 4, 2020.

And now let us look at the graph for Connecticut:

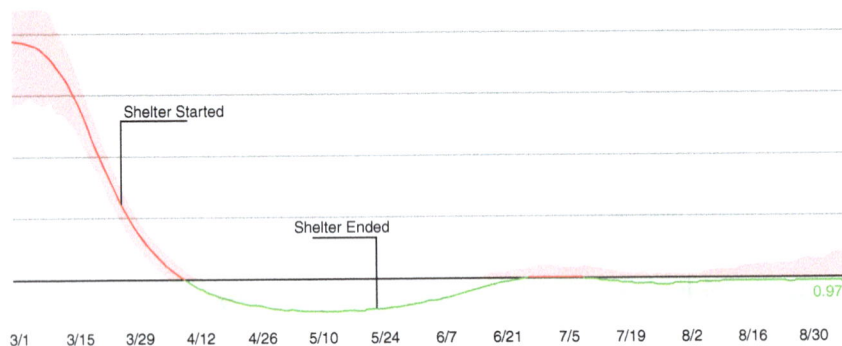

Fig. 28.4   Change of R in Connecticut between March 1 and September 4, 2020.

Bob: Why did some states have much smaller bumps than others?

Alice: The most important factor may have been how seriously people were concerned about the infection. Connecticut had a terrible outbreak in April, and people in this state have been cautious ever since. In other states, too many people may have believed that the pandemic was practically over and have become careless.

Cindy: They should have been more cautious!

Bob: I agree, but you cannot blame the people, Cindy. I recall that at the time there was a lot of talk about the pandemic being behind us.[149] Perhaps in some states more people believed it more than in others. If they thought that the outbreak was practically over, they would have seen no reason to remain cautious.

Alice: Good point, Bob! Coming back to Frank's question of why I'm cautiously optimistic: In the vast majority of our states, the reproduction number R had been brought back down below 1 again at least at some time after these initial bumps.[150] So it is possible to achieve this with a combination of relatively mild restrictions. Pennsylvania needed to impose new mandates about mask wearing in late June to make it happen. Nevada needed to close bars in some counties. New Hampshire and Connecticut achieved the same without any new mandates or restrictions [3].

Cindy: But in both Pennsylvania and New Hampshire, the reproduction number R has crept up above 1 again!

Alice: This shows that we need to keep up our vigilance and cannot let down our guard. Even when the reported numbers of cases are decreasing, we still need to practice social distancing, wear masks, and frequently wash our hands. We should not be paranoid about becoming infected, but use common sense. And we need to be prepared to maintain these inconvenient practices for a long time. If we do, we will avoid an increase in new cases. Then very disruptive control measures will not be necessary. Right now this is working in Connecticut, Nevada, and 18 other states. It can work everywhere.

Bob: But is it really working? Nevada still reports on average over 136 daily new cases per million people. For Connecticut, this number seems to be around 35 [1]. Why are the daily numbers still so large even in Connecticut, where R has been below 1 for a long time?

Alice: When the reproduction number R falls below 1, the daily number of new cases will decrease over time. But when R is only slightly less than 1, this process will take a long time. Even with $R = 0.9$, it would take about one month to decrease the daily new infections by 50%. Both in Nevada and Connecticut, the reproduction numbers are currently larger than 0.9; so this process will take even longer.[151] The big problem in the U.S. is that we have not brought down the numbers enough.[152] We have been living with the consequences ever since.

Cindy: Are there countries where the numbers are super low?

Alice: Yes, there are.[153] For example, Vietnam is a next-door neighbor of China, with many people traveling between the two countries. The first case of Covid-19 in Vietnam was reported on January 23, 2020. The country acted very early and decisively with strict quarantine measures. As of today, they reported 1,045 total cases and 35 deaths from Covid-19. And Vietnam is a large country of over 97 million people, almost one third of the population of the U.S.

Another example is New Zealand, with 1,772 total cases and 24 total deaths. It is a much smaller country than Vietnam. But their number of 354 total reported cases per million people is less than 2% of the 19,409 total cases per million that the U.S. reported as of today.

South Korea also had an outbreak early on. It was much bigger than the one in Vietnam. They quickly brought it under control, and their total number of 413 reported cases per million people as of today is close to New Zealand's.

Similarly, Rwanda also reported some cases in mid-March, but managed to keep their total at 334 cases per million so far.

Most European countries have been very successful. Italy and Spain had large outbreaks early on, but brought them under control with drastic and sufficiently long lockdowns. In June, their daily numbers were somewhere around 6 new cases per million, less than 10% of what they are now in Connecticut.

Other European countries never had large early outbreaks. Germany has reported 2,995 total cases per million people so far. In neighboring Poland, the number is 1,872, less than 10% of what we had in the U.S. until now. And in Greece it is only 1,093, less than 6% of the number in the U.S.

And closer to home: Our neighbors in Canada and Mexico have so far reported 3,479 and 4,872 total cases per million people, respectively. In the same ballpark as Germany.

Cindy: What did all these countries do right?

Alice: This is an important question. Covid-19 is a new disease, and we learn only gradually how it really spreads. Countries need to learn from each other's experiences.

We need to be careful though to not over-generalize. Every country made some mistakes. At least small ones. But the countries who were successful made fewer mistakes than others.

Also, with the exception of Canada and Mexico, in all of the countries I have mentioned, there already have been second waves. A big one in Spain; smaller ones in the other countries. Remember what I said earlier: Even if the numbers are low or decrease, people cannot let down their guards.

It is interesting that different things worked in different countries. South Korea responded to the initial outbreak with extremely vigorous testing and contact tracing. Vietnam is not as rich as South Korea and had fewer resources for testing. So they mostly relied on strict quarantines. New Zealand was helped to some extent by the fact that the country consists of two fairly remote islands. Both in New Zealand and neighboring Australia, drastic travel restrictions actually helped a lot.

It is fascinating to study the details of the many different approaches that worked in the most successful countries. I encourage you to read more about this on the web. Wikipedia has a separate page for the Covid-19 outbreaks in each of the countries I mentioned, and you can start there. Let me only say that there is no one-size-fits-all response to the Covid-19 outbreak that worked equally well everywhere.

Bob: Did cultural differences make it easier for some countries to control the pandemic?

Alice: Such factors certainly played a role. For example, in many Asian countries, there had already been a long tradition of wearing face masks to protect others from infections like the flu. And in some countries, people will more readily comply with government directives than in others.

But again, we should not jump to conclusions. In Poland, for example, people are proudly individualistic and generally skeptical of government regulations. But still the country has reported significantly fewer cases per million than neighboring Germany.

Frank: Interesting.

Bob: But are there things that all of these relatively successful countries have in common?

Alice: Yes, there are. In all of them the central government took decisive action. Very early in Vietnam, a little later in other countries. In none of them has the response to Covid-19 been politicized nearly as much as in the U.S.

Most importantly, in the most successful countries there has been clear and consistent messaging[154] at all levels of the government: Covid-19 is a dangerous disease. Here is how we can protect ourselves. If we don't, or if we let down our guard too soon, we will be in trouble.

This messaging was based on the best available scientific evidence. And most people in these countries had enough trust in science and scientists to accept the message.

Endnotes

[148] The information on timelines for imposing and lifting control measures in individual states was obtained from [3].

[149] Messaging by the White House and conservative media outlets that led to a false sense of security has been a problem in the U.S. throughout most of 2020. A detailed discussion of this issue is beyond the scope of this book. Some information can be found in [4].

[150] According to the graphs at [2], Kansas and Montana were the only states where the reproduction number did not drop below 1 at any time between the post-lockdown bump and September 5.

[151] Alice's estimate is based on a serial interval of 4.5 days, so that one month would correspond to approximately $\log_{0.9} 0.5$ serial intervals. Under the same assumption about the serial interval, but with $R = 0.95$ instead of $R = 0.9$, it would take about two months to decrease the numbers of new infections by 50%. Published estimates of the serial interval for Covid-19 vary[51] and the median length of the serial interval may change as a result of control measures being in place. The values of one and two months given here should be treated only as intuitive ball-park figures.

[152] Compare, for example, the graphs for Italy and the U.S. in Chapter 17. One factor that contributed to the problem was that some states did not adhere to federal guidelines and started re-opening too soon. Examples were discussed in Chapters 13 and 22.

[153] The numbers of infections in various countries in the next few paragraphs were quoted from [1].

[154] A few days prior to this conversation, New York Times posted a video about Covid-19 messaging in various countries [5].

References

[1] Worldometers.info. Dover, Delaware, U.S.A. COVID-19 coronavirus pandemic. [cited 2020 Sep 5].
https://www.worldometers.info/coronavirus/

[2] Krieger M, Systrom K, Vladeck T. R_t COVID-19. [cited 2020 Sep 5]. https://rt.live/

[3] Johns Hopkins University of Medicine. Coronavirus Resource Center. Critical Trends. Impact of opening and closing decisions by state. [cited 2020 Sep 5].
https://coronavirus.jhu.edu/data/state-timeline

[4] Leonhardt D, Leatherby L. The unique U.S. failure to control the virus. The New York Times 2020 Aug 6. [updated 2020 Aug 8; cited 2020 Sep 5]. https://www.nytimes.com/2020/08/06/us/coronavirus-us.html

[5] Dosani S., Dingari C. The three rules of coronavirus communication. The New York Times 2020 Sep 2. [cited 2020 Dec 20]. `https://www.nytimes.com/2020/09/02/opinion/coronavirus-communication.html`

Chapter 29

What does the future hold?

Alice, Bob, Cindy, and Frank meet on December 21, 2020, after the end of their Fall Semester. Daily reported Covid-19 cases in the U.S. have been on the order of 220,000 over the preceding week, and daily reported deaths from the disease on the order of 2,650.[155] Hospitals in parts of the country are running out of capacity [1]. European countries had also seen large waves of new infections in the fall. In France, it peaked in early November after a second lockdown had been imposed.[156] Neighboring Germany is still struggling to get the outbreak under control and will remain under lockdown into January 2021 [2]. Emergency approval for two Covid-19 vaccines was given in the U.S. on December 11 and December 18, 2020. Vaccines are also already in use in several other countries.[157] Clinical trials have shown these vaccines to be highly effective. Vaccinating sufficiently large numbers of people to achieve coverage close to herd immunity is expected to take at least several months.[158] A new variant of the coronavirus has emerged in Great Britain, and several countries have banned entry of travelers from the U.K.[159]

Alice: Welcome back everyone!

Cindy: So nice to see you all again!

Bob: Has been a while. The semester got busy really fast. Glad it's over.

Frank: You can say that! Insane amount of homework, especially in that linear algebra class I took. Not much time left for doing anything else. How fair is that? But at least I got an A; first time for me in a math class.

Alice: Congratulations, Frank! My grades weren't good this semester. I contracted Covid-19 in early October. For a while, it made me too tired to study.

Frank: You caught it, Alice? With all your knowledge about preventing infections?

Alice: It can happen to anybody. We had a spike of cases on campus right after many students came back to campus in Phase 2 of the re-opening. When there's spread in the community, nobody can perfectly protect her- or himself.

Cindy: I'm so sorry to hear that! Are you are feeling all right now, Alice?

Alice: Thank you, Cindy, for asking. I'm back to normal by now and feel fine.

Bob: I'm glad to hear about your recovery. I had told my parents and sibs about the things I had learned from you, and we all stayed healthy. Thanks again for all these meetings with us.

Cindy: I now think it was for the better that all my classes were online. I didn't like how some of them were taught, but I stayed home as much as possible and was super-careful all the time. So I didn't catch the virus.

Alice: I'm happy for you, Cindy. Overall, I'm also quite pleased with the response to Covid-19 at Ohio University. There were many infections among students, but fewer than the median for universities of comparable size, at least in Ohio.[160] After the initial spike in early October, new infections dropped a bit. Then they increased again, but very slowly.

Bob: Would that mean that the reproduction number R at Ohio University was close to 1 in the later part of the semester?

Alice: It must have been below 1 when we saw that drop in new infections. Over the last weeks of the semester, the increase in the number of cases looked more linear than exponential, so the reproduction number R seems to have been very close to 1.

It seems to me that after the first wave of infections and quarantines, most students had gotten the message. When I walked around campus and in town after I could leave my isolation, I saw that almost everyone was wearing masks.

Frank: Perhaps so. I was just too busy to go out much. Didn't catch anything.

Bob: Tell us, Alice, what's going on right now? New infections have been going up a lot in the U.S., and some places are running out of hospital beds. I've read that in California, they are already discussing rationing hospital care [1].

Frank: And in Europe they aren't doing any better. Germany, of all places, is under lockdown again.

Cindy: I've also read about the lockdown in Germany. Families will not be allowed to get together over Christmas. People will feel so lonely!

Alice: All of this is very disturbing. When we talked about preventive measures, we said that a combination of wearing masks, testing, contact tracing, frequent hand-washing, social distancing, limiting the size of social gatherings, and moving them outdoors can lower the reproduction number R from close to 3 to less than 1. But only to just a little below 1, it seems.

Bob: So, when we omit one component from this list, the combination of the other measures would not be sufficient and R would remain above 1. And then new infections will increase nearly exponentially. Is this what you want to say, Alice?

Alice: Exactly! The biggest factor that drives the recent waves of infections is cold weather. With winter approaching, outdoor social gatherings are no longer an option in most of Europe and in many parts of the U.S.

We can see the effects very clearly when we study the current wave of new infections in our country. It first hit in the northern parts, where the weather gets cold early in the fall. In Minnesota, it peaked on November 18. Further south, in Indiana, the peak was reached on December 6; still further south, in Tennessee, it seems to have peaked two days ago, on December 19. And in Florida, new infections still appear to be increasing. In this state with its hot and humid climate, things aren't as bad yet as they were in the summer when people wanted to be in air-conditioned buildings as much as possible.[161]

Bob: Seems that meeting outdoors instead of indoors really makes a big difference. This might also explain why Chile in the southern hemisphere had a huge wave that peaked on June 16, a few days before the start of their winter. When we looked at their data in early July, their total reported Covid-19 infections per million people were higher than in the U.S. But Chile has kept daily infections at a fairly constant level since mid-July, while ours went up. Now our total infections per million people are almost twice as high as theirs.[162]

But does cold weather alone explain all the recent increases?

Cindy: I think many people have become careless and don't follow the recommendations anymore.

Frank: What do you expect, Cindy? Who would want to wear these damn masks forever?

Alice: Yes, people are becoming impatient. We saw this over the Thanksgiving holiday in late November.[163] It was strongly recommended not to travel for family visits, but too many people did. I am afraid the same may happen over Christmas. It's only natural that people want to be with their extended families on holidays that are important to them. But it's dangerous.

Bob: Well, I can see why they recently imposed mask mandates in most of our states. I'm glad they worked and reversed the increase of new cases in most of them. Only a few states needed to close businesses on a large scale again.[164]

They just approved two vaccines in the U.S., and I've read that they are very effective. I guess we need to just sit it out for a few more months. Can you tell us more about the vaccines, Alice?

Alice: Yes. The vaccine developed by Pfizer-BioNTech was the first that got emergency approval in the U.S. and the vaccine developed by Moderna was the second.[157] Both vaccines appear to be around 95% effective, which is better than many epidemiologists had expected.

Frank: How do these companies know their vaccines are that effective?

Alice: Let me explain how the vaccine developed by Moderna was tested.[165] It was similar for the one developed by Pfizer.

In their clinical study of 30,000 volunteers, Moderna gave two doses of the vaccine to half of the volunteers and an injection with a placebo to the other half. Neither the volunteers nor the researchers who monitored them for symptoms knew who got the vaccine and who got the placebo. After some time, 196 among the volunteers developed symptoms of Covid-19 and tested positive. It turned out that 185 of these volunteers had been given the placebo.

Bob: A placebo is a fake vaccine that doesn't have any effect, right? So it seems among the 15,000 volunteers who did get the vaccine, also around 185 should have become infected and developed symptoms had they not gotten the real vaccine.

Alice: Right. But only 11 did. So it seems that the vaccine has prevented 174 out of 185 expected infections, or 94.1% of them.

Frank: So that's why they claim the vaccine is 94.1% effective. I wouldn't trust that precision of 0.1% though.

Alice: Me neither. A sample size of 185 is fairly small, and the true effectiveness may a few percent lower or higher than the result from the study. But even an effectiveness of 90% would be very high.

Cindy: But are the vaccines safe?

Alice: I can only say that so far, the clinical studies of the vaccines approved in the U.S. have not found major side effects.

Bob: So how many people will need to get vaccinated to achieve herd immunity?

Alice: This depends on the exact values of the basic reproduction number R_0 for Covid-19 and on the exact effectiveness of the vaccines. For a 94% effective vaccine and $R_0 = 3$, we would need to vaccinate at least 68% of all people, which is still very close to two thirds.

We talked about why it may be difficult to convince enough people to get vaccinated for achieving this much vaccine uptake.[166] But public confidence in the vaccines seems to have recently improved; that's an encouraging sign.[143]

Bob: So how long will it take until everybody who wants to get vaccinated can get a shot?

Alice: Two shots, actually, several weeks apart [3]. And then it may still take some time until immunity fully develops after the second shot. It will probably take until the summer before we will have the full benefits of the vaccines.[158]

And this is just in the U.S. The Covid-19 pandemic can only be eradicated on a worldwide scale, and this will require mass vaccinations also in countries with much more limited resources than we have.

Frank: Sounds we may need to keep up social distancing and wear these damn masks for a while longer.

Alice: Unfortunately, this may remain necessary at least through much of 2021 even under the most optimistic assumptions.

Bob: The way you say this sounds like a lot of things could go wrong.

Alice: There may not be enough vaccine uptake. We already talked about this. Logistics may also be a problem, as the vaccines that have been approved in the U.S. must be stored at very low temperatures. And we don't know yet for how long vaccinated people will remain immune before they need another shot.

Another question is whether people who are immune from developing the disease really cannot infect others. It seems rather unlikely that they could, but the clinical trials so far have not run long enough to rule out this possibility.[167] So we may need to continue wearing masks even after we have been vaccinated.

Also, viruses constantly mutate. Chances are that sooner or later some variants of coronavirus will evolve that are immune to the existing vaccines so that we will need develop and test new ones. It's an uphill struggle.

Cindy: That sounds so scary. I've read there is a new variant of the coronavirus in Great Britain that's even worse. Is it more deadly? What if the vaccines don't work against this variant?

Alice: The new variant in Great Britain has a number of mutations, but it is believed that our current vaccines will still be effective against it. There is no evidence that it would be more deadly than the previous variants. The main reason it is believed worse is that this variant is now more common in some areas of the U.K. than the older ones. This would suggest that it is more contagious and spreads faster.[159]

Bob: Would this mean that the basic reproduction number R_0 is larger for this variant than for the older ones?

Alice: This is what it boils down to in epidemiological terms.

Frank: They should ban all travel from Britain. France and some other European countries did it. Why does the U.S. still let flights come in from London?

Alice: Travel bans are very disruptive to the economy and have only limited effect; we talked about this. The new variant has been circulating in Britain since September and has already been found in other countries. It seems too late for stopping its global spread.

Even if R_0 is really larger for the new variant, we may need to bring the reproduction number down below 1 from somewhere like 4 instead of somewhere around 3, which would mean avoiding about 4 out of 5 effective contacts instead of 3 out of 4. So we may need to become even more conscientious about social distancing, limiting the size of gatherings and meeting outdoors weather permitting, wearing masks, frequent hand-washing, getting tested, and quarantining. It won't be easy, but if we all work on it together, we can do it.

Cindy: Can we keep meeting next semester, Alice? So that we can ask you how to best protect everybody if things really get worse?

Bob: That would be great. I've learned so much already and still have more questions.

Frank: I don't completely agree with everything Alice is telling us. But I like talking with you all. If Alice can spare the time, count me in.

Alice: Will be my pleasure to keep meeting with you. Enjoy the break, stay safe and healthy, and see you next semester!

Endnotes

[155] On December 20, the 7-day moving averages for the U.S. were 218,478 new cases and 2,643 deaths per day [4].

[156] The 7-day moving average of daily cases in France peaked on November 8 at 56,377 and then decreased steeply [4]. The second lockdown in France started on October 30 [5] and ended on December 14, with an overnight curfew remaining in place [6].

[157] On December 11, 2020, the FDA approved the vaccine developed by Pfizer-BioNTech for emergency use in the U.S. [7]. On December 18, 2020, the agency did the same for the vaccine developed by Moderna [8]. For continuously updated information on development and approval of Covid-19 vaccines, see [9].

[158] For detailed information about the planned time line of vaccine distribution in the U.S. and potential hurdles, see [10].

[159] For a description of the new variant, see [11]. Travel bans from the UK were being announced right at the time of this conversation. By December 22, 2020, some 40 countries had imposed such restrictions [12]. Experts remained skeptical whether they would work [13].

[160] A New York Times survey of more than 1,900 colleges and universities in the U.S. has revealed more than 397,000 cases and at least 90 deaths since the pandemic began [14]. Ohio University reported 882 cases total on all of its campuses, which corresponds to about 3% of its total student population. The corresponding percentage was higher for five of the ten largest universities in Ohio, including Miami University and Ohio State University, where it was several times higher.

[161] Based on 7-day moving averages reported by Worldometer [4]. In Florida this average was 11,943 on July 17 and 10,805 on December 20, 2020.

[162] As of December 20, Chile had reported a total of 30,507 Covid-19 infections per million people, while the corresponding number for the U.S. was 55,054 [4].

[163] Thanksgiving is an important holiday in the U.S. that is traditionally celebrated in large family gatherings.

[164] According to the New York Times [15], at the time of this conversation, masks were mandatory in 35 of the 50 states of the U.S. and businesses were mostly closed in 7 states.

[165] The description of these trials is based on [16]. See also [17] for more information on Moderna's vaccine.

[166] See Chapter 27.

[167] See [18] or [19] for an explanation why this possibility cannot yet be ruled out.

References

[1] Weber C. California hospitals discuss rationing care ss virus surges. Huffpost 2020 Dec 21. [cited 2020 Dec 22].
https://www.huffpost.com/entry/california-hospitals-coronavirus-surge_n_5fe17b04c5b6ff74797cbc60

[2] Eddy M. Germany locks down ahead of Christmas as coronavirus deaths rise. The New York Times. 2020 Dec 13. [cited 2020 Dec 22]. https://www.nytimes.com/2020/12/13/world/europe/germany-lockdown-christmas-covid.html

[3] Birkinbine B. Here's a list of how the Moderna & Pfizer vaccines compare. ABC 13 Eyewitness News 2020 Dec 17. [cited Dec 22 2020]. https://abc13.com/moderna-and-pfizer-vaccine-whats-the-difference-between-side-effects-effectiveness/8815593/

[4] Worldometers.info. Dover, Delaware, U.S.A. COVID-19 coronavirus pandemic. [cited 2020 Dec 22].
https://www.worldometers.info/coronavirus/

[5] BBC News. Coronavirus: Macron declares second national lockdown in France. 2020 Oct 29. [cited 2020 Dec 22].
https://www.bbc.com/news/world-europe-54716993

[6] France 24. Coronavirus pandemic: France eases some restrictions while imposing new curfew. 2020 Dec 15. [cited 2020 Dec 22]. https://www.france24.com/en/video/20201215-coronavirus-pandemic-france-eases-some-restrictions-while-imposing-new-curfew

[7] U.S. Food and Drug Administration. FDA takes key action in fight against COVID-19 by issuing emergency use authorization for first COVID-19 vaccine. 2020 Dec 11 [cited 2020 Dec 22]. https://www.fda.gov/news-events/press-announcements/fda-takes-key-action-fight-against-covid-19-issuing-emergency-use-authorization-first-covid-19

[8] U.S. Food and Drug Administration. FDA takes additional action in fight against COVID-19 by issuing emergency use authorization for second COVID-19 vaccine. 2020 Dec 18 [cited 2020 Dec 22]. https://www.fda.gov/news-events/press-announcements/fda-takes-additional-action-fight-against-covid-19-issuing-emergency-use-authorization-second-covid

[9] Wikipedia: The free encyclopedia. Wikimedia Foundation, Inc. COVID-19 vaccine; [cited 20202 Dec 22]. https://en.wikipedia.org/wiki/COVID-19_vaccine

[10] Danner C, Stieb M. What we know about the U.S. COVID-19 vaccine distribution plan. Intelligencer. 2020 Dec 18. [cited 2020 Dec 22]. https://nymag.com/intelligencer/2020/12/what-we-know-about-u-s-covid-19-vaccine-distribution-plan.html

[11] Doucleff M. What we know about the new U.K. variant of coronavirus—and what we need to find out. National Public Radio. 2020 Dec 22 [cited 2020 Dec 23]. https://www.npr.org/sections/goatsandsoda/2020/12/22/948961575/

[12] Landler M, Castle S. Concerns about coronavirus variant cut off U.K. from Europe. The New York Times. 2020 Dec 21 [updated 2020 Dec 22; cited 2020 Dec 23]. https://www.nytimes.com/2020/12/21/world/europe/coronavirus-variant-uk.html

[13] Santora M. Can Travel bans really stop the spread of coronavirus variants? Experts are skeptical. The New York Times 2020 Dec 22. [updated 2020 Dec 24; cited 2021 Jan 5]. https://www.nytimes.com/2020/12/22/world/europe/travel-bans-coronavirus-variants.html

[14] Tracking the Coronavirus at U.S. Colleges and Universities. The New York Times. [cited 2020 Dec 23].
https://www.nytimes.com/interactive/2020/us/covid-college-cases-tracker.html

[15] The New York Times. See Coronavirus Restrictions and Mask Mandates for All 50 States. [cited 2020 Dec 22].
https://www.nytimes.com/interactive/2020/us/states-reopen-map-coronavirus.html

[16] Herper M, Garde D. Moderna to submit Covid-19 vaccine to FDA as full results show 94% efficacy. STAT. 2020 Nov 30. [cited 2020 Dec 22]. https://www.statnews.com/2020/11/30/moderna-covid-19-vaccine-full-results/

[17] Corum J, Zimmer C. How Moderna's vaccine works. The New York Times. 2020 Dec 18. [cited 2020 Dec 22].
https://www.nytimes.com/interactive/2020/health/moderna-covid-19-vaccine.html

[18] Koerth M. Once you get the COVID-19 vaccine, can you still infect others? FiveThirtyEight 2020 Dec 18. [cited 2020 Dec 20]. https://fivethirtyeight.com/features/once-you-get-the-covid-19-vaccine-can-you-still-infect-others/

[19] Mandavilli A. Here's why vaccinated people still need to wear a mask. The New York Times 2020 Dec 8. [updated 2020 Dec 9; cited 2020 Dec 23]. https://www.nytimes.com/2020/12/08/health/covid-vaccine-mask.html

Index

www.ingramcontent.com/pod-product-compliance
Lightning Source LLC
Chambersburg PA
CBHW061232220326
41599CB00028B/5400